# Practice Management in Neurology

*Guest Editor*

ORLY AVITZUR, MD, MBA

# NEUROLOGIC CLINICS

www.neurologic.theclinics.com

*Consulting Editor*
RANDOLPH W. EVANS, MD

May 2010 • Volume 28 • Number 2

SAUNDERS an imprint of ELSEVIER, Inc.

**W.B. SAUNDERS COMPANY**
*A Division of Elsevier Inc.*

1600 John F. Kennedy Boulevard ● Suite 1800 ● Philadelphia, Pennsylvania 19103-2899

http://www.theclinics.com

**NEUROLOGIC CLINICS Volume 28, Number 2**
**May 2010 ISSN 0733-8619, ISBN-13: 978-1-4377-1919-2**

Editor: Donald Mumford

*Neurologic Clinics* (ISSN 0733-8619) is published quarterly by Elsevier Inc., 360 Park Avenue South, New York, NY 10010–1710. Months of issue are February, May, August, and November. Periodicals postage paid at New York, NY, and additional mailing offices. Subscription prices are $247.00 per year for US individuals, $401.00 per year for US institutions, $124.00 per year for US students, $310.00 per year for Canadian individuals, $482.00 per year for Canadian institutions, $344.00 per year for international individuals, $482.00 per year for international institutions, and $175.00 for Canadian and foreign students/residents. To receive student/resident rate, orders must be accompanied by name of affiliated institution, date of term, and the *signature* of program/residency coordinator on institution letterhead. Orders will be billed at individual rate until proof of status is received. Foreign air speed delivery is included in all *Clinics* subscription prices. All prices are subject to change without notice. **POSTMASTER:** Send address changes to *Neurologic Clinics*, Elsevier Health Sciences Division, Subscription Customer Service, 3251 Riverport Lane, Maryland Heights, MO 63043. **Customer Service: Telephone: 1-800-654-2452 (U.S. and Canada); 314-447-8871 (outside U.S. and Canada). Fax: 314-447-8029. E-mail: journalscustomerservice-usa@elsevier.com (for print support); journalsonlinesupport-usa@elsevier.com (for online support).**

*Reprints.* For copies of 100 or more of articles in this publication, please contact the Commercial Reprints Department, Elsevier Inc., 360 Park Avenue South, New York, New York, 10010-1710; Tel.: (+1) 212-633-3812; Fax: (+1) 212-462-1935, and E-mail: reprints@elsevier.com.

*Neurologic Clinics* is also published in Spanish by Nueva Editorial Interamericana S.A., Mexico City, Mexico.

*Neurologic Clinics* is covered in *Current Contents/Clinical Medicine, MEDLINE/PubMed (Index Medicus), EMBASE/Excerpta Medica, and PsycINFO, and ISI/BIOMED.*

Printed and bound in the United Kingdom
Transferred to Digital Print 2011

# Contributors

## CONSULTING EDITOR

**RANDOLPH W. EVANS, MD**
Clinical Professor, Department of Neurology, Baylor College of Medicine, Houston, Texas

## GUEST EDITOR

**ORLY AVITZUR, MD, MBA**
Editor-in-Chief, American Academy of Neurology Website; Clinical Assistant Professor of Neurology, New York Medical College, Valhalla, New York

## AUTHORS

**ORLY AVITZUR, MD, MBA**
Clinical Assistant Professor of Neurology, New York Medical College, Valhalla, New York

**J.D. BARTLESON, MD**
Associate Professor of Neurology, Department of Neurology, Mayo Clinic College of Medicine, Rochester, Minnesota

**AMANDA BECKER, BA**
American Academy of Neurology, St Paul, Minnesota

**JAMES L. BERNAT, MD**
Professor of Neurology and Medicine, Dartmouth Medical School, Hanover, New Hampshire; Attending Neurologist, Department of Neurology, Dartmouth-Hitchcock Medical Center, Lebanon, New Hampshire

**NEIL BUSIS, MD, FAAN**
Chief, Division of Neurology, Department of Medicine, UPMC Shadyside Hospital; Director, Neurodiagnostic Laboratory, UPMC Shadyside Hospital; Practice Management and Technology Editor, Pittsburgh Neurology Center, Pittsburgh, Pennsylvania

**OKSANA DROGAN, MS**
American Academy of Neurology Professional Association, St Paul, Minnesota

**GREGORY J. ESPER, MD, MBA**
Assistant Professor, Department of Neurology, Emory University School of Medicine, Atlanta, Georgia

**W. DAVID FREEMAN, MD**
Assistant Professor, Mayo Clinic College of Medicine, Jacksonville, Florida

**WILLIAM S. HENDERSON, MA, FACMPE**
Administrator, Upstate Neurology Consultants, LLP, Albany, New York

**JOHN W. HENSON, MD**
Neurology Division, Swedish Neuroscience Institute, Seattle, Washington

**DANIEL B. HIER, MD, MBA**
Neuroscience Center, University of Illinois at Chicago, Chicago, Illinois

**ANDREA N. LEEP HUNDERFUND, MD**
Instructor in Neurology, Department of Neurology, Mayo Clinic College of Medicine, Rochester, Minnesota

**JAMES C. JOHNSTON, MD, JD, FCLM, FACLM**
Consultant Neurologist and Attorney, Seattle, Washington; Barrister of the High Court of New Zealand, Auckland, New Zealand

**RALPH F. JÓZEFOWICZ, MD**
Professor of Neurology and Medicine, Associate Chair for Education, Department of Neurology, University of Rochester School of Medicine and Dentistry, Rochester, New York

**LILY K. JUNG, MD**
Neurology Division, Swedish Neuroscience Institute, Seattle, Washington

**JOEL M. KAUFMAN, MD, FAAN**
Executive Director and Chief Executive Officer, Lifespan/Physicians Professional Service Organization; Clinical Associate Professor of Clinical Neurosciences (Neurology), Department of Neurology, The Warren Alpert Medical School of Brown University, Providence, Rhode Island

**BRETT KISSELA, MD**
Associate Professor, Co-director, Neurology Residency Program, Vice-Chair of Education and Clinical Services, Department of Neurology, University of Cincinnati, Cincinnati, Ohio

**DANIEL G. LARRIVIERE, MD, JD**
Academic Instructor, University of Virginia School of Law; Assistant Professor of Neurology, Department of Neurology, University of Virginia School of Medicine, Charlottesville, Virginia

**STEVEN L. LEWIS, MD**
Professor and Associate Chairman, Department of Neurological Sciences, Rush University Medical Center, Chicago, Illinois

**JANIS M. MIYASAKI, MD, MEd, FRCPC, FAAN**
Co-Chair, Technology and Therapeutics Assessment Subcommittee, American Academy of Neurology; Deputy Physician-in-Chief, The Morton and Gloria Shulman Movement Disorders Centre, Toronto Western Hospital, University Health Network, University of Toronto, Toronto, Ontario, Canada

**EMILY B. RUBIN, JD, MD**
Medical Resident, Departments of Internal Medicine and Pediatrics, Massachusetts General Hospital, Boston, Massachusetts

**JUSTIN A. SATTIN, MD**
Assistant Professor of Neurology, Department of Neurology, Clinical Science Center, University of Wisconsin, Madison, Wisconsin

**BRUCE SIGSBEE, MD, MS, FAAN**
Medical Director, Pen Bay Physicians and Associates, Penobscot Bay Medical Center, Rockport, Maine

**BARNEY J. STERN, MD**
Professor of Neurology, Department of Neurology, University of Maryland, Baltimore, Maryland

**JAMES C. STEVENS, MD, FAAN**
Associate Professor of Neurology, Indiana University School of Medicine, Indianapolis; Chair of the Practice Committee for the American Academy of Neurology, St Paul, Minnesota; Department of Neurology, Fort Wayne Neurological Center, Fort Wayne, Indiana

**DAVID E. THIESS, JD**
American Health Lawyers Association, Washington, DC

**KENNETH A. VATZ, MD**
Private Practice, Winnetka, Illinois

# Contents

near-instantaneous dissemination of the latest developments in neurologic knowledge, although their value is dependent on the degree of awareness of neurologists and is limited by the reluctance of some sources to make information readily accessible. The encyclopedic nature of the Internet, with its vast resources of online information, may be diminished by issues of access, variable quality and reliability, and a lack of intelligent retrieval systems. A major hindrance, for example, is seen with restrictions on archival, but proprietary, neurologic literature. Neurologic patients and their caregivers use the Internet heavily, but for somewhat different reasons. It is important for neurologists to understand these differences. The emergence of the online Personal Health Record will become increasingly valuable as these sites evolve and more medical providers incorporate electronic applications and medical records into their practices. Online groups for neurologists with similar interests, often referred to as "networks," have the potential to catalyze the natural organizing tendencies among those seeking solutions to shared problems. Networking can function well for neurologists, neurologic patients, and for focused efforts in an area such as advocacy. These considerations are discussed in this article.

Smartphones make mobile computing at point of care practical. Smartphones can think, sync, and link. Built-in and user-installed applications facilitate communications between neurologists and their medical colleagues and patients and augment data acquisition and processing in the core medical information domains of patient data, clinical decision support, and practice management. Mobile telemedicine is becoming practical in certain scenarios. Smartphones can improve neurologic diagnosis and treatment, teaching, and research. Patients can benefit from smartphone technology. In addition to enhanced communication, patient education, and social networking, these devices can promote healthy lifestyles, preventive medicine, and compliance and even serve as monitoring and prosthetic devices.

The tipping point for electronic health records (EHR) has been reached and universal adoption in the United States is now inevitable. Neurologists will want to choose their electronic health record prudently. Careful selection, contracting, planning, and training are essential to successful implementation. Neurologists need to examine their workflow carefully and make adjustments to ensure that efficiency is increased. Neurologists will want to achieve a significant return on investment and qualify for all applicable financial incentives from payers, including CMS. EHRs are not just record-keeping tools but play an important role in quality improvement, evidence-based medicine, pay for performance, patient education, bio-surveillance, data warehousing, and data exchange.

**THE CLINICS ARE NOW AVAILABLE ONLINE!**

Access your subscription at:
**www.theclinics.com**

# Preface

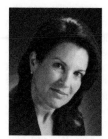

Orly Avitzur, MD, MBA
*Guest Editor*

*It was the best of times, it was the worst of times, it was the age of wisdom, it was the age of foolishness…*
*A Tale of Two Cities, Charles Dickens*

Neurology exists today in a dichotomous world evocative of Charles Dickens. Neurology's catalog of triumphs, both scientific and clinical, over the past 40 years has been counterbalanced, from the perspective of practitioners, by a burdensome, if not oppressive, economic, regulatory and medicolegal climate still undergoing rapid change.

This issue of *Neurologic Clinics*, the first devoted to practice, attempts to establish the current state of neurology and address the issues the authors consider to be most important to current and future neurologists.

In 1970, practicing neurologists, trained in classical neurology and armed with reflex hammers and pins, along with ophthalmoscopes, stethoscopes, and a couple of tuning forks, usually spent at least an hour with new patients, made handwritten notes in the chart, sent typewritten consultation letters with an impression and plan to referring physicians, and had a few ancillary tests at their disposal. Medical treatment options were limited and many neurologic conditions had no cures. When neurologists had questions about diagnosis or treatment, they would consult colleagues, look in *Merritt's Textbook of Neurology*, or go to the nearest medical library to search through Index Medicus for relevant articles in the journals. Neurologists charged on a fee-for-service basis, and were covered by most insurance plans. Malpractice was beginning to be an issue, but the premiums were still fairly low, and no one considered the situation to be in crisis. There was virtually no regulatory oversight of the practice of medicine, other than by state licensing boards. Medicare had been in place for about 5 years and, despite early fears by physicians, it served to facilitate good care for retired and elderly patients. Also, overall, the lifestyle for neurologists in solo or small group practice was comparable to that of physicians in other medical fields.

Neurol Clin 28 (2010) xiii–xv
doi:10.1016/j.ncl.2009.12.001
0733-8619/10/$ – see front matter © 2010 Elsevier Inc. All rights reserved.

neurologic.theclinics.com

A quick perusal of the 14 chapter headings in this issue of *Neurologic Clinics* tells the reader that over the past 40 years something has happened on the way to the office. The patient who consults the neurologist now has wide access to medical information about his or her symptoms, disease, and treatment options from a plethora of Internet sources. We take histories, perhaps entering them electronically into the record, and perform neurologic examinations essentially unchanged from those in 1970, albeit under pressure from tighter time constraints. Following this, we formulate a differential diagnosis and treatment plan, order laboratory studies, perform electrophysiological testing, and request various imaging studies, taking into account not only what is medically reasonable and necessary for the insurers, but also what is required to achieve the highest degree of certainty of diagnosis and appropriate treatment, because that is, in reality, the standard to which we will be held by the legal system should there be a less-than-optimal outcome. Proper informed consent will have to be obtained for any procedures or treatments that entail risk. We are also expected to provide sufficient educational materials to the patient such that the patient can make informed decisions about care options.

If we require additional information about the patient or the patient's presumed diagnosis or treatment, we now have available a wealth of electronic resources, including possibly an electronic health record from the primary care physician or hospital, and the medical Internet, using the numerous medical information databases that can be accessed by computer or through a mobile smartphone. We are encouraged to use evidence-based medicine in our practices, not only in the best interest of care, but in recognition that credentialing bodies, such as hospitals and third-party contracted carriers, as well as the medicolegal system, will look at the degree to which we do so.

We submit bills for our services not to the patient, but rather to a third party, either private or governmental or both, using a fee schedule that has either been negotiated or determined by them. Beginning in 2010, fee structures themselves will be predicated to a greater or lesser degree upon demonstrated performance, although the methodology for such determination is still under development.

A neurologist may be in a solo practice, but more likely is in a small or medium-sized group of subspecialized neurologists in competition for referrals with other similarly constituted groups within the same geographic area. The group practice needs to benchmark its performance against those of competing groups and try to achieve efficiencies that will enable its long-term financial viability. Within the group, the partners and associates need to work out and agree upon a fair and equitable distribution of income according to the quality and quantity of work performed by each neurologist, factoring in practice management time, teaching, and promotional work.

Approximately 40% of neurologists practice within an academic setting or multispecialty clinic, the business structures of which vary from the group practice model described above to those with full-time or modified salaried positions. There may be both clinical and teaching responsibilities, depending upon the venue and degree of academic affiliation. Medical school clerkships and neurology residency programs are labor intensive from the teaching standpoint, and are even more onerous now for academic neurologists due to the restrictions on resident workloads and hours. Furthermore, there has been little increase in the numbers of students choosing neurology as a specialty, and the future is uncertain as to whether there will be sufficient numbers of neurologists to handle the ever-growing demand.

Medicine, and neurology in particular, will have to cope with some difficult problems and trying times over the next several years. The future is bright in terms of research and advancements in the science of neurology but less certain with respect to day-to-day practice. It is hoped that this issue, which addresses the operational, financial, and legal aspects of the practice of neurology, will enable the reader to function more efficiently and at a higher level of performance in the current climate.

I want to express my gratitude to the authors for their valuable contributions. They have succeeded in presenting complex issues in practical terms and in a manner that is clear and informative. I would like to thank Dr Kenneth A. Vatz, in particular, for his extensive input and review of this project. My special thanks go to Don Mumford for his guidance throughout the preparation of this issue, as well as to my family and those of the contributing authors for their patience and support.

Orly Avitzur, MD, MBA
55 South Broadway
Tarrytown
NY 10591, USA

E-mail address:
oavitzur@earthlink.net

# Physician Compensation: Approach and Models in Neurological Practice

Bruce Sigsbee, MD, MS, FAAN

## KEYWORDS

- Physician compensation • Salary • Incentive
- Productivity • Model

Compensation methodology has always challenged physician groups. The highly complex system of physician reimbursement for services in the rapidly changing environment of health care makes the choice of a compensation model even more problematic. Any methodology should reflect the underlying philosophy and culture of a group, and have the flexibility to accommodate the variability of interests, expertise, energy levels, and practice styles of its members. Further, compensation models must strike a balance between the financial viability of the practice and fair compensation for all its physicians. This article describes the most common compensation structures and addresses the strengths and weaknesses of each.

Any compensation model should reward behaviors and values considered important by the group. For example, does the group want most to protect lifestyle, maximize compensation, or reward its physicians for high patient satisfaction? The design of the model will vary according to the weighted goals of the practice. External issues relevant to compensation include the recruitment of physicians, retention of physicians already employed, the potential for part-time work, and the nonfinancial rewards of medical practice.

The following principles are critical when designing a compensation model. The model must be simple, clear, and transparent. Any sense of a lack of fairness is likely to engender dissatisfaction and may lead to the failure of the group. Complexity erodes the incentive value of the model because physicians may find it difficult to understand incentive provisions, consider them arbitrary, or try to take advantage of the complexity of the model to "game" the incentives. For example, the highly complex compensation systems that evolved from the managed care and capitation

Penobscot Bay Medical Center, 4 Glen Cove Dr, Suite 102, Rockport, ME 04856, USA
*E-mail address:* bsigsbee@tidewater.net

Neurol Clin 28 (2010) 339–348
doi:10.1016/j.ncl.2009.11.012
0733-8619/10/$ – see front matter © 2010 Elsevier Inc. All rights reserved.
neurologic.theclinics.com

models so prevalent in the 1990s were often arbitrary, difficult to understand, time-intensive, burdensome to administer, and therefore, counterproductive.

Compensation methodology is equally important to both employer and employee. John A. Fromson, MD, advised in a medical employment Web site: "Even more important [than compensation] is whether a job is one that the physician truly feels will contribute to his or her professional development and provides satisfaction and enjoyment."[1] Whereas aspects of the practice, such as call, collegiality, emphasis on continuing education, opportunities for teaching, and other qualitative features of the day to day functioning of the group may be more relevant to retention, it is critical, particularly for a physician joining a group, to fully comprehend the compensation model.

## COMPENSATION. WHAT DOES IT REPRESENT?

Practices tend to have distinct characteristics that make up the personality of the group. Whereas some practices emphasize quality of life rather than maximization of compensation, others are more focused on generating maximum income. Many groups are close and have frequent social interactions, whereas others are cordial at work but go in different directions after hours. Whatever the culture, clinicians who are reasonable in every other respect often become agitated, anxious, uneasy, and even angry when dealing with compensation and finance issues. Physicians have little or no preparation in negotiating compensation or understanding practice finances. Compensation is often considered a proxy for "How much do you value me?" Although group traits may vary, fairness and transparent finances, of which compensation methodology is an integral part, represent essential characteristics of any successful group.

Physician productivity generally determines the success of a group. Medical services have high fixed, relative to marginal, cost structures. The ability of the group to compensate its members is therefore highly dependent on physician productivity. Factors influencing productivity include a clear understanding of this dependency and the basic economics of a service business, peer pressure from within the group, and personal financial incentives. The absence of any of these factors in individual physicians may threaten the continued viability of the group.

The mid-1990s saw a rush on the part of hospitals to purchase practices, in particular primary care practices, to obtain an assured market share. The purchase price was often high and the compensation model was not necessarily well thought out. The resultant lowered productivity of the physicians led to severe financial stress on the system, and in some circumstances, complete failure. In the past five years, there has been a new wave of employment of physicians. This trend is driven by the increasingly complex nature of practice-management (including the mandated transition to information technology), escalating regulations, and increased oversight. Physicians have been driving this change, causing employers to focus more on the engagement of physicians within the entity to avoid the failures of the past. Compensation models are critical in establishing engagement.

The incentives inherent in the compensation model can be viewed from another perspective. Physicians may focus on their own behavior to maximize personal productivity however it is calculated, even to the detriment of others in the same group or specialty; alternatively, they may consider their behavior in the context of benefit to the medical community, the group, or the specialty. Most often, a balance must be drawn between individual performance and the performance of the group as a whole.

In the compensation methodologies examined in this article, the key principle is that the model must reward what the physician does rather than who the physician is. The end product must place value on productivity, patient satisfaction, quality, and other characteristics of a high-performing practice. From inception, the model should not include a component that reflects the importance of the individual physician. Otherwise, contract negotiations become a vain and fruitless exercise in addressing the concept that particular physicians are "more special" than the others down the hall.

## EQUAL SHARE

In this model all of the physicians receive an equal share of the revenues. Physicians vary substantially in their practice styles and there will be substantial differences in productivity. One physician may commit time that is carved out of revenue-producing hours to the management of the practice. Another physician may have a particular interest in electromyography (EMG), perform a large number of studies, and generate a substantial amount of revenue. The managing physician contributes substantially to the success of the group, but may not generate the same income. The electromyographer often is able to commit time to these studies only because another physician covers the emergency room or provides other services that generate far less revenue. Although the generated revenue may vary substantially, all the physicians contribute to the success of the group.

The distinct advantage of this method is that individuals have a sense of shared purpose and that it emphasizes the group to the exclusion of individual performance. The physicians are not working for themselves as individuals but for the group as a whole. This methodology does, however, require that individuals commit to the process. If the managing physician takes advantage of that position and devotes excessive time to management in lieu of clinical work, or if another physician elects to leave early on a frequent basis, these actions disadvantage the group. If another physician is particularly efficient, stays late, and books patients through the lunch hour, his extra efforts are diluted across the whole group. He does not receive much recognition for these efforts. In this model, peer pressure is a key incentive for high productivity. This formula obviates the need to attach specific values to economically differing skill sets, such as neurophysiology or financial management.

This format can work well in small groups. However, if the practice has more than a few physicians, the group as a whole may suffer from the lack of perceived individual benefit from extra work. This burden may start to weigh heavily on the physicians who are hardworking and highly productive. Physicians who generate a substantial part of extra revenue may believe that they deserve extra financial recognition. They may not understand the support given by the group to high-revenue generators such as electromyographers. There is also a strong risk that some members of the group will develop a "civil servant attitude." (ie, "It's 5 o'clock and it is somebody else's problem"). In larger groups and certainly in multispecialty groups, therefore, the "equal share" methodology tends not to work.[2]

The problems experienced in the rush to employ physicians during the mid-1990s resulted in large part from fixed salaries and declines in real productivity. Individual incentives may be effective in increasing productivity, but group incentives are not.

Consider that you are a highly productive physician. You see 20% more patients in a day than the average members of the group. Often, you fit patients into the noon hour, and if on call, you do not shorten the office day. Next to you is a physician who schedules more time with each patient and even at that rate cannot get records done. When on call, his last scheduled appointment in the office is 3 PM. He sees 20%

fewer patients than the group average. If you both receive the same compensation, would you tolerate that differential? Or would you become cynical and reduce your productivity? You may even become upset to the point that you would look for a position whereby your efforts would be better recognized and appreciated. At a time of marked difficulty in recruiting neurologists, the loss of a physician, generally preventable, can be very harmful to a group.

In some groups the disparity in productivity can exceed 50%. Unless this inequality, which "… penalizes high producers and allows low producers to 'coast'"[3] is specifically addressed, it puts the survival of the group at substantial risk. Even if productivity is not a component of compensation, the measurement of individual productivity provides some reassurance that there is reasonable equality across the group—a concept that may be critical to the functioning of the group.

To effectively execute the shared model of compensation, the performance of each physician must be reviewed on a regular basis. There must be enough personal comfort within the group to enable differences to be discussed openly to address the problems outlined earlier.

## VARIABLE COMPENSATION

There are many possible methods of varying compensation. These include the recognition of special contributions, such as the management of the practice or valuing particular skills, for example, neuroimaging or electrophysiology. Some groups will reward "senior members" with increased compensation, as is common in the legal profession and accounting. In law practices, there may be justification for the senior partners being considered "rain makers," that is, in recognizing that they are responsible for attracting the most business to the firm. In medicine this is less the case, at least in nonsurgical practices. New physicians try to develop their own referral base, although they still depend on senior members for support. Although issues of seniority and other special circumstances need to be considered by the group, any differential must be carefully weighed to avoid an "I am more special" argument. Unless there is sound justification, differential compensation based on who a physician is rather than what the physician is producing, challenges the concept of fairness.

Variable compensation is, or should be, based predominantly on some measure of productivity. The most commonly used metrics are charges, receipts, and work relative value units (wRVUs). The advantage of variable compensation is that it both encourages greater productivity and recognizes the value of that increased productivity. Historically, large institutions including academic departments have compensated physicians on the basis of fixed salaries. Today fixed salaries without productivity standards rarely exist. As one department chair put it, his physicians needed to support themselves. There was no subsidy available from the department or the institution. A system in which the physician's income will vary according to productivity and includes the possibility of compensation going down will often result in a 20% to 30% increase in productivity. If it can be accomplished, a mechanism should be created for decreasing compensation if targets are not met.

Capitation still exists in some markets and is included in many of the proposed models for reform of the health care system. A variable compensation plan may be based in part on the incentives surrounding capitated care. It is also likely that other methods of reimbursing physicians will evolve in the future. As the market changes, novel methods will provide opportunities for alternative, productivity-based compensation models.

## INCENTIVE-BASED COMPENSATION

The threshold question is whether incentives work. There is a body of literature that supports the concept that incentives do work effectively in all environments including primary care,[3] academic departments,[4] and hospital departments.[5] The formula for compensation incentives is a key element in physician engagement, satisfaction, and retention.

It is important that any productivity measurement be transparent, easily obtained, simple in concept, and perceived to be free of bias, error, or evidence of manipulation. Charges and receipts can be easily retrieved from the financial systems of the practice, and should be readily verifiable. wRVUs are numbers determined by the Centers for Medicaid and Medicare Services and are tied to individual service codes, with spreadsheets available online. Each physician can verify the calculations provided by the practice without difficulty.

Emphasizing productivity can also create problems. Such emphasis carries the potential to encourage competition among physicians for patients who will provide a higher return, based on the measurements used. There is also the risk that the physician may "cherry pick" the services that provide the greatest reward, based on the defined incentive. A pure productivity incentive recognizes individual performance exclusively and does not recognize community or group performance. In any specialty, there are services for which the charges per unit of time are higher. For example, the charges for reading electroencephalograms (EEGs) represent a very high return on time invested compared with most other services that neurologists provide. In terms of gross receipts, the better private insurers in most areas reimburse more for similar services than Medicare and Medicaid. In any specialty there are some services that provide more wRVUs per unit of time than others. EEGs and even EMGs are in this category.

Because of such disparities, incentives have the potential to reduce quality or impair service to the community. It may be difficult to get physicians to commit to caring for underinsured patients or to provide services that are not cost effective, such as emergency room visits or inpatient consults. Most groups handle this well because individual physicians recognize the need to provide various services. However, some physicians will game the system to the detriment of their colleagues. Thus, if not well designed, the incentive formula may serve to encourage negative behavior rather than improved productivity. Often, it is just a few physicians who are problematic. In the long run it may better to move ahead without these physicians, because they have the potential of being "poison pills" that sabotage efforts to engage the other physicians, and consequently thwart the group's goals of job satisfaction, mission, and service to the community.

In the author's own experience, groups operating in a salary-based compensation system tend to decompensate with the introduction of a productivity model of compensation. The new model is such a major change in the physicians' view of their practice and their interaction with their colleagues that it can create major destructive behaviors. For example, on analysis of a group of specialists, productivity was more or less even across the members of the practice, although low compared with national standards. The group clearly had the capacity to increase productivity. If the introduction of a productivity model had led to a cooperative effort to increase productivity for all physicians, it would have been a positive force. Unfortunately, individual physicians began to round on their days off. Obstetricians, for example, tried to avoid passing deliveries to colleagues or nurse midwives, and were unwilling to continue to share responsibilities as they had in the past. This self-serving behavior developed despite active discussions of the goals prior to adopting the compensation model and ongoing physician counseling following its introduction. As a result, the model was changed to a less obvious and group-oriented productivity model.

It is not unusual for physicians with low productivity to express the attitude that their stature or reputation and the business they bring to the institution in the form of admissions and ancillary testing justify their (higher) level of compensation. This disregard for meeting the goals of productivity, quality metrics, and patient satisfaction can become the basis for turmoil between the physician and the institution, whether it is a hospital, group, or other entity. Although the status the physician brings to the institution is important and should be recognized, this recognition should not be inherent to the contract. The emphasis must always be on the physicians' accomplishments, not on who they are or what other revenues their patients generate. Unless effectively countered, this attitude, along with shrinking health care revenues and pending health care reform, risks a death spiral for the institution.

Although beyond the scope of this article, at the core of this problem is the effective engagement of physicians. Individual physicians must be part of the governance and day-to-day functioning of the entity. Although there is often a tendency is to establish a task force or to "empower" a group of physician leaders, these efforts alone will not accomplish the intended engagement unless individual physicians know what is going on and believe that they are part of the process. This engagement necessitates senior management meetings with individual physicians and small groups. It is time consuming and often frustrating, but it is a necessary commitment. Persons charged with this responsibility must have the necessary support, including access to relevant data analyses and allocation of the time required.

In considering variable compensation, there are several important aspects to take into account. First, the measurements need to be fair, objective, and readily verifiable or, in a word, transparent. Not only should the formula be simple and easy to manage, the physicians should have ready access to the data and be able to ask questions and challenge the calculations. Second, incentive components need to be chosen carefully to encourage positive rather than destructive competitive behaviors. Third, productivity is a team effort. The staff should contribute materially to office efficiency and productivity; for example, a physician should be supported by one of his partners in providing low-cost patient care, such as emergency room consults. Because of all these variables, a pure productivity model may not be the best choice for certain groups and their physicians.

It is worth reviewing specific models of variable compensation. One of the most popular methods is to use wRVUs as the basis for determining compensation. Within a single specialty, the wRVU is probably the best measure of productivity. In neurology, EEG and EMG carry wRVU levels that may be higher than is reasonable in comparison with difficult evaluation and management work, making some adjustments necessary. A second method of compensation, using total charges, has the same problem and may be even more disproportionate across various services than wRVUs. A third parameter, gross receipts, is another basis for measurement, but insurance companies vary substantially in the remuneration made for a given service, and some physicians may attempt to "cherry pick" the best payers. It is also notable that none of these measures takes into account adequately the expense side of practice finances. The author's single, preferred measure of productivity from the three described above is the wRVU. However, all these methods represent incentives to increase revenue-generating activities.

It is possible to develop a compensation method based on the bottom line that also factors in expense considerations, making the entire economic success of the group inherent in the incentive. The bottom line can be distributed based on individual physician productivity, perhaps as represented by wRVUs. Many national compensation consultants are now advising clients to adopt this method of determining compensation, although it is not directly related to the physician's individual performance. The adoption of this type of incentive needs careful consideration because it is a less effective personal motivator.

Finally, an incentive method needs to include qualitative contributions that are not revenue generating, such as committee work. In general, physicians are expected to participate in these activities as a condition of employment. However, there are some positions that are so valuable to the entity and so time-consuming that they require special consideration. Rather than contaminate the incentive system, activities involving substantial time, such as leadership positions, can be recognized with a stipend.

## BLENDED MODEL

Blended models can avoid some of the problems seen in the extremes of either equal pay for all physicians or a 100% productivity model. Such a model may also provide increased flexibility, in that behavior and characteristics other than productivity alone can be recognized as part of the incentive system. A blended model can achieve a balance between individual performance and community success. This model includes a fixed base compensation and in addition, a variable amount based on one or more measures or incentives.

The initial base compensation may vary, depending on previous productivity. This method readily accommodates part-time physicians. The method also recognizes physicians who are willing to work longer hours, and those who respond to the requests of their patients or referring physicians by scheduling in the noon hour or by staying late. For example, a group of six physicians may include three who work hard and who have had similar historical productivity. They may all be highly productive and may be offered the same base salary. A fourth physician's productivity may be approximately 85% of his colleagues' output despite working full-time, and his salary is 85% of the other physicians' base salary. The remaining two physicians are part-time and will receive pro rata base compensation.

This model adopts the view that there is a floor, representing the minimum compensation the physician would receive if he did not meet any of the incentive measures. That floor varies between 60% and 85% of the anticipated salary based on historical performance. The actual payments on a weekly or biweekly basis are based on anticipated, historically based performance, with the possibility that financial compensation could go down or could be set at the base, with settlement predicated on performance related to the incentive characteristics. It is widely accepted that regular payments are based on historical performance; however, if this structure is instituted, the contract must allow for a decrease if performance lags.

The largest component of the variable amount remains productivity, which is often in the neighborhood of 20% but may be higher. For well-defined groups, charges and receipts can remain effective bases for the productivity component. In groups employed by hospitals or in multispecialty groups, perhaps the most effective compensation method is wRVU based. It should be noted that wRVUs across a single specialty, despite the caveats discussed earlier, best represent the relative work of individual services. But across specialties, the comparison breaks down. If wRVUs are to be used, specific thresholds should be defined for each specialty. The physician's base salary is paired with a specific wRVU level. Every wRVU in excess of this base is converted into a specific dollar amount. To be competitive, the compensation model must recognize national benchmarks.

Additional incentive measures can include other aspects of medical practice that are important, such as quality of performance, patient satisfaction, or "good citizenship." As health care reform moves ahead, such metrics may become more important than productivity. Good citizenship can be a blend of satisfaction and quality, but often includes attendance at meetings, contribution to group efforts, and other more subjective facets of performance. Their measurement should be easily determined with a high degree of reliability. Some institutions include subjective components, but these should be kept to a minimum.

Whatever the basis for variable compensation, it is important that physicians have rapid and frequent feedback regarding their performance. This would be in the form of monthly reports and should take place shortly after the close of the month. If the variable compensation is viewed as an incentive, that incentive is most effective with frequent, accurate and timely evaluations. Failure to adhere to any of these principles rapidly degrades the effectiveness of the incentive measure. It is also important to be careful about the choice of incentive. Behaviors or activities which are not included in the incentive program, but are nevertheless important to the entity, may erode its potential for success.

## RECRUITMENT

Neurology has been identified as one of the most difficult specialties in the country for recruitment. In Massachusetts it takes two years, on average, to recruit a neurologist to a practice (personal communication, 2009). Compensation is even more important in recruitment than in the retention of neurologists.

There are many sources for obtaining national compensation levels for specific specialties. Perhaps the best is the survey conducted and published by the Medical Group Management Association (MGMA).[6] Sometimes only a few practices participate in this survey, mainly the best-performing practices. Although recruitment and retention are not solely based on compensation, the offered salary does needs to be competitive. Recruitment and retention are national and not regional considerations. Recruiters and recruitment efforts reach out to a national audience.

The competitive nature of recruitment leads to inducements beyond the level of compensation. Offers commonly include a sign-on bonus, payment of educational debts, payment of relocation costs, and even the inclusion of a monthly stipend until training is completed. Noneconomic incentives must also be considered, including time off, scheduling flexibility, and job sharing. These inducements vary, depending on the specialty and the region.

## ESTABLISHING AN INCENTIVE-BASED COMPENSATION SYSTEM

There is now a thriving and growing national industry geared to assist with the issue of physician compensation. This industry uses consultants, courses, and published materials. Its very existence indicates that establishing a formula is difficult and complex, and that no one answer fits all situations. In fact, it is unlikely that any group adopts the identical formula to another.

This review establishes some critical principles. It is important that the model selected is fair, competitive, simple, and transparent.

The first step is to determine the expected level of compensation. The MGMA salary levels represent the best available information, but specialty societies, recruiters, and colleagues are also sources for data on levels of compensation. A method for placing a cap on expectations should be included in the compensation package. In particular, in a multispecialty group the differences in specialty compensation are substantial and represent a potential source of conflict. Unless a group is mature and has a firm understanding of medical economics, allowing the physician leadership to establish specialty-specific compensation is likely to be counterproductive. The compensation model should be applied uniformly across the specialties, and the model should be flexible enough to adapt to specialty-specific differences.

The second step is to establish the actual incentives and determine how they affect compensation. The physicians themselves must participate in this step. Physician buy-in and physician engagement are much more likely, although not guaranteed, with physician involvement. Decisions to be made include the selection of the incentive method (ie, wRVUs), and the actual formula. The base salary may vary from 50% to 80% of the expected income, with the balance at risk dependent on production. For wRVUs, the base salary is linked to a wRVU threshold; wRVUs in excess of this threshold are paid out at a certain dollar value. These decisions should not be made by an isolated group of physician leaders, but should involve the entire group on a regular basis. An effort to effectively engage all physicians is important. Isolation of the physician leadership will lead to the same "them versus us" mentality that occurs when the administration makes decisions in isolation.

The model should also address other issues to avoid any perception of unfairness or privilege. These issues include compensation for continuing education and time off. Some specialties, like radiology, expect, as a standard, substantial time off, such as one week in a month. Uniformity across all specialties should be the goal, but in practical terms this may not be achievable.

Once decided upon, all physicians should be transitioned to the new model over time. The process should include multiple educational efforts to explain the model and physician-specific performance information to indicate how their prior productivity would fare in the new model. There will be winners and losers. Strategies to help the losers are important. Any transition for a group of physicians is difficult, particularly in the highly charged area of compensation.

Once established, attention must be paid to continued transparency. Although specific compensation levels may not be shared across the board, it is strongly suggested that individual productivity be shared within groups or specialties, and across the entire group. The group should reassess the model on a regular basis to ensure that there are no unintended consequences resulting in destructive behaviors or changes in health care reimbursement that require a modification of the model.

## SUMMARY

It is important to view any compensation method as an incentive. Both experience and studies demonstrate that unless individuals recognize that their efforts are closely tied to their compensation, productivity falls. Equal compensation can be effective if physicians view their efforts as contributing to the group as a whole, and if they benefit from the success of the group. As a group increases in size, it becomes less likely that physicians will adopt this view. Variable compensation requires some form of metric involving charges, receipts or wRVUs. It is important to recognize that the adoption of the variable compensation principle can cause destructive behaviors, such as unhealthy competition and attempts to game the system.

Fairness as represented by compensation and equality in responsibilities, such as call, is critical to the success of any group. Successful groups pay continuous attention to ensure that individuals are fairly treated and information is frequently shared in an understandable format.

Other aspects of employment share equal importance with compensation in contributing to the effectiveness of the group and its ability to recruit and retain high-quality physicians. Respect, recognition, professional satisfaction, a good fit with the group philosophy, and spousal happiness all constitute important aspects of professional satisfaction. The selection of a group by a new physician, and recruitment and retention efforts, must look beyond compensation alone.

Physician compensation remains a complex and difficult topic, and models of compensation continue to evolve. Health care reform may change medical economics in unpredictable ways. A model should be designed with careful consideration of its advantages and disadvantages, and with appropriate attention to physician involvement; the entity must also accept that flexibility and frequent modification are required.

## REFERENCES

1. Available at: http://www.nejmjobs.org/career-resources/physician-compensation-basics.aspx. Accessed June 13, 2009.
2. Conrad DA, Sales A, Linag SY, et al. The impact of financial incentives on physician productivity in medical groups. Health Serv Res 2002;37(4):885–906.
3. Greenfield WR. In search of an effective physician compensation formula. Fam Pract Manag 1998. Available at: www.aafp.org/fpm/981000fm/cover.html. Accessed June 13, 2009.
4. Reece EA, Nugent O, Wheeler RP, et al. Adapting industry-style business model to academia in a system of performance-based incentive compensation. Acad Med 2008;83(1):76–84.
5. Reich DL, Galati M, Krol M, et al. A mission-based productivity compensation model for an academic anesthesiology department. Anesth Analg 2008;107(6): 1981–8.
6. Medical Group Management Association. Physician compensation and production survey: 2008 report based on 2007 data. Glacier Publishing Services, Inc; 2008.

# Negotiating with Payers

Joel M. Kaufman, MD[a,b,]*

KEYWORDS

- Negotiations • Payer contracts • Insurer contracts
- Practice management

Physicians, particularly those practicing in smaller practices, often feel powerless to negotiate with payers for better reimbursement or changes in policies and procedures that impact their practice. By not negotiating, practitioners give up an opportunity to convince payers of their point of view. If one does not ask, one will never know what is possible. Negotiation can cover more than reimbursement issues. For example, a practice may want protective language in the contract, support for practice enhancements such as an electronic health record (EHR), or changes in payer policies or procedures. Even without immediate success, by negotiating, practitioners send the payer a message that they care, are interested and should be listened to. In taking this step, one will be surprised what can be achieved over time, both for an individual practice and colleagues.

This article discusses keys to successful negotiating and several specific areas beyond reimbursement that deserve the reader's attention.

## NEGOTIATING

The key to successful negotiations, like with most endeavors, is preparation, expectation, presentation, and attitude. Unfortunately, some physicians believe that they can be successful by relying on bluster and entitlement. The person, and more likely the team, across the table from the physician, consists of professionals who negotiate contracts all the time. They are prepared with data regarding the economics and efficacy of the physician's care of their members, as well as stories about the physician's or office staff's interaction with company representatives. Therefore, physicians should be prepared to discuss the economics and efficacies of the care provided to patients and provide verifiable data to support such positions. Similarly, physicians

[a] Lifespan/Physicians Professional Service Organization, 167 Point Street, Suite 3A, Providence, RI 02903, USA
[b] Department of Neurology, The Warren Alpert Medical School of Brown University, 110 Lockwood Street, Suite 324, Providence, RI 02903, USA
* Lifespan/Physicians Professional Service Organization, 167 Point Street, Suite 3A, Providence, RI 02903.
E-mail address: jkaufman@lifespan.org

Neurol Clin 28 (2010) 349–364
doi:10.1016/j.ncl.2009.11.009
0733-8619/10/$ – see front matter
**neurologic.theclinics.com**

also should be prepared with specific examples of the payer representative's behavior and responses to certain situations.

The payer is able to agree to some items on the spot, but often also must articulate the physician's points to others before responding. The physician is looking out for his or her practice; they are keeping in mind what is best for the payer, knowing that any special arrangements for one practice may have implications for others down the line.

The goal of negotiation should not be to trick the other party. It is unlikely that the physician will out-smart the other side. Nor is the purpose of negotiating to bend to every whim of the payer. What follows are suggestions on maximizing the physician's ability to succeed.

This article only touches the surface of the art of negotiation. There are several recommended books that are listed at the end of the article. It is a good idea to read several of them, as they differ in terms of approach; for example, who should make the first offer, or where meetings should be held. One also will learn how these skills will help the physician with everyday matters. And as with all skill development, practice makes a difference.

## DEFINITIONS
### Payer

In this article, the term payer is used for anyone with whom the physician has a contract or agreement to provide services. This includes insurers, such as Blue Cross plans, and also others such as the Center for Medicare and Medicaid Services, which manages Medicare. Large companies that self-insure for health care are also payers. The term third party commonly is used to refer to the payer, with the first party being the patient, and the second party being the provider of service.

### Insurer

Although one traditionally thinks of an insurer as an entity that assumes some financial risk for a service based on underwriting, companies such as United Healthcare or local Blue Cross plans also provide administrative services for self-insured employers. For the purpose of this article, insurer is defined as a company whose primary purpose is to reimburse a provider for certain services provided to an insured person.

### Current Procedural Terminology

Current Procedural Terminology (CPT) is a systematic listing of codes and descriptions that classify medical services and procedures. It is maintained and copyrighted by the American Medical Association. CPT codes are mandated by federal law for Medicare, Medicaid, and other federal programs, and accepted or required by all other third-party payers.

### Relative Value Units

Relative value units (RVUs) are standard units that place a value to each unit of service assigned to each CPT code that is covered by Medicare. To learn more, please read the article by Busis and Becker.[1]

### The American Academy of Neurology Professional Association

The American Academy of Neurology (AAN) is a professional medical association made up of more than 20,000 members in 97 countries. The American Academy of Neurology Professional Association (AANPA) is a companion organization focusing on practice-related issues, the type noted in this article.

*Member and Patient*

Payers and insurers have members with whom they have a financial responsibility to pay for benefits. Physicians and other providers of health care have patients. The physician's patient is the payer's member. Payers do not make medical decisions. They make decisions about what they will pay for or cover under the contract they have with their member.

## PREPARATION

Nothing enhances the likelihood for success more than the work one does before sitting down with the payer.[2] Knowledge regarding one's own practice and the other party is power at the table. In this section, the most important one of the article, the data and concepts that should be addressed well before face-to-face meetings will be reviewed.

*Determine the Relationship*

It is vital to consider the physician's relationship with his or her local payer as a long term one. The payer needs the physician, and the physician needs them. The success of each is truly dependent on the other. Without a comprehensive network, payers do not have a product to sell. Practices succeed best when they are paid promptly and fairly for their services, with a minimum of administrative overhead.

When the physician chooses to negotiate with someone, it can be on a onetime basis, such as for a renovation to the office, or with someone with whom the physician will have a long-term relationship, such as a payer or billing company. With the former, one is not interested in the contractor becoming a friend. For the latter, assuming the physician wants continued service and attention, a cooperative, respectful, and professional relationship is desired. This does not mean that the payer or vendor must be a best friend, or that both parties must be equal winners in the process. It does, however, mean that success, both as negotiations are completed and going forward, requires a working relationship.

The relationship the physician chooses also is determined by what he or she accomplishes or hopes to accomplish. If one has minimal volume with a payer who does not pay very well, and one must follow onerous and expensive procedures to get paid, it may be time to end the relationship or not invest much of the practice's time to enhance the relationship. On the other hand, if 40% of a physician's practice volume is with one payer, it is necessary to invest considerable time to make that relationship work.

*Who are the Players?*

Payers are either governmental or private entities. Governmental payers include federal programs such as the Centers for Medicare and Medicaid Services (CMS) and state-directed programs such as Medicaid. Private programs include national companies such as United Healthcare, Aetna, Cigna, and Wellpoint, and local or regional insurers, such as many Blue Cross plans, Harvard Pilgrim Health Care, and others.

Can one negotiate with CMS regarding Medicare? Perhaps not as an individual; however, organized medicine, such as the AANPA, negotiates all the time with CMS over coverage issues and reimbursement. Most recently, for example, the AANPA and other specialty societies collaborated to seek coverage of the canalith repositioning procedure.

Negotiation with state agencies regarding Medicaid also is done best via your local medical society and local specialty society.

Remember that in quite a number of locations, private insurers have managed Medicare and Medicare products, and one can negotiate for favorable terms. The insurers, either through CMS or state agencies, sign contracts to provide comprehensive management of populations of local residents in exchange for a set per member-per-month fee, and for Medicare plans, often an additional monthly premium from the member. If the cost of caring for the population is less than what is received, then the insurer has a surplus. If the cost is greater than what is received, then there is a loss, which the insurer absorbs. The local insurer is responsible for maintaining a local network and is able to negotiate its own fees and enhancements, such as risk-based contracts and gainshare arrangements, to align clinicians to provide better and more efficient care.

### Early and Ongoing Preparation

Preparation begins months before formal negotiation and is an ongoing process. Because the physician and the payer are both going to be in the community for a while, developing personal contacts is important from the get-go. One wants to identify the right people, those who make or influence policy, such as the medical director, chief executive officer, director of case management, or chief quality officer. Participating in physician advisory groups or on expert panels helps shape policy and creates personal relationships with key management.

### When to Begin

Set a timetable working back from the contract renewal date. This needs to be done whether one is a solo practitioner or part of a large group. This allows the physicians to assign preparation tasks and set a schedule so that he or she is ready when the time comes to meet with the payer. **Table 1** presents a schedule for a contract with a renewal date of January 1.

### PRACTICE DATA

The physician needs to have his or her practice data to know exactly what he or she is being paid by the insurer on a stand-alone and comparison basis with other payers. The physician's product is his or her time and expertise, which are sold to several sources. Knowing the basic data, such as those items in **Box 1**, as well as what each payer pays, lets the physician know where and how to focus negotiating efforts.

**Table 1**
**Contract schedule**

| Task | Due | By |
| --- | --- | --- |
| Prepare financial analysis | June 15 | Billing or practice manager |
| Schedule meetings with payer | July 1 | Practice manager |
| Nonreimbursement issues identified with staff | July 5 | Practice manager and staff |
| Group meets to review analysis | July 10 | Practice manager and physicians |
| Ask-and-walk away position articulated | July 18 | Negotiating team |
| Unique practice characteristics and quality data assembled | July 18 | All |
| First offer presentation finalized | July 25 | Negotiating team |
| First meeting with payer | August 1 | Negotiating team |
| Sign new agreement | December 1 | |

| Box 1 |
|---|
| **Practice data** |
| Total revenue |
| Number of unique patients |
| Number of visits by CPT |
| RVU total by CPT |
| Compute $/RVU by insurer |
| Accounts receivables–less than 30 days |
| Accounts receivables–greater than 90 days |

One of the best ways to do this is by CPT code and RVUs. The physician will need his or her practice data by CPT code for each payer, the Medicare RVUs for each CPT, and Medicare reimbursement for each CPT code. The Medicare data are available on the Medicare Web site (http://www.cms.hhs.gov), from the physician's billing company or staff, or from the AANPA.

One will need three tables (**Tables 2–4**) that either the physician or his or her billing company can set up. The first will demonstrate for a payer the frequency and payments per RVU of each CPT code and total number of RVUs for the practice. This should be done for all payers with meaningful volume. **Table 2** is an example of how this may be done for one payer.

Separately compute the average payment per RVU by dividing the total payments (sum of column E) by total number of RVUs (sum of column D). This will be used in **Table 4**.

**Table 3** will normalize each CPT code compared with Medicare. This will allow one to see if the payer under- or overweighs some codes relative to others. Payers may reimburse less for codes used frequently by the physician's practice and more for

| Table 2 | | | | | | |
|---|---|---|---|---|---|---|
| **Frequency and payments per RVU of each CPT code and total number of RVUs for a payer** | | | | | | |
| A | B | C | D | E | F | G |
| CPT Code | Frequency | RVU | Number of RVUs (Column B × Column C) | Total Payments for this CPT | Payments Per RVU (Column E/Column D) | Payment Per RVU as a % of Medicare[a] |
| 99213 | 65 | 1.70 | 110.5 | $5260.45 | $47.606 | 132% |
| 99214 | 75 | 2.56 | 192.0 | $9002.25 | $46.887 | 130% |
| 99215 | 35 | 3.46 | 121.1 | $5590.55 | $46.165 | 128% |
| 95819 | 50 | 6.42 | 321.0 | $10,535.50 | $32.821 | 91% |
| 95860 | 50 | 2.23 | 111.5 | $5429.03 | $48.691 | 135% |
| TOTAL | | | 856.1 | $35,817.78 | $41.8383 | 116% |

99213 Office visit for evaluation and management (E&M), expanded level/low complexity.
99214 Office visit for E&M detailed level/moderate complexity.
99215 Office visit for E&M comprehensive level/complex.
95819 Routine EEG, awake and sleep.
95860 Needle electromyography, one extremity.
See CPT manual for full code descriptions.
[a] Divide column F by the same year's Medicare Conversion Factor adjusted to local area.
One should use the same year's RVUs in column C. The unadjusted Medicare Conversion Factor for 2009 is $36.0666.

**Table 3**
**CPT code compared with Medicare**

| A | B | C | D |
|---|---|---|---|
| CPT | Payer 1 Payment | Medicare | Percent Medicare |
| (See Table 2 for Descriptions) | | Payment | (For Each Row, Column B/Column C × 100) |
| 99213 | $80.93 | $61.31 | 132% |
| 99214 | $120.03 | $92.33 | 130% |
| 99215 | $159.73 | $124.79 | 128% |
| 95819 | $210.71 | $231.55 | 91% |

less commonly used codes. For example, getting paid 125% of Medicare for 99233 (subsequent hospital care, per day, detailed/high complexity), when you get paid 105% for a 99213 (office visit for evaluation and management expanded level/low complexity) is not a good deal unless one is a hospitalist.

**Table 4** should be helpful to compare the total for each payer, and each payer product, again normalized against Medicare. One should use this table to determine where to aim for each payer and which payers require greater attention overall.

As one negotiates reimbursement, also use these worktables to see what has been accomplished. Payers may increase fees strictly in certain families of codes or minimize charges for certain procedures. For example, the payer may offer a 7% overall increase for all providers in one's area, with some codes increasing 10% and others only going up 2%. If this increase is not uniform across the entire fee schedule and is less for codes the physician commonly uses, he or she may only see a 2% or 3% change. Insurers also may suggest smaller increases for lower level evaluation and management codes (level 1, 2 and 3) than for the higher level 4 and 5 codes.

Other preparation would include knowing how the practice does with various quality initiatives, such as Medicare's Patient Quality Reporting Initiative, or insurer-specific programs, such as United Healthcare Premium Designation program.

The AANPA makes data available on average coding. If one codes 99221 (Initial hospital care, problems of low severity), 30% of the time, chances are the coding is being done in a manner consistent with peers. If one is coding 99222 (Initial hospital care, problems of moderate severity) 50% of the time, chances are the coding is being done in a manner consistent with peers. If one is coding 99233 (Initial hospital care, problems of high severity) 80% of the time one should be prepared to document why. Note that even if one has a general neurology practice, one's coding profile will have higher-level codes (more comprehensive history and examination and

**Table 4**
**Total for each payer normalized against Medicare**

| Payer | Payment Per RVU | As a Percent of Medicare |
|---|---|---|
| Medicare | $36.0666 | 100.0% |
| Payer X Commercial | $41.8383 | 116.0% |
| Payer X Managed Medicare | $33.5419 | 93.0% |
| Payer Y | $37.8699 | 105.0% |

more complex decision making) than an internal medicine or other practice. Use of national data will help make that point. All this, of course, assumes that one's coding and documentation are proper and complete.

The physician also should be aware of the level of difficulty of dealing with each payer, as assessed by the items in **Box 2**, and how those characteristics affect his or her practice. Time spent chasing down claims or seeking help has a cost to it. Sitting down with one's office staff and billing staff should provide this information. Try to assign a value to each item. Be prepared to present your list when sitting down with the payer, not to whine about things but as points of negotiation that one may achieve or trade for something else.

## HOW IS AN INDIVIDUAL PRACTICE SPECIAL?

Aspects of the physician's patient panel or practice differentiate it from other practices, and will make the case for either enhanced reimbursement, supplemental support services paid for by the payer, or waiver of other requirements or reviews. Indignantly informing the payer of this without documentation and expecting immediate acceptance of one's demands will not go very far. Putting together the story of one's practice, with facts and figures, has a better chance of helping the physician meet his or her goals.

This section contains some items that should be included in the story.

### Which Patients are Seen

What is the average age of patients? Does the physician have a subspecialty practice, or are many patients seen who require extra time either during the visit or between visits? And if so, is this different for this particular payer versus others? Knowing the why is also helpful.

### Quality Measures and Use of Evidenced-based Medicine and Guidelines

There are emerging measures of quality as developed by the American Quality Alliance and used by CMS and others. Having systems in place to measure a practice's performance is important in itself. Demonstrating to patients and the payers that one does a good job will be an important chapter in the story of one's practice as enhancements in one's contract are negotiated. Systems to collect quality data need not be complex, although it is easier to measure performance with an EHR.

---

**Box 2**
**Payer issues to review**

Are claims paid correctly and promptly?

Are the evidence of payment forms accurate and understandable?

Is it easy to verify insurance coverage?

Is one able to reach provider relations staff who are knowledgeable and can help solve problems quickly and efficiently?

Does the plan medical director return the physician's calls?

Are care management staff available to help with complex patient needs?

Is there an imaging referral management program, and if so, how much professional time and staff time are involved in the interaction?

### Service and Patient Satisfaction

Tracking patient satisfaction, telephone responsiveness, wait for appointment, and test results notification are important parameters in their own right. Demonstrating that one measures these and other items is helpful. Payers want satisfied members, and if the physician can demonstrate that he or she takes patient satisfaction seriously, that further aligns him or her with the payer for the long term. As a neurologist, referring physician satisfaction is also a key with attention to items such as ease of referral, timeliness of a note back, helpfulness of the note, use of resources, ability to reach, and patient management. Demonstrating one's value to the community differentiates one physician from others, and ultimately may contribute to the determination of what one should be paid.

### Investments in Technology and Other Services

Does the physician have an EHR or, if not, is he or she planning on investing in one soon? Does the practice have a nurse practitioner with an emphasis in a particular clinical area? Does the practice have additional educational or counseling services? Does the practice have patients who participate in the payer's disease management or case management programs? Demonstrating that one's practice is forward thinking is another way to engage the payer and encourage sharing the investment.

### Insurer Strategic Plans

Learn the payer's plans for the individual's area, both from a business and clinical program standpoint. Is the payer interested in expanding its reach into new areas? How does the physician's practice support the payer's plans for growth? If the payer has a managed Medicare program, does the physician see a lot of seniors, or does he or she have a strong referral relationship with geriatricians or nursing homes?

Is the payer rolling out new disease management or chronic care programs in areas that the physician has an interest in, such as dementia or multiple sclerosis? Are advisors for programs needed, or offices to pilot initiatives? It is best to have some idea of this before sitting down, but it is certainly acceptable to make this part of the meeting, as long as the physician asks that the payer bring staff members who are knowledgeable about these programs to the meeting. If the physician is interested in participating in payer programs, he or she should think about what to ask for in return.

It is easier to obtain this information than one might think. Consider calling the medical director, planning department, or director of case management. Background intelligence gives the physician power at the table and when used judiciously demonstrates that homework has been done.

### Investments in Practice

Did the physician invest in an EHR? How has this affected the practice, both positively and negatively? Although there is a return on investment (ROI) to the practice, most of the savings from EHR adoption goes to the payer in terms of reductions in redundant testing and better compliance with practice guidelines.

### EXPECTATIONS
#### Determining What is Wanted and the Minimum that Can Be Agreed Upon

One of my favorite stories is about the pilot who announces to the passengers midflight that he has good news and bad news. The bad news is that they are lost. The good news is that they are making great time. Going into a meeting without having articulated to oneself the specific goal is a waste of everyone's time.

According to the Medical Group Management Association (MGMA), the median collections for professional charges for a neurologist in 2008 were $387,027.[3] If one is able to obtain an additional 1% increase from private payers (assume half of one's business), that is an additional $1939 that the physician can take directly home for doing the same amount of work.

A key concept in negotiating is to know if and when to walk away. If one cannot walk away from the table, and the other party knows that, then the physician's negotiating position is weak. Unfortunately, a large number of physicians are in this position because of the dominance of large insurers in many places. Ideally, one would like no more than 15% to 20% of one's practice with any one insurer. In a market dominated by one or two insurers, developing a unique niche either clinically or programmatically will serve the same purpose, if one is able to tell that story.

If one can walk away, as part of the physician's strategy, he or she needs to determine when before sitting down.

### Important Nonfinancial Issues

The practice's financial success is determined by the difference between revenue and expenses. Most physicians concentrate on the revenue side and ignore the impact payer operations have on their expense side. The need to hire an additional person for insurance verifications, authorizations, or chasing down incorrect payments has a substantial economic impact on an individual's practice.

### How to Identify Contract Language Issues

This should be a formal process with the entire staff, with particular input from the billing and collections area. Often, payment denials are caused by insurance verification problems, which may be due to front office inefficiencies. For example, does the practice's intake staff verify coverage with each visit and collect copays and deductibles on presentation? Does staff confirm coverage using online tools? Complaining to the insurance company when office procedures are lacking is not useful.

On the other hand, for example, if the physician's staff registration and coverage verification processes are all in line, yet the office must spend considerable time resubmitting or appealing claims because the payer does not maintain their records, there is a strong case to be compensated for that extra time.

### PRESENTATION

The physician's contract proposal should be prepared in writing in a professional and clear manner, and presented orally in a confident, concise, and assertive manner (practice beforehand). The written proposal avoids confusion and misinterpretation later, and provides an opportunity to provide reasoning or data supporting the request, which the physician may highlight during his or her oral presentation. This also demonstrates that the physician has done his or her homework and is prepared; both are strong messages. For example, one's request for a 10% increase in rates may be in the context of a $35,000 investment in an EHR. Or one's 9% request may reflect additional staff to handle (successful) claims appeals or referral management requirements imposed by the payer. Remember that more often than not, the payer representative will need to take the proposal to his or her director; telling the story concisely and accurately is important so that it may be relayed clearly.

Similarly, any proposal or response from the payer should be in writing or summarized soon after meeting. Ask the payer representative to do this. If he or she refuses or does not seem enthusiastic about responding, the physician should offer to summarize his or her understanding of the proposal or response and provide it in writing. The physician should make sure that he or she understands every detail of what is presented, and not be shy about seeking clarification about inconsistencies or omissions in the proposal. For example, does the term "yearly increase" mean January or later in the year?

## ATTITUDE
### Keeping Emotions in Check

Does anyone really believe that yelling and screaming works? The physician always should remember that he or she wants something from the people on the other side of the table. Belittling them, their relatives, coworkers, or company is not a good way to achieve this goal. If the physician is perceived as professional, he or she will be treated as a professional. Like them or not, the payer staff members have a job to do, and just like anyone else, they will prioritize whom they will call back first or for which practice they will push for some flexibility in the contract.

### Whining—Be Prepared Not to

The people on the other side of the table likely have heard every complaint the physician is prepared to make at least 100 times (if not, they are too junior). Remember, the goal is to get these individuals to tell the physician's story to their supervisors in a positive way. Interacting and telling one's story in a positive and factual manner makes their job easier, and helping the physician easier. They want to be perceived as helpful and appreciated.

### Who Should Be at the Table?

It is a good idea not to go alone, whether one is representing oneself or a larger practice. Having at least two people hear a conversation helps avoid misinterpretations later and serves as a check on what is said by both parties. Certainly, before the meeting, one should determine who is the principal presenter. If the physician wishes to confer with a partner, one should not hesitate to ask for a break to caucus to meet alone. This is a good way to ensure that the physician's side has the same understanding as to what is being said and what are the next steps.

If at all possible, the physician wants the payer's representative to be someone who has the authority to make decisions. If one has developed a solid relationship with the payer over the years, or if the group is large and has a unique position in the community, this is more likely to happen. Even so, chances are the payer's representative will take new items and significant financial requests back to the office to review with a higher authority. This is a common technique in negotiations, which the physician also can employ ("I have to discuss this with my other partners..."). If the person with whom the physician is meeting does not have final authority, determining who does, making sure one's message is delivered properly, and insisting on timely response times are all important. If talks stall or the physician feels he or she is getting the run-around despite good faith efforts, one should insist on including the decision maker in meetings.

## THE CONTRACT

The payer may include sections in contracts that the physician may not like but that the payer considers standard, core language. This may include a requirement to participate in all payer products, a prohibition against criticizing the payer (gag clauses), agreement to follow all new policies and procedures even though the physician does not have an opportunity to review and approve them, or mandatory arbitration in the case of a disagreement. One's local medical society can often be very helpful with these issues. Because of restrictions in the antitrust laws, physicians who are not economically or clinically integrated cannot negotiate together with payers or discuss payer participation decisions with each other. However, either through one's independent practice association (IPA) or medical society, or some other trusted neutral third party, one can use a messenger model to pass comments back and forth between the payer and the groups. The negotiating advantage with this approach is that if there is concern regarding language that one would like to change, there is a good chance that others feel the same way and that a joint message will have greater impact. Also, the IPA or medical society may have legal or other resources that the individual physician does not.

The American Medical Association (AMA) developed a model managed care contract, the most recent version of which is available to members on its web site (http://www.ama-assn.org/ama1/x-ama/upload/mm/368/nmcc-2009.pdf).[4] In addition the AMA has twelve issue briefs on such topics as common managed care contract clauses, coordination of benefits, overpayments and underpayments, and alternative dispute resolution (http://www.ama-assn.org/ama/pub/advocacy/current-topics-advocacy/private-sector-advocacy/national-managed-care.shtml).[5] Please see references for complete list. These are excellent documents and resources and worth reading.

### Railroads Cannot Do It, and Neither Can the Physician

As mentioned previously, federal antitrust law dictates that physicians cannot jointly negotiate or discuss participation decisions, reimbursement or contract terms unless economically or clinically integrated. Economically integrated means one is part of the same practice, which commonly is manifested by all the providers in a group billing under the same tax identification number. Clinically integrated means a very stringent standard for care of patients has been met. There are only a few clinically integrated practices in the United States that meet the federal government's standard for clinical integration. Failure to follow these guidelines is a per se violation of antitrust laws, which means that the federal government will not consider the facts and circumstances relating to the activities, but rather simply apply the prohibition. Antitrust rules do not differentiate between a billion dollar company and two solo physicians. Despite the absurdity that an insurance company with 70% of the market can make unreasonable demands, and two solo physicians cannot negotiate jointly with the same payer about their contracts, these rules must be taken seriously.

### Read the Contract

Before signing the contract, make sure that all of it is read, and that all the terms and conditions are understood. It is important that if the physician does not understand something that he or she seek clarification at this point and not sign the contract. Although having an attorney or someone else read the contract may be useful, that is not a substitute for the physician reading the contract as he or she will have a perspective that is different from external advisors.

I have been surprised about the number of times when, in response to questions on standard contracts from physicians, large insurers go back and make changes. They say, "no one noticed that before."

Similarly, it is important to read policies and other documents that are referenced in the contract that one is agreeing to follow, such as payment policies, how to determine what services are not covered by the payer, or how disputes are handled. If one signs the contract and only then finds out what has been agreed to, the opportunity to negotiate has been missed. One should consider working with his or her local medical society, the AAN, or IPA to change policies or procedures that are burdensome.

### Use of an Attorney or Other Advisor

Legal questions may arise after one has read the proposed contract prepared by the payer. The contracts that payers are presenting have been thoroughly reviewed by the payer's attorneys. It is expensive for an attorney to review a contract for a small practice, and depending on the physician's comfort level, this may not be necessary. One option is via the messenger model in which the physician asks his or her IPA or medical society to have its attorney review the standard contract to identify problematic terms and conditions on behalf of the members, and pass comments back and forth between parties, but without the ability to negotiate changes. The physician's accountant also may be helpful.

### Contract Language that is Worth Particular Attention

#### Terms and definitions

One should make sure that all the terms used in the contract are understood. These should be spelled out in the definition section. Terms generally are capitalized later on in the contract.

#### Audit rights

Although payers likely have policies and procedures regarding their right to review the physician's documentation of the services performed, this is one area that should be discussed carefully. How far back can they go? Are payments suspended during the audit? If one must supply copies of records, will they pay copying costs, and if so how much? What is the physician's right of appeal? If an expert does the review, is it another neurologist? Are there guidelines, and if so, are they proprietary and unique to the payer, or more generally available? Can the physician see them?

#### Payment terms

This should include not only how much one will get paid, but when. As part of the physician's preparation, he or she should know the accounts receivable history with the payer. Money has value that is lost over time. If one is not paid in a timely manner, what is that worth, and how will the payer make that up? Some states have timely payment laws in place.

#### Timely filing

The contract will specify how soon one needs to submit a claim to get paid. However, a claim may be denied if another payer is rightfully responsible, or a claim may be pended and ultimately denied because of work or other legal issues, and determined to be the responsibility of another payer. The defined period to submit may easily pass. Language that states that the filing period commences from either the date of service or the denial date from another payer will address this issue. Remember, errors on the practice side, even if covered by this language, will result in significant cash flow problems.

#### Evergreen clauses

Consider eliminating automatic renewals that extend the contract term to term. A hard stop to the contract term, whether 1 year or 3 years, forces the opportunity to examine what is working in the relationship and what is not. That may include if the physician is being paid on time, denials, additional administrative hassles, and other issues. As mentioned previously, the physician's relationship with the payer is a long-term one. There may be items the physician was unsuccessful in achieving in negotiations last time, which he or she may achieve now. Also as noted previously, the only way to receive is to ask.

### All products

Most insurers have different products that they sell to companies or the public. This may include Managed Medicare, Managed Medicaid, preferred provider organizations (PPOs), and point of service plans, among others. The physician wants the right to participate in these plans, and to know how much he or she will be paid. The physician also would like the right not to participate in some products if the fee schedules or procedures are unacceptable. Some insurers make their PPO network available to other payers without the physician's knowledge (silent PPOs) such that one finds oneself discounting services to entities that have little volume in one's area, and, to add insult to injury, from which one may have difficulty collecting.

### Pay-for-performance, bonus or risk-sharing arrangements

Getting additional revenue for meeting quality or utilization goals is an important trend over recent years. These programs sound great. After all, physicians provide the right care at the right time. However, it is important to articulate the details of these programs in the physician's contract.

Measures should be objective, based on available data, specialty specific, with a defined measurement period, program duration, and set payout date. The contract should allow verification of data to ensure completeness and some language that will address unanticipated quirks. Payments may be either lump sums as a bonus or base increases.

It is also important to understand how the data will be reported both to the physician and others, as well as who will have access to the data. Will the physician's results be on the Internet? Will the payer's members have access to it? Will it be used to direct members to preferred providers?

The AMA and the AANPA in 2008 adopted policies regarding physician tiering and the use of quality or cost data to direct patients toward certain providers using member financial incentives. These policies are available on the AMA and AANPA Web sites. Both call for transparency in how the payers set up these programs, sharing of data sufficiently ahead of publication to allow physicians to review the information and seek corrections, and the use of specialty-specific criteria.

Be cautious of accepting bonus or performance payments in lieu of a rate increase, as the amount one receives does not go into the base that will be used for future rate increases. The 5% increase one receives now will grow each year because of compounding, while the performance payment, which is not a sure thing, must be earned each year. As can be seen in **Table 5**, accepting a 3% rate increase and a 2% performance bonus is 1% less than a straight 5% rate increase.

### Lesser of

Payers may have language that they will pay the lesser of one's charges or the fee schedule in the contract. If one is not vigilant in reviewing and updating his or her fee schedule every year, charges may fall behind otherwise negotiated reimbursement. Eliminating lesser of language from the contract is the best way to eliminate this "gotcha" problem.

**Table 5**
**5% Rate increases versus 3% rate increases and 2 % annual performance payments**

|  | 5% Annual Rate Increase | 3% Annual Rate Increase | 2% Annual Performance Bonus |
|---|---|---|---|
| Year 1—base | $50,000 | $50,000 | $1000 |
| Year 2 | $52,500 | $51,500 | $1030 |
| Year 3 | $55,125 | $53,045 | $1061 |
| Year 4 | $57,881 | $54,636 | $1093 |
| Subtotal | $215,506 | $209,181 | $4184 |
| Total | $215,506 | $213,365 | |
| Difference | $2141 less or approximately 1% of total over the 4 years | | |

## NONCONTRACTURAL NEGOTIATIONS WITH PAYERS
### Coverage for New Technology

Payers, on behalf of their subscribers, evaluate new technologies, including drugs, devices, and procedures and decide if they will pay for their use. Payers want to be prudent and not cover technologies or procedures that are unproven or may harm their members. Expensive new technologies receive considerable attention. Cost to the payer, member, and employer clearly play a significant role in which items are covered or limited. Specialty societies, such as the AANPA, take the lead in working with CMS and national payers. Most decisions, however, are made at the local level, including most Blue Cross plans, and regional Medicare intermediaries.

When making a request for coverage, it is important to present data, including credible studies from peer-reviewed literature, and if available, guidelines from specialty societies. There are technologies that start off full of promise that do not pan out. There are also advocates who have a stake in the technology and who promote adoption based on anecdotal reports or personal investment.

The following series of three questions will be helpful to answer in one's presentation. First, does the technology do what it says that it does? If the answer is no, there is no need to proceed. Second, does it perform equal to, better than, or worse than existing technologies? This should include outcomes, adverse effects, and complications. If worse, then no need to proceed. If better, then a direct request can be made for coverage. If equal to, then a third question needs to be answered: what is the cost to the payer, the patient and society?

One's presentation to the payer should be in writing, focused and factual. It should include a brief summary of what the physician is requesting, clinical summaries of one or two paragraphs per patient, a summary of relevant literature, and supporting references, including copies of the articles. A call in advance to the plan medical director is important. Guidelines or restrictions should be suggested when appropriate.

## IMPORTANT QUALIFYING STATEMENT

I am neither an attorney nor an accountant. For specific legal or financial advice, one should not rely on any statements in this article and should seek qualified professional advice.

## SUMMARY

Negotiating with payers for better reimbursement, contract language, support for practice enhancement, or changes in policies and procedures is a critical function that may greatly enhance a practice's success over time. This article reviewed aspects of preparation, setting expectations, presentation, and attitude. Several specific contract items also were reviewed, as well as noncontractual negotiations with payers. Although negotiating with payers is often difficult and frustrating, being as well prepared as possible when approaching discussions enhances the likelihood of a positive outcome for a practice.

## ACKNOWLEDGMENTS

My thanks and appreciation to Avi N. Kaufman, MBA, Carol Goodman Kaufman, PhD, Judy Randal, and Attorney Stephen Zubiago, for their thoughtful and thorough reviews and suggestions, and to Diane DaCosta, for her ongoing assistance and suggestions in the preparation of the manuscript.

## REFERENCES

1. Busis NA, Becker A. Primer to payment for neurology services and procedures. Neurol Today 2007;7(5):30.
2. Mayse CA. Physician practice and ASC managed care contracting, MGMA smart pack, getting paid what you deserve medical group management association; payer contracts & reimbursement. 2005.
3. Physician compensation and production survey: 2009 report based on 2008 data. Medical Group Management Association. pg 72: Table 16.
4. 2009 American Medical Association/Federation National Managed Care Contract; Available to AMA members at: http://www.ama-assn.org/ama1/x-ama/upload/mm/368/nmcc-2009.pdf. Accessed 1/25/2010.
5. The following issue briefs are also available to AMA members via the AMA web site http://www.ama-assn.org/ama/pub/advocacy/current-topics-advocacy/private-sector-advocacy/national-managed-care.shtml. Accessed 1/25/2010. Issue brief topics are: Physicians Beware of these Common Managed Care Contract Clauses; Medical Necessity and Appeals of Medical Necessity Denials; Rental Networks; "All Products" Provisions; Disclosure of Payment-Related Information; Claims Submission, Processing, Payment and Remedies; Coordination of Benefits; Verification of Eligibility and Preauthorization or Pre-notification of Proposed Services; Overpayments and Underpayments; Alternative Dispute Resolution-Arbitration; Amendment; Term, Termination and Nonrenewal

## FURTHER READINGS

Donaldson MC. Negotiating for dummies. 2nd edition. Hoboken (NJ): Wiley Publishing; 2007.

Dawson R. Secrets of power negotiating. 2nd edition. Franklin Lakes (NJ): Career Press; 2001.

Fisher R, Ury W, Patton B. Getting to yes, negotiating agreement without giving in. 2nd edition. New York (NY): Houghton Mifflin; 1991.

Harvard Business Essential; Negotiation. Your mentor and guide to doing business effectively. Boston (MA): Harvard Business School Press; 2003.

Babitsky S, Mangraviti JJ. The physicians' comprehensive guide to negotiating. Boston (MA): SEAK; 2007.

Nelson R. Knowledge of third-party-payer contracts critical. MGMA e-Connection, Issue 37, August 2003.

Mertz MG. Case study: negotiating higher reimbursement from an insurance company. MGMA Connection, Vol 4, Issue 9, October 2004.

Simons AB. Know-how expanding knowledge for the practice administrator. MGMA Connection, Vol 3, Issue 9, October 2003.

Weymier RE. MGMA focus on managed care, what payers want. MGMA e-Connection, Issue 42, November 2003.

Stampiglia T. Getting the most from your payor contracts. Group Pract 2008;33–6.

# Benchmarking the Neurology Practice

William S. Henderson, MA, FACMPE

**KEYWORDS**

• Benchmark • Finances • Practice management
• Physician production

During the first decade of the twenty-first century, health care in the United States has been in the throes of change that has not been seen since the initial rollout of the Medicare insurance program for the elderly. President Barack Obama, working in conjunction with the US Congress in 2009, has promised to provide an overhaul of the current health care system. This initiative follows years of increasing administrative demands on physicians by insurers, decreasing reimbursement for the care provided to patients, increasing costs of running a medical practice, and, in some cases, poorer patient outcomes than would be anticipated.[1] Since 1998, revenues per unit of physician work have not risen as quickly as medical practice expenses. From 2001 to 2009, operating costs in the average medical practice increased 50.1%, compared with the Consumer Price Index that increased just 19.2% during that same time period.[2] In 2008, according to the Medical Group Management Association (MGMA), that percentage rose to 63%.[3] It is certain that factors such as these and the rising costs associated with providing health care to Medicare recipients and to those Americans without insurance will be a political focus in the next few years.

Although no professional medical society or association keeps statistics on the number of failed medical practices per year, it is commonly known that the number of solo and small physician practices (3 or less providers) has been shrinking since the mid-1980s. Since about 16% of neurologists in private practice, according to 2008 numbers kept by the American Academy of Neurology (AAN), work in solo practices (Gina Gjorvad, AAN Staff, personal communication, 2008), their future viability is at greatest risk. Solo practitioners and neurologists in small groups are in greater jeopardy of making a costly financial or operational blunder from which they cannot recover as compared with those working in larger groups or for hospitals or academic institutions. Solo and small practice physicians often lack alternative revenue streams and good information technology systems that would warn them of impending financial problems. The economic reality affects neurologists more than most physicians. According to the 2008 Physician Practice Information survey done by the American

Upstate Neurology Consultants, LLP, 3 Atrium Drive Suite 200, Albany, NY 12205, USA
*E-mail address:* whenderson@upstateneurology.com

Neurol Clin 28 (2010) 365–384
doi:10.1016/j.ncl.2009.11.003
0733-8619/10/$ – see front matter © 2010 Elsevier Inc. All rights reserved.

**neurologic.theclinics.com**

Medical Association (AMA), it cost neurologists more to provide care to their patients than most other physicians—$127.21 per patient as compared with $116.96 for all physicians.[4]

Although many medical schools have introduced a business course or two into their curriculum, new physicians are most often unprepared to face the rigors of running a medical business. Physicians must learn not only patient care but also the business principles that will ensure success. All this begs the question: can a neurology practice survive in times such as these? More to the point, can the practice thrive? There are tools available that can help a practice better understand its business dynamics as well as its effectiveness and efficiency. The key tool, often overlooked by harried physicians, is benchmarking. While not a panacea for the problems of health care in general, benchmarking can act as a warning alert, a measurement of progress toward established performance goals, and a clarifier of the dynamics of medical practice performance. In fact, this is not optional. As Gans and Feltenberger[5] note: "The current state of health care ....dictates more elaborate and accurate methods of measurement, analysis, comparison and improvement. Because long-term success is directly related to a practice's ability to identify, predict and adjust for changes, benchmarking, when used properly, is the best tool for overcoming these challenges."

## WHAT IS BENCHMARKING?

In 1979 the Xerox Corporation lost 80% of its market share in copiers to Japanese companies. As a result Xerox executives sought to determine what they were doing wrong and how they could improve their performance. The process they created developed into "benchmarking" as we know it today.

The American Productivity & Quality Center (APQC) defines benchmarking as "the process of identifying, learning, and adapting outstanding practices and processes from another organization to help improve performance." Benchmarking, simply put, is the process of identifying best practices in an industry and seeking to implement those practices in a specific business. Benchmarking involves measuring, comparing, and evaluating data from your business. It does the measurement over time, comparing one year to the next (internal benchmarking) and also against data of businesses in the same business field (external benchmarking).

In health care, benchmarking specifically measures data sets that are applicable to a medical care provider; it includes finances, practice operations, and the delivery/quality of patient care. Benchmarking can involve measuring everything from patient satisfaction to the number of days a bill for patient services sits in accounts receivable (AR) before it is collected. While there are literally hundreds of data points that could be measured in a medical practice, there is neither the time nor necessity to measure them all.

What does a practice benchmark? Each medical practice has to define what its goals are. A practice needs to describe in words, through a mission statement, what it means to those in the practice to be a "good medical practice." The mission statement lays out what the group wants to be or achieve. The benchmarking process then identifies the crucial data that should be measured to enable the group to know that it is making progress in meeting its goals, which grow out of the mission statement. Not all neurology practices are the same; the culture of how medicine is practiced can differ dramatically between groups. Benchmarking can benefit diverse medical practices, but it is most useful when the group identifies what it wants to be.

## STANDARD BENCHMARKING CATEGORIES FOR MEDICAL PRACTICES

Each neurology practice is unique; its vision and goals define the relationship of the physicians to their patients, their staff, and their community. However, each practice needs to benchmark itself in three areas: financial performance, operational/staff measures, and clinical measures.

Unless a practice is profitable, it will not be able to provide care to its patients. That is why financial measures are so crucial. Financial measures include far more than the income a neurologist makes. The key measures are fee schedules, coding, billing, revenue collection, and insurance claims denials. These measures even delineate how the revenue in the practice is spent to "do the business of medicine."

Operational and staff measures look at the work that is being done by each employee, including physicians, as compared with national measures. Measures can be as diverse as the amount of time it takes a patient to go from check-in to actually seeing the physician (patient flow), the number of new patient registration phone calls a scheduling secretary should be able to complete per hour, or even the number of work relative value units (RVU) that a physician does. This type of benchmarking can help identify if a practice has too few or too many staff members or whether it has the right or wrong type of staff members.

Clinical measures look at clinical care outcomes and clinical care costs. While still in its developmental infancy for most specialties, since 2005 there has been an intensive effort by both medical specialty societies and insurers to measure the value of patient care based on its cost and the actual health condition of the patient before and after treatment. This evaluation can also include measures for encouraging patient safety, such as "e-prescribing."

## EXTERNAL AND INTERNAL BENCHMARKS

For medical practices much work has been done to identify benchmark statistics in the areas of financial measures and operational/staff measures. The major organization that collects these data is the MGMA, located in Englewood, Colorado. Since the 1990s the MGMA has done annual surveys for physician compensation and production,[6] as well as a cost survey.[3] These data can be analyzed both from a conglomerate perspective (all medical specialties, sizes, regions of the country) or from a specialty perspective (neurologists or neurology groups in the United States). **Table 1** shows the type of neurology-specific data that the MGMA collected from 2006. The results of better-performing groups are also presented annually by the MGMA.[7]

Although the data provided by the MGMA are the best available for comparison purposes, there are several caveats that must be noted. First, the MGMA tends to gather data from the more sophisticated, better-run practices (ie, usually larger practices). Second, for neurology in particular, the number of groups participating in the annual cost survey is often less than 30.[3] (This is in contrast to the more than 400 neurologists who participated in the compensation survey in 2008).[6] Third, MGMA surveys give median numbers but they do not show the confidence intervals for the data. Fourth, there can be confusion in what a benchmark item actually means. For example, what does the full time equivalent (FTE) support staff ratio to physician actually mean? How does one know if the staff person is being used efficiently? Fifth, what happens if a practice meets or exceeds an external benchmark? For some groups, this can lead to "post-success" inefficiencies. Sixth, there are tremendous revenue variations (and resulting income differences) based on the size of the medical practice, the ancillary services it may own, and its ability to undertake major capital purchases such as a magnetic resonance imaging scanner or a building. Furthermore, the low

**Table 1**
MGMA neurology data

**Medical Group Management Association**

**Cost Survey: 2007 Report Based on 2006 Data**

**1.1 Staffing and Practice Data for All Neurology Practices**

| Staffing and Practice Data | Practice Type Neurology | | | | | | | |
|---|---|---|---|---|---|---|---|---|
| | Count | Mean | Standard Deviation | 10th Percentile | 25th Percentile | Median | 75th Percentile | 90th Percentile |
| Total physician FTE | 14 | 9.44 | 4.47 | 4.43 | 5.38 | 8.00 | 13.43 | 16.55 |
| Total support staff FTE | 14 | 47.99 | 45.19 | 11.00 | 20.58 | 32.00 | 59.88 | 143.20 |
| Number of branch clinics | 14 | 1.14 | 1.83 | 0.00 | 0.00 | 1.00 | 1.25 | 4.50 |
| Square footage of all facilities | 11 | 18,703 | 12,974 | 3,951 | 7,918 | 15,000 | 28,949 | 41,303 |

**1.2 AR Data, Collection Percentages and Financial Ratios for All Neurology Practices**

| AR Data, Collection Percentages, and Financial Ratios | Practice Type Neurology | | | | | | | |
|---|---|---|---|---|---|---|---|---|
| | Count | Mean | Standard Deviation | 10th Percentile | 25th Percentile | Median | 75th Percentile | 90th Percentile |
| Total AR/physician | 13 | $125,535 | $63,236 | $56,825 | $82,322 | $101,€28 | $174,929 | $241,242 |
| 0–30 days in AR | 14 | 57.32% | 14.76% | 26.26% | 53.88% | 61.46% | 67.11% | 71.66% |
| 31–60 days in AR | 14 | 15.48% | 5.59% | 9.72% | 11.93% | 14.00% | 16.71% | 27.27% |
| 61–90 days in AR | 14 | 8.24% | 2.67% | 5.31% | 6.21% | 7.53% | 9.72% | 13.04% |
| 91–120 days in AR | 14 | 4.25% | 1.57% | 1.88% | 2.97% | 4.26% | 5.32% | 6.68% |
| 120+ days in AR | 14 | 14.72% | 12.32% | 4.91% | 7.22% | 10.17% | 18.60% | 37.07% |
| Months gross fee-for-service charges in AR | 14 | 1.24 | 0.41 | 0.58 | 1.00 | 1.21 | 1.48 | 1.93 |
| Days gross FFS charges in AR | 14 | 37.57 | 12.56 | 17.68 | 30.49 | 36.67 | 45.05 | 58.58 |
| Gross FFS collection % | 14 | 54.91% | 11.32% | 36.83% | 47.14% | 55.38% | 64.67% | 70.83% |
| Adjusted FFS collection % | 13 | 99.33% | 5.46% | 88.91% | 98.21% | 99.75% | 101.88% | 106.57% |

**1.4b Charges and Revenue per FTE Physician for All Neurology Practices**

| Charges and Revenue per FTE Physician | Practice Type Neurology | | | | | | | |
|---|---|---|---|---|---|---|---|---|
| | Count | Mean | Standard Deviation | 10th Percentile | 25th Percentile | Median | 75th Percentile | 90th Percentile |
| Net fee-for-service revenue | 14 | $812,477 | $419,863 | $399,000 | $552,281 | $703,332 | $985,089 | $1,616,115 |
| Gross FFS charges | 14 | $1,663,593 | $1,424,670 | $665,421 | $938,954 | $1,199,308 | $1,880,165 | $4,371,300 |
| Adjustments to FFS charges | 13 | $837,152 | $1,057,839 | $205,412 | $372,734 | $563,127 | $843,836 | $2,979,969 |
| Adjusted FFS charges | 13 | $831,332 | $474,287 | $391,804 | $516,877 | $645,408 | $1,097,718 | $1,773,269 |
| Bad debts because of FFS activity | 12 | $20,376 | $25,566 | $2,795 | $5,880 | $8,135 | $28,711 | $76,720 |
| Net other medical revenue | 10 | $58,060 | $92,280 | $1,863 | $16,718 | $30,379 | $51,615 | $290,269 |
| Gross revenue from other activity | 10 | $56,079 | $93,599 | $667 | $10,880 | $26,129 | $57,269 | $290,269 |
| Other medical revenue | 10 | $55,717 | $93,776 | $123 | $10,535 | $26,129 | $57,143 | $290,218 |
| Total gross charges | 13 | $1,308,408 | $534,284 | $647,848 | $913,129 | $1,194,351 | $1,725,148 | $2,264,873 |
| Total medical revenue | 13 | $769,764 | $303,533 | $407,327 | $527,909 | $671,783 | $1,015,578 | $1,267,276 |

**1.4c Operating Cost per FTE Physician for All Neurology Practices**

| Operating Cost per FTE Physician | Practice Type Neurology | | | | | | | |
|---|---|---|---|---|---|---|---|---|
| | Count | Mean | Standard Deviation | 10th Percentile | 25th Percentile | Median | 75th Percentile | 90th Percentile |
| Total support staff cost | 13 | $189,786 | $77,082 | $102,773 | $112,947 | $183,925 | $235,847 | $328,056 |
| Total business oper. staff | 13 | $45,570 | $14,769 | $25,565 | $31,518 | $45,871 | $58,642 | $67,504 |
| Total front office support staff | 13 | $54,422 | $12,041 | $33,985 | $48,750 | $52,068 | $64,288 | $71,490 |
| Total clinical support staff | 8 | * | * | * | * | * | * | * |
| Total ancillary support staff | 11 | $39,013 | $34,395 | $2,269 | $13,424 | $27,486 | $56,614 | $102,419 |
| Total empl. supp. staff benefits | 12 | $33,785 | $11,999 | $18,071 | $24,196 | $33,419 | $40,168 | $55,807 |
| Total general operating cost | 13 | $240,682 | $167,227 | $77,449 | $141,372 | $197,226 | $261,844 | $596,443 |
| Information technology | 13 | $12,412 | $6,388 | $3,682 | $8,059 | $10,941 | $16,243 | $23,867 |
| Drug supply | 13 | $68,500 | $92,621 | $2,987 | $7,043 | $46,424 | $86,168 | $266,658 |
| Medical and surgical supply | 12 | $12,024 | $19,883 | $1,523 | $2,893 | $4,391 | $6,846 | $58,328 |
| Building and occupancy | 13 | $39,578 | $18,916 | $10,627 | $26,552 | $37,510 | $53,834 | $68,243 |

(continued on next page)

**Table 1**
*(continued)*

**Medical Group Management Association**

**Cost Survey: 2007 Report Based on 2006 Data**

| | Count | Mean | Standard Deviation | 10th Percentile | 25th Percentile | Median | 75th Percentile | 90th Percentile |
|---|---|---|---|---|---|---|---|---|
| Furniture and equipment | 9 | * | * | * | * | * | * | * |
| Administrative supplies and services | 13 | $18,919 | $12,312 | $5,400 | $9,394 | $17,328 | $23,850 | $43,722 |
| Professional liability insurance | 13 | $17,350 | $8,154 | $7,442 | $10,761 | $13,329 | $26,177 | $28,860 |
| Other insurance premiums | 12 | $3,439 | $3,233 | $480 | $1,025 | $2,292 | $4,628 | $9,733 |
| Outside professional fees | 13 | $6,056 | $4,806 | $1,146 | $1,359 | $5,416 | $8,300 | $15,077 |
| Promotion and marketing | 13 | $2,845 | $2,444 | $461 | $774 | $2,245 | $4,418 | $7,360 |
| Clinical laboratory | 3 | * | * | * | * | * | * | * |
| Radiology and imaging | 5 | * | * | * | * | * | * | * |
| Other ancillary services | 8 | * | * | * | * | * | * | * |
| Miscellaneous operating cost | 12 | $14,560 | $13,584 | $1,150 | $3,147 | $8,734 | $30,736 | $35,614 |
| Total operating cost | 13 | $430,468 | $232,174 | $186,822 | $283,499 | $355,877 | $511,851 | $900,617 |

**1.4d Provider Cost per FTE Physician for All Neurology Practices**

| Provider Cost per FTE Physician | Practice Type | | | | | | | |
|---|---|---|---|---|---|---|---|---|
| | Neurology | | | | | | | |
| | Count | Mean | Standard Deviation | 10th Percentile | 25th Percentile | Median | 75th Percentile | 90th Percentile |
| Total medical revenue after operating cost | 13 | $339,296 | $129,387 | $186,600 | $262,660 | $313,601 | $407,683 | $588,116 |
| Total physician cost | 13 | $300,668 | $103,937 | $169,088 | $250,131 | $277,098 | $334,895 | $510,854 |
| Total physician compensation | 13 | $251,894 | $75,681 | $154,222 | $201,785 | $239,674 | $293,132 | $394,544 |
| Total physician benefit cost | 11 | $57,643 | $47,581 | $12,005 | $37,165 | $48,626 | $57,500 | $167,385 |

**1.5b Operating Cost as % of Total Medical Revenue for All Neurology Practices**

| Operating Cost as % of Total Medical Revenue | Practice Type Neurology | | | | | | | |
|---|---|---|---|---|---|---|---|---|
| | Count | Mean | Standard Deviation | 10th Percentile | 25th Percentile | Median | 75th Percentile | 90th Percentile |
| Total support staff cost | 14 | 23.75% | 5.42% | 13.18% | 21.80% | 24.30% | 27.44% | 29.68% |
| Total business oper staff | 14 | 6.06% | 2.18% | 2.82% | 4.06% | 6.09% | 7.85% | 9.00% |
| Total front office support staff | 14 | 7.52% | 2.32% | 4.63% | 5.61% | 7.51% | 9.17% | 11.26% |
| Total clinical support staff | 10 | 3.12% | 1.54% | 0.38% | 2.17% | 3.29% | 4.27% | 5.44% |
| Total ancillary support staff | 11 | 4.30% | 2.73% | 0.54% | 2.00% | 4.52% | 7.14% | 8.19% |
| Total empl. supp. staff benefits | 12 | 4.57% | 1.31% | 2.42% | 3.73% | 4.52% | 5.33% | 6.66% |
| Total general operating cost | 14 | 28.39% | 10.65% | 14.73% | 21.62% | 27.28% | 32.36% | 48.24% |
| Information technology | 13 | 1.88% | 1.49% | 0.50% | 0.97% | 1.51% | 2.42% | 4.85% |
| Drug supply | 13 | 7.81% | 9.46% | 0.67% | 1.49% | 5.48% | 8.73% | 28.09% |
| Medical and surgical supply | 13 | 1.52% | 2.73% | 0.20% | 0.27% | 0.76% | 1.17% | 7.30% |
| Building and occupancy | 14 | 5.43% | 2.15% | 1.73% | 3.97% | 5.62% | 6.87% | 8.43% |
| Furniture and equipment | 9 | * | * | * | * | * | * | * |
| Administrative supplies and services | 13 | 2.45% | 1.35% | 1.09% | 1.48% | 2.16% | 3.25% | 5.07% |
| Professional liability insurance | 13 | 2.59% | 1.52% | 0.83% | 1.30% | 2.20% | 4.09% | 4.95% |
| Other insurance premiums | 12 | 0.46% | 0.44% | 0.07% | 0.19% | 0.31% | 0.51% | 1.41% |
| Outside professional fees | 14 | 0.99% | 1.05% | 0.18% | 0.30% | 0.75% | 1.29% | 2.90% |
| Promotion and marketing | 13 | 0.35% | 0.24% | 0.08% | 0.16% | 0.28% | 0.55% | 0.76% |
| Clinical laboratory | 3 | * | * | * | * | * | * | * |
| Radiology and imaging | 5 | * | * | * | * | * | * | * |
| Other ancillary services | 8 | * | * | * | * | * | * | * |
| Miscellaneous operating cost | 12 | 1.75% | 1.46% | 0.16% | 0.64% | 1.35% | 2.62% | 4.62% |
| Total operating cost | 14 | 52.14% | 12.64% | 31.34% | 45.33% | 53.28% | 57.69% | 72.65% |

(continued on next page)

**Table 1**
*(continued)*

**Medical Group Management Association**

**Cost Survey: 2007 Report Based on 2006 Data**

**1.5c Provider Cost as % of Total Medical Revenue for All Neurology Practices**

| Provider Cost as % of Total Medical Revenue | Practice Type Neurology | | | | | | | |
|---|---|---|---|---|---|---|---|---|
| | Count | Mean | Standard Deviation | 10th Percentile | 25th Percentile | Median | 75th Percentile | 90th Percentile |
| Total medical revenue after operating cost | 14 | 47.86% | 12.64% | 27.35% | 42.31% | 46.72% | 54.67% | 68.67% |
| Total physician cost | 14 | 42.76% | 11.63% | 28.30% | 34.19% | 40.48% | 47.10% | 65.47% |
| Total physician compensation | 13 | 34.47% | 7.42% | 25.05% | 28.65% | 34.53% | 38.09% | 48.07% |
| Total physician benefit cost | 11 | 7.44% | 4.17% | 1.21% | 3.70% | 7.26% | 10.26% | 14.46% |

*Abbreviations:* FFS, fee-for-service; FTE, full time equivalent.

*Reprinted from* the Medical Group Management Association. Available at: http://www.mgma.com; Copyright 2007; with permission. For current information go to www.mgma.com.

response rate of neurologists to the MGMA cost surveys likely indicate that neurology groups overall are not as sophisticated or as focused as they should be in collecting details of (and thereby measuring) their own business performance.

Additional sources for external benchmarking data include the AMA's annual surveys[8] and the biannual surveys done by the AAN of its physician members.[9] Again, as with MGMA surveys, it is important to understand the limitations of the data that are collected. Despite those limitations, the data from all these surveys can still provide helpful insight and ideas for neurologists who wish to improve the financial and operational performance of their medical practice.

But it is precisely because of the limitations of these external benchmarking data that many experts stress that physicians should benchmark their own practice against itself over time.[10] This process constitutes internal benchmarking. A physician group decides on measures it wants to use, and then keeps track of how those measures change over time. This method is in many ways more realistic for each group and allows a clearer perspective on improvements that are made.

The first part of the process of internal benchmarking involves a gap analysis. Gap analysis shows the difference between where the physician or practice is today and where that individual or the group wants to be. It asks the hard questions—What will it take to reach that goal? What must the group do differently from what it does now?

## MANAGEMENT AND BENCHMARKING

The American College of Medical Practice Executives (ACMPE), the certification body of MGMA, has created a "body of knowledge" that defines the unique knowledge and skill sets required for the medical practice management profession. Included here are the following items that stress the importance of benchmarking to the successful operation of a medical practice:

- Conduct financial benchmarking, including revenue, expenses, adjusted collection rate, collection rate by payer, payer mix, reimbursement, productivity, AR, and profitability
- Benchmark staff performance reviews and establish professional development plans
- Identify, develop, and maintain benchmarks for establishing practice performance standards
- Develop effective benchmarking reports, such as dashboards and scorecards
- Identify appropriate internal and external benchmark data to guide strategy performance.[11]

Benchmarking is not optional for the office manager or administrator of a medical practice; it is considered absolutely necessary to successfully carry out the responsibilities of managing a medical practice.

## FINANCIAL MEASURES

Many of the benchmarking measures for medical practice are tied to finances. The reason is straightforward: a practice that is not profitable cannot provide the quality of care that patients require. Frank Cohen, a health care consultant with MIT Solutions, has told physicians: "Your number one responsibility is to be profitable. If you're not profitable, you cannot provide quality care. If you're not willing to do what it takes to make money, you're going to go out of business, and the community is going to suffer as a result."[12]

In surveying experts in the benchmarking field, the following are the financial elements that should be measured in a neurology practice:

- *Days in AR*: Total AR divided by (12 months of gross charges/365). Each time this number is generated, it looks at the total AR on that day as well as the previous 12 months of gross charges.
- *Net collection ratio:* Collections (less refunds and unapplied credits; also called net revenue) divided by net charges (actual charges less contractual adjustments)
- AR greater than 120 days
- *Overhead rate*: Operating expenses (personnel, facility, supplies, and marketing — everything but physician wages and benefits) divided by net revenue
- *Copayments collected at time of service:* Copayments collected at the time of service divided by copayments due at the time of service (this can also be done for coinsurance and deductible amounts)
- *Claims denial percentage* (number of claims that are denied in a month divided by the number of claims filed).[13–16]

If a practice does a baseline analysis (the initial measurement of these metrics), all future financial activity can be monitored and compared with the baseline. While there will be some variation in what an efficient practice should seek to achieve in each of the above-listed categories, reasonable goals suggested by a range of researchers are

- Days in AR: 50 to 60 days
- Net collection rate: 95% or better
- AR greater than 120 days 15% to 18%
- *Overhead rate*: Less than 47% if office based; neurology, however, exceeds 50% based on MGMA data
- Co-pays collected at time of service: 98%
- *Claims denied*: 4%; claims denied due to late filing: 0%.[17–19]

These measures, when benchmarked regularly, allow the physician to know the trends of the practice before a specific trend has too much of a negative impact on the practice. The overall focus of these measures is to assist the medical practice in getting the money it is owed as quickly as possible for the least cost possible. That is why some trends are more important than others. For example, the actual amount of AR in a practice is not important in itself; and there will be variations in AR each month caused by vacations or weather or even the act of installing a new computer system. What does matter is how quickly that AR is "turned over" or turned into revenue for the practice. The longer it takes to collect what is owed, the greater the financial strain on the practice.

If there are financial concerns that the benchmarking process raises, the general areas to review are as follows.

The problems could be on the "charge side" of the process. It will be necessary to look more carefully at measures, such as patient volume (is it decreasing), charge entry (accuracy and timeliness), fee schedule (is it set correctly), coding practices (are they accurate, reflecting the actual work that was done), contract negotiation (is insurance reimbursement adequate for all payers).

On the reimbursement side, examine the following: payer mix (has it changed in the last 6 months, and if so, why), adjustment percentage (are adjustments appropriate), denials (what are the 10 top reasons for claims not being paid), account follow-up (how many accounts are being followed up on and how successful are the follow-up efforts), front-end processes (is information incomplete at registration or is the registration error rate too high), payment posting (is it being done quickly), claims processing (how long does it take to get the bill "out the door" after the service is performed).

Financial measures lend themselves most easily to dashboard analysis. Sophisticated data mining products are now relatively easy to use and provide "quick glance" analysis of the key measures. As shown in **Fig. 1**, this sample dashboard lets physicians know what their current AR are as well as the days in AR. The dashboard is updated at least daily. When looking at monthly trends of charges and revenues, as seen in **Fig. 2**, the physician can easily see how this year's charges compare with those of the previous year. Variances can be noted and reviewed. The underlying data can be reviewed for detailed explanation by using the built-in drill-down features of this product.

## STAFF PRODUCTIVITY

In a medical practice, apart from significant capital investments, the largest expense item is staff wages and benefits. For this reason it is critical that neurologists understand their staff costs in comparison to the work the staff does. Employees can appear busy but can have work capacity that is untapped. But how does a busy physician judge if a staff member is "busy enough" or, more accurately, productive enough?

The following are key data points that a practice should consider benchmarking, with a recommended range of work for an 8-hour workday as noted by Walker and Gans[20]:

- Telephone calls with message taking (180–200)
- Appointment scheduling with full registration (75–100)
- Patient office check-in with registration check and verification (75–85)
- Checkout, collection of money owed and charge entry (70–90)
- Payment posting (500–600 manual payment items)
- Insurance follow-up (60–75)
- Patient inquiries (125–150)
- Claim submission time (within 48 hours for in-office; within 5 days for hospital work)
- Action on unpaid account (at least once every 30 days)
- Professional coders' coding office visits and procedures for providers (108).[21]

One critical operational area to measure relates to scheduling. Most physicians think in terms of how long a patient has to wait to get either a new or follow-up visit. Actually other indicators are far more important[22]:

- Time to next available new patient appointment (another concept is "time to third next new appointment", which reveals more about provider "schedule density")[23]
- Time to next follow-up visit appointment
- Appointment no-show rate
- Appointment bump rate (ie, need to move patient due to physician schedule change)
- Converted canceled appointments (when the appointment slot is successfully filled).

In many small offices an employee may do many things (eg, answer telephones, prepare charts, and collect co-pays); such employees are in a multi-tasking role. To evaluate their productivity, it is necessary to divide up the daily responsibilities of the employee, assign a time allowance to each task per day, and take the total measure of their combined work.

Walker and Gans have also coined, for the medical community, the term "rightsizing": "The right staff in the right place with the right skills at the right cost with the right behavior with the right rewards with the right outcomes, no more, no less."[20] By

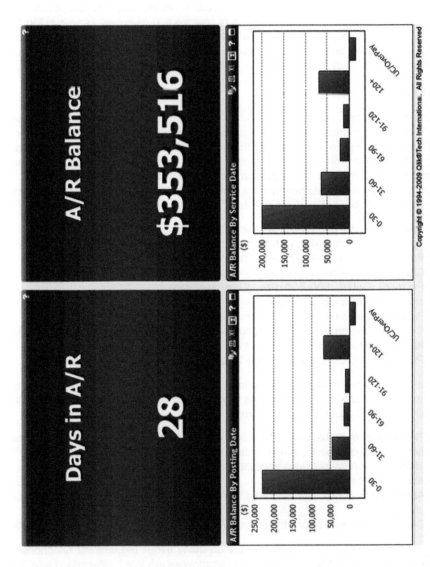

**Fig. 1.** Sample dashboard. Copyright contained on slide. (*Courtesy of Qlik Tech International 1994–2009; with permission.*)

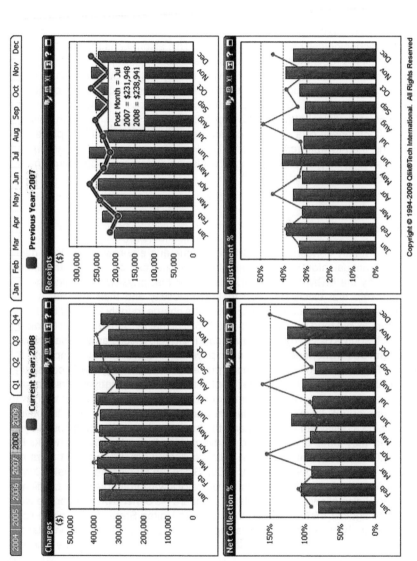

**Fig. 2.** Monthly trends of charges and revenues. Note in right upper graph how underlying data are shown when hovering over the data point on the graph. Copyright contained on slide. (*Courtesy of* Qlik Tech International 1994–2009; with permission.)

monitoring productivity the physician shows the staff that he or she values employees' work and will enlist their help to become more efficient in how they work. In fact, many future productivity gains in a practice will depend on the synergistic relationship that physicians establish with staff for reducing costs and increasing productivity.[24]

Benchmarking staff operations result in decreased rework, increased automation, and increased productivity. As health care grows more sophisticated, with an increasing use of the Internet and information technology, it is also clear that a neurologist needs to hire staff members whose skills and experience match the current demands for technologically productive workers. This also means that staff must be provided with all the tools they need to be successful.

Poor performance can result from not having the right staff. But it is also possible that a practice's "work culture" hurts staff morale. In 2004, according to MGMA, the staff turnover rate was 20% for receptionists and those who work in medical records, 12.5% for clinical staff, and 8% for billing staff.[25] Rates this high severely impact the effectiveness of a smaller practice because it takes time to replace staff who leave and then to train replacements. The loss of good employees can be prevented by fostering, as part of the practice's mission statement, a culture of mutual respect and celebration of successes.[26]

## PHYSICIAN PRODUCTIVITY

Physicians are rightly concerned about their income and any reductions they might face. Accurate annual information on neurologist income can be found in the annual surveys done by the MGMA.[6] However, it is crucial that physicians understand the direct relationship that exists between their productivity and their income. A poor measure to use is the AR, because most physicians charge roughly 200% of the Medicare fee schedule, but tend to collect closer to 115% of that fee schedule. But Medicare is tied to the Resource based relative value scale (RBRVS), which can provide a means to compare the true work performed by each physician in a practice by comparing the annual work RVU from each of the current procedural terminology (CPT) codes that a physician bills annually.[10] This is a true "apples to apples" comparison, which allows physicians to compare themselves against other providers in the group as well as to compare their productivity over time using the same methodology. Beyond this value, RBRVS can help a physician to understand the fundamental methodology used by all insurers when they offer a contract to participate in their physician network. For instance, in 2008 the national average of dollars collected per RVU was $41 (personal conversation with Frank Cohen, January 2009). Since the Medicare conversion factor was $36.0666, a practice could be profitable overall if it was profitable under Medicare.

Using RBRVS also allows a neurologist to compare his or her own work or the work of the practice against that of all neurologists in the United States in any given year. **Table 2** charts a physician's use of initial inpatient hospital consultations in relationship to that of all other neurologists in the same state in the same year by using all neurologists' insurance claims submitted to the Centers for Medicare and Medicaid Services (CMS). The CMS data are available free of charge on the CMS Web page. While there are inexpensive programs that can create the reports like those shown in **Table 2**,[27] more sophisticated analytical programs exist. For example, Comprehensive Medical Practice Analysis (CMPA) is one that offers additional analysis capability, such as how one practice compares to all other neurology practices in terms of the most common procedures done, as shown in **Table 3**. CMPA also can provide alerts to enable a practice to review certain aspects of its practice as in **Fig. 3**. This can help

**Table 2**
Initial inpatient consultations

| Code | Current Annual Frequency | Current/ Calculated Fee | Current Gross Charges | Current Practice Dist. % | Control Dist. % | Variance Practice vs Control | ReDist Annual Frequency | Redist Gross Charges | Charge Differential |
|------|------|------|------|------|------|------|------|------|------|
| 99251 | 0 | 71 | $0 | 0.00% | 0.50% | -100.00% | 10 | $676 | $676 |
| 99252 | 3 | 113 | $339 | 0.16% | 2.21% | -92.84% | 42 | $4,735 | $4,396 |
| 99253 | 145 | 168 | $24,360 | 7.63% | 16.95% | -54.98% | 322 | $54,110 | $29,750 |
| 99254 | 1332 | 243 | $323,676 | 70.11% | 54.11% | 29.56% | 1,028 | $249,827 | ($73,849) |
| 99255 | 420 | 302 | $126,840 | 22.11% | 26.23% | -15.73% | 498 | $150,518 | $23,678 |
| Totals | 1900 | | $475,215 | 100.00% | 100.00% | | 1,900 | $459,865 | ($15,350) |

Courtesy of MIT Solutions, Inc. Available at: http://www.mitsi.org; with permission.

**Table 3**
**CMPA analysis of a neurology practice**

| Neurology | | National | | Practice | |
|---|---|---|---|---|---|
| CPT Code | Description | Rank | Percent | Rank | Percent |
| 95904 | Sensory nerve conduction test | 1 | 7.62% | 2 | 12.91% |
| 99214 | Office/outpatient visit, test | 2 | 7.15% | 1 | 18.71% |
| 99213 | Office/outpatient visit, test | 3 | 5.77% | 6 | 8.14% |
| 99232 | Subsequent hospital care | 4 | 5.13% | 3 | 10.48% |
| 95903 | Motor nerve conduction test | 5 | 4.70% | 5 | 8.39% |
| 95900 | Motor nerve conduction test | 6 | 3.31% | 7 | 5.00% |
| 99231 | Subsequent hospital care | 7 | 2.30% | 17 | 0.91% |
| 99233 | Subsequent hospital care | 8 | 2.06% | 19 | 0.60% |
| 99254 | Inpatient consultation | 9 | 1.90% | 8 | 4.82% |
| 99244 | Office consultation | 10 | 1.89% | 4 | 9.90% |
| 99215 | Office/outpatient visit, test | 11 | 1.80% | 11 | 2.48% |
| 99255 | Inpatient consultation | 12 | 1.32% | 14 | 1.52% |
| 99245 | Office consultation | 13 | 1.25% | 13 | 1.54% |
| 95819 | EEG, awake and asleep | 14 | 1.21% | 15 | 1.33% |
| 95816 | EEG, awake and drowsy | 15 | 1.02% | 9 | 2.87% |
| 95861 | Muscle test, 2 limbs | 16 | 0.86% | 16 | 1.10% |
| 95934 | H-reflex test | 17 | 0.86% | 2 | 0.16% |
| 95860 | Muscle test, one limb | 18 | 0.71% | 10 | 2.65% |
| 99212 | Office/outpatient visit, test | 19 | 0.63% | 18 | 0.62% |
| 93880 | Extracranial study | 20 | 0.52% | | |
| 97110 | Therapeutic exercises | 21 | 0.47% | | |
| 99253 | Inpatient consultation | 22 | 0.44% | 21 | 0.52% |
| 99243 | Office consultation | 23 | 0.38% | 12 | 1.60% |
| 95920 | Intraop. nerve test add-on | 24 | 0.31% | | |
| 97140 | Manual therapy | 25 | 0.27% | | |

*Abbreviation:* EEG, electroencephalogram.
*Courtesy of* MIT Solutions, Inc. Available at: http://www.mitsi.org; with permission.

alert a physician to coding patterns that should be reviewed in light of the annual guidance given by the Office of Inspector General on behalf of CMS.

All of these data allow physicians both to reflect on their coding accuracy for services and to identify opportunities to increase revenue. However, charts and summary reports alone do not reflect the accuracy of the physician's coding; that can only be tested by doing regular internal prospective audits of medical services. Such benchmarking information can help neurologists to formulate a plan to make better use of their time so as to become more productive.

## THE FUTURE DIRECTION OF PRACTICE IMPROVEMENT: NEW METHODS, BETTER PERFORMANCE

While the importance of benchmarking a medical practice becomes more commonly publicized,[28] the focus of the emphasis has shifted to improving profitability by improving processes in a medical practice. In many industries Six Sigma was pioneered as a disciplined methodology of defining, measuring, analyzing, improving,

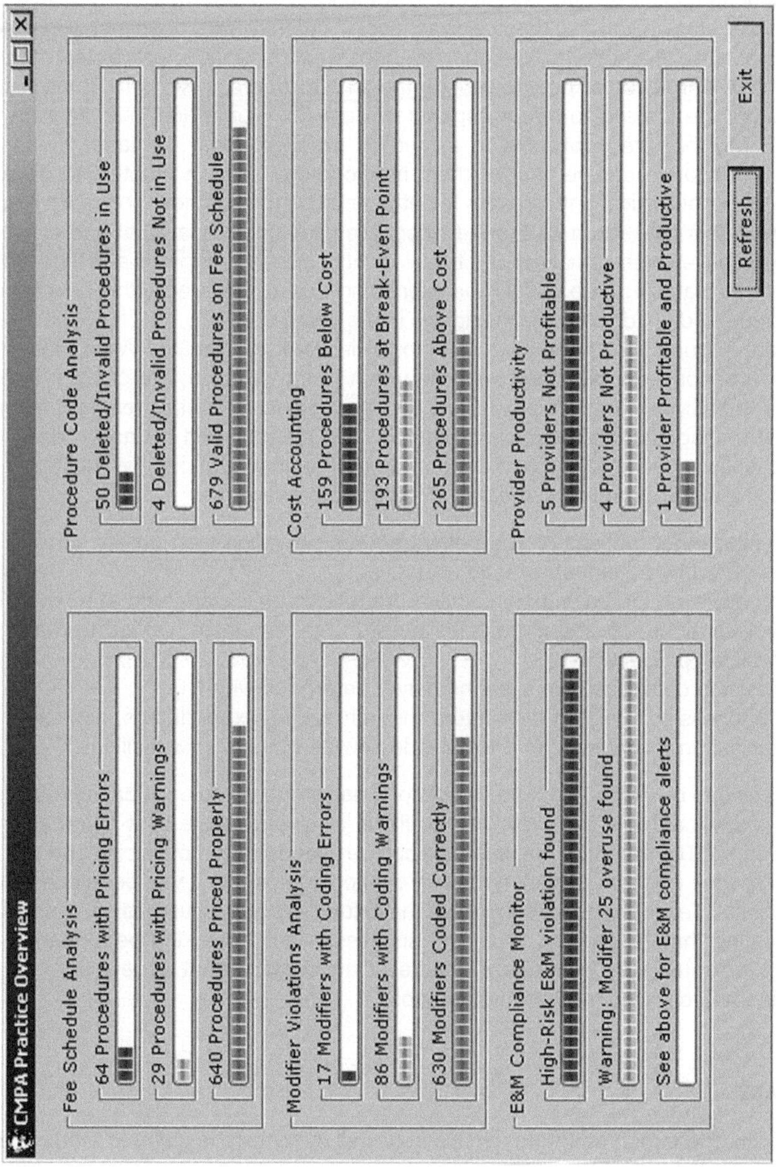

**Fig. 3.** CMPA practice overview. (*Courtesy of CMPA ©, copyright 2009 MIT Solutions, Inc, Available at: http://www.mitsi.org; with permission.*)

and controlling the quality in every one of a company's products, processes, and transactions. The key methodology used is DMAIC: define, measure, analyze, improve, and control cycle. Although Six Sigma is successful for many businesses, the problem in applying it to health care is that it was never intended to work in such a transactional business. Six Sigma is, however, effective in eliminating defects in a production business such as car manufacturing. Some attempts have been made to seek to apply Six Sigma to medical practices,[29] but they have been met with limited success outside of a hospital environment. Another continuous improvement method is "Lean," which looks at how to reduce the time to deliver a service. Some recent researchers are looking to adapt aspects of both Six Sigma and Lean to take the best of both that are applicable to a medical practice under the label "Lean Six Sigma." This total practice improvement methodology helps a practice to develop a strategy, set of tactics, and logistics to better improve the practice. Some of the early pioneers in this field, such as Frank Cohen, are developing analytical and mapping tools to enable even the smallest practice to identify places to improve and to measure the changes that are made.[30] It will be interesting to see how readily this new benchmarking method is adopted by physicians in the years ahead.

It is not enough to survive as a neurologist in medical practice. What matters is striving to become, in alignment with the vision of the practice, a better performing group. The MGMA measures physicians and their groups in these areas: profitability and cost management; productivity, capacity and staffing; and AR and collections. With extensive years of data collection from medical groups, the MGMA now describes a better performing medical practice as one with:

- A culture that focuses on the patient and on providing high-quality services as measured by patient satisfaction surveys
- Emphasis on increasing productivity from both physicians and staff even if it involves higher operating costs to invest in the resources needed to maximize physician productivity
- Physician compensation systems based on productivity
- Willingness to invest in their future through capital expenditures, especially for information technology, and to provide new services or new facilities.[31]

Success can be measured. Even a solo or small group neurologist can take advantage of analytical tools that were not available at a reasonable cost as recently as 5 years ago.[32] The data that are collected can be used to help a physician and a practice to improve and thrive even in difficult economic times. Will you be successful in this process? Tesch and Levy concluded their study of successful medical institutions by observing that "ultimately, to ensure success in benchmarking performance, an organization must fully embrace a culture of accountability at all levels."[23] In the end, it is that commitment that matters most.

## SUMMARY

There is no one benchmark that reveals how well everything is going in a practice. A practice with the highest-paid neurologists may be a practice that is on the verge of bankruptcy or may have the lowest patient satisfaction scores. The practice with the best business intelligence software may fail to understand and make use of their data. The practice may do an excellent job of benchmarking and identifying areas for improvement, but the physicians or staff may fail to embrace necessary changes and follow the action plan. Benchmarking as a process can help a neurology practice improve and thrive. But as in any business, its ultimate success depends on the commitment of the owners to make sure it succeeds.

Undergirding the concepts discussed in this article are steps that have been highlighted, which should be followed when a neurology practice commits itself to benchmarking its work[33]:

- Establish a group practice mission/purpose and objectives
- Identify performance indices—what will be measured
- Identify benchmark sources—if using external sources
- Collect data
- Establish baseline reference points
- If comparing to external sources, do a gap analysis
- Communicate findings to practice owners, physicians, and staff
- Develop an action plan
- Implement plans and monitor progress toward measurable goals
- Calibrate as needed to achieve goals
- Repeat the process.

## REFERENCES

1. Reforming American Health Care. London: The Economist;  2009. p. 75–7.
2. Margolis J. Medical practice today. Englewood (CO): MGMA Connexion; 2009. p. 32.
3. Cost Survey Questionnaire Based on 2007 Data. Englewood: MGMA; 2008. For additional information on the research MGMA does see Margolis J. Surveys, Research, Polls and Evaluations. MGMA Connexion 2009. p. 42–4.
4. 2008 Physician Practice Information Survey, American Medical Association, PowerPoint Presentation. Chicago, April 23, 2009.
5. Feltenberger GS, Gans DN. Benchmarking success: the essential guide for group practices. Englewood (CO): MGMA; 2008. p. 1.
6. Physician Compensation and Production Survey. 2008 report based on 2007 data. Englewood (CO): MGMA; 2008.
7. Performance and Practices of Successful Medical Groups. 2008 report based on 2007 data. Englewood (CO): MGMA; 2008.
8. American Medical Association. Physician socioeconomic statistics: Chicago: AMA. Published annually.
9. Neurologists HK. 2004: AAN Member demographic and practice characteristics. St. Paul (MN): American Academy of Neurology; 2005. This is updated every 3 years. Available at: http://wwwaan.com/go/about/statistics/report. Accessed August 5, 2009.
10. Cohen F. Mastering RBRVS. Gaithersburg (MD): Decision Health; 2003.
11. American College of Medical Practice Executives. Body of knowledge for medical practice executives. 2nd edition. Englewood (CO): MGMA; 2008.
12. Berry E. How to set your fee schedule. Available at: http://www.ama-assn.org/amednews/2009/05/04/bisa0504.htm. Accessed May 16, 2009.
13. Woodcock E. Practice benchmarking. In: Wolper L, editor. Physician practice management: essential operational and financial knowledge. Englewood (CO): MGMA; 2005. p. 293–316.
14. Woodcock E, Browne R, Jenkins J. A physicians due: measuring physician billing performance, benchmarking, healthcare financial management 2008;62:94–9.
15. Ayers C. Employ these indicators to rev your A/R engine. Part B News: 20.40(10/16/2006): 5–6.

16. Fiegl C. Benchmarking can improve your practice's revenue stream. Part B News. 23.5. (2/2/2009).
17. Walker DL, Larch SM, Woodcock EW. The physician billing process: avoiding potholes in the road to getting paid. Englewood (CO): MGMA; 2004. p. 185–219.
18. Mourar M, Compiler. Experts answer 101 tough practice management questions. Englewood (CO): MGMA; 2007.
19. Pavlock EJ. Financial management for medical groups. 2nd edition. Englewood (CO): MGMA; 2000.
20. Walker DL, Gans DN. Rightsizing – Appropriate staffing for your medical practice. Englewood (CO): MGMA; 2003.
21. Dunn R. Putting productivity plans to work. J AHIMA 2001;61.
22. Woodcock E. Mastering patient flow. 2nd edition. Englewood (CO): MGMA; 2003.
23. Tesch T, Levy A. Measuring service line success. the new model for benchmarking. Healthc Financ Manage 2008;62:68–74.
24. Gaulke R. Engage staff, set benchmarks, think lean. Englewood (CO): MGMA Connexion; 2009. p. 20–21.
25. Baird K. Customer service in health care. Chicago: Jossey-Bass; 2000.
26. Performance and Practices of Successful Medical Groups: 2005 report based on 2004 data. Englewood (CO): MGMA; 2005.
27. E/M Template for Neurology. Available in Excel or book format. Gaithersburg (MD). Decision Health. Annually updated.
28. Lessons for Financial Success. Available at: http://www.mgma.com/about/article.aspx?id=27386. Accessed July 7, 2009.
29. Snee RD, Hoerl RW. Six sigma beyond the factory floor – deployment strategies for financial services, health care, and the rest of the real economy. New York: Prentice Hall; 2005.
30. Cohen F. Improving profitability through improving processes. powerpoint presentation, New York Medical Group Management Association Annual Meeting, Saratoga Springs (NY), June 24, 2009 and Cohen F. Lean Six Sigma for the medical practice. Baltimore: Greenbranch; 2009.
31. Gans D. The seven habits of highly effective medical groups. Englewood (CO): MGMA Connexion; 2008. p. 20–2.
32. Nunez A, O'Malley T. Outpatient access metrics: a new approach to aggregation and presentation of data. Group Pract J 2009;16:30–4.
33. Walker, DL. Rightsizing staff to improve practice profitability. powerpoint presentation. New York Medical Group Management Association Annual Meeting. Saratoga Springs (NY), June 26, 2003; modified by William S. Henderson.

# Neurology on the Internet

John W. Henson, MD[a],*, Lily K. Jung, MD[b]

**KEYWORDS**

- Internet • World Wide Web • Social network
- Advocacy • Personal heath record

## ALERTING RESPONSES

It can be a major challenge to keep current with the rapidly growing body of scientific and clinical neurologic knowledge. Fortunately, there are several tools available for neurologists to gain access to this information, almost all of which are now available online. Email alerts, RSS (Really Simple Syndication) and XML (Extensible Markup Language) feeds, and mashups (Web pages that display continuously updated information simultaneously from multiple sources, using RSS and XML) are among the most important of these alerting methods. Podcasts (multimedia files that are transferred over the Internet for playback on a mobile device or a personal computer) are another good way to obtain organized presentations of in-depth information on new topics. Other sources of current neurologic information include major media outlets, academic society Web sites, proprietary medical news sites, neurology news magazines (eg, *Neurology Today* and *Clinical Neurology News*), the National Library of Medicine's PubMed data service, and traditional peer-reviewed journals.

Various online tools facilitate access to these information sources. So-called push technologies such as RSS and XML allow media sources to send recipients selective updated information, including late-breaking news or newly published articles, along with links to more detailed information. RSS and XML feeds have come into wide use among media sources, and are identified on Web sites of these sources by the symbols 🔊 and XML.

Early versions of the special Web browsers required to view RSS and XML feeds, called readers, were limited in that they could only display one information source at a time. Internet Explorer, Firefox, Safari, Opera, and Chrome all have the ability to display individual RSS/XML feeds. Various readers, or aggregators (eg, Google Reader), allow more efficient viewing of multiple RSS/XML feeds on a single screen.

[a] Neurology Division, Swedish Neuroscience Institute, 550 17th Avenue, Suite 500, Seattle, WA 98122, USA
[b] Neurology Division, Swedish Neuroscience Institute, 550 17th Avenue, Suite 540, Seattle, WA 98122, USA
* Corresponding author.
*E-mail address:* john.henson@swedish.org (J.W. Henson).

Neurol Clin 28 (2010) 385–393
doi:10.1016/j.ncl.2009.11.004
0733-3619/10/$ – see front matter © 2010 Elsevier Inc. All rights reserved.
**neurologic.theclinics.com**

Mashups permit constant desktop display of multiple RSS or XML feeds. Examples include *i*Google (**Box 1**, **Fig. 1**) and Netvibes, both of which simultaneously display multiple RSS feeds in small boxes, called modules or gadgets, on a single screen. The mashup can be set as the browser's home page, providing the neurologist with a tremendous array of frequently updated news sources. One advantage of mashups is the ability to create a module, or gadget, based on any RSS or XML feed, in addition to the vast number of predefined modules from commercial sources, such as BBC News World Edition. These are powerful tools for organizing information that is being updated constantly.

### Email Alerts

Several media outlets with a large reporting staff monitor breaking health-related news and offer real-time email alerts. The advantage of email alerts is that they actively place news in front of the neurologist's eyes, compared with more passive information sitting on a Web site to which the viewer must refer frequently. Sources such as http://www. CNN.com, Reuters, and major newspapers can all send health-related news to registered individuals. Registration is generally free, with the email alert function activated by a link at the bottom of the home page. Unfortunately, only a few media sites (eg, http://www.CNN.com) allow prefiltering of information specific to neurologists' interests through the use of key words (eg, "neurology," "stroke," and so forth), thus generating an email when a news story containing one of the key words is published. Other sites, including the New York Times and Reuters, send email alerts from a category called "Health," but these cannot be further filtered. Several journals, including the *Annals of Neurology* and *Neurology*, send email alerts containing the table of contents for each new issue to subscribers who request them, and these, too, can be viewed on a mashup page (see **Fig. 1**).

MedWatch Safety Alerts (http://www.fda.gov/Safety/MedWatch/default.htm), a service of the US Food and Drug Administration (FDA), provides email alerts, also available as RSS feeds, regarding new safety information for human medical products. Each contains a summary of the safety alert and a hyperlink to more detailed information. Items of interest to neurologists are sufficiently common to make this a worthwhile

---

**Box 1**
**Creating a custom gadget in *i*Google**

Use the following steps to create a custom gadget in *i*Google:

- Open a free Google account
- On the Google Accounts page, click on *i*Google and follow the instructions to create a mashup page
- Find an RSS or XML feed of interest (eg, see the symbols on the home page of http://www. AAN.com)
- Click on the RSS or XML icon
- Copy the URL for the RSS feed from the address box at the top of the browser
- Click on the "Add stuff" link in the upper right of the *i*Google screen
- On the next page, click on the "Add feed or gadget" link in the left-hand column
- Paste the URL into the address box
- The RSS gadget will automatically appear on the *i*Google mashup page. The gadgets can be organized on the page by drag and drop.

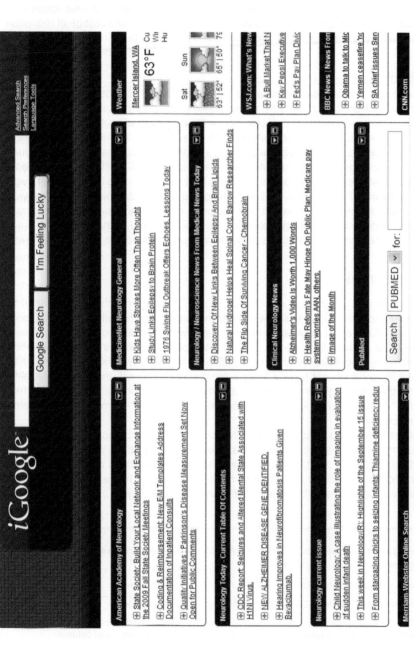

**Fig. 1.** A mashup is a Web page that displays constantly updated information from several media sources, using RSS or XML feeds. Each of the small boxes, or gadgets, contains a summary of several news items, with a link to more detailed information. The *i*Google mashup shown here can be set as a home page, allowing the neurologist to follow multiple news sources in real time.

service, maybe even a necessity, because clinicians may be held legally responsible for the information that applies to the clinical use of the products discussed.

The National Library of Medicine's PubMed database offers a useful email alerting system based on newly indexed medical literature of interest. With this system it is possible, for instance, to receive a daily or less frequently updated list of all new publications detected with a specific set of search terms (**Box 2**).

### Podcasting

Podcasts are media files downloaded from the Internet for playback on personal computers or Portable on Demand media players such as iPods, iPhones, BlackBerry phones and other handheld devices. These files typically offer 10 to 30 minutes of audio recordings, playable at the listener's convenience, that feature a review of a neurologic topic or newly published paper, and often with continuing medical education credits offered. Some podcasts are enhanced by inclusion of images or video. A list of podcast sites for neurologists can be found by downloading iTunes player, registering with the iTunes Store, and searching the store's database using the word "neurology" in the "Titles" search box. Tailoring of Web sites for the Web browsers on smart phones is increasingly common. A good example of this is the AAN's site, http://m.aan.com/m/, which can also be viewed on a desktop or laptop computer.

## PUBMED CENTRAL

When faced with an unusual or puzzling clinical, imaging, or laboratory finding, the modern neurologist might enter several key terms into search engines such as Google Scholar or PubMed. A publication is discovered with the title and abstract promising precisely the information needed, but on attempting to click through to the article, a splash page appears requesting a $30 payment to download the paper. If the hospital library does not have a license for the online journal, the neurologist either pays for the article sight unseen, sends an email to the author requesting an electronic "reprint," or simply concedes defeat, frustrated that crucial information was so close but inaccessible.

In an attempt to address such restricted access to research publications, and thus speed the rate of research discoveries, the National Institutes of Health (NIH) has mandated that from April, 2008, all peer-reviewed publications describing research supported by NIH funds or authored by an NIH-funded researcher be deposited into a freely available online site called PubMed Central (PMC) within one year of

---

**Box 2**
**Email updates from PubMed for newly published medical literature on a specific topic of interest**

- Go to the PubMed Web site (http://www.ncbi.nlm.nih.gov/pubmed)
- Register for a free "My NCBI" account in the upper right hand corner
- After logging in, return to the PubMed home page and enter the desired search term(s). Click on "Search". This will return all articles relevant to the search term
- Click on "Save search". Confirm the search terms on the next page
- Follow the directions on the following page to receive updated searches at any desired time interval (eg, daily or weekly)

publication (see http://www.pubmedcentral.nih.gov/). Unfortunately, many clinical papers are not controlled by this regulation.

*NIH Public Access Policy. The Director of the National Institutes of Health shall require that all investigators funded by the NIH submit or have submitted for them to the National Library of Medicine's PubMed Central an electronic version of their final, peer-reviewed manuscripts upon acceptance for publication, to be made publicly available no later than 12 months after the official date of publication: Provided, That the NIH shall implement the public access policy in a manner consistent with copyright law. Division G, Title II, Section 218 of PL 110–161 (Consolidated Appropriations Act, 2008).*

NIH granting agencies now require investigators to document submission of their papers to PMC, and therefore it is the author, rather than the journal, who bears the responsibility of implementing the new rule. Author instruction pages for many journals no longer discuss this requirement, implying that most publishers assume authors will be submitting their own papers. Moreover, in the first year of the program, the firm one-year deadline has seemingly been reduced to only a suggested deadline. A review of the current PMC database finds that approximately 100 papers published by a large US neurology journal were submitted between April and September of 2008 (from inception of the policy to one year before this writing). This number likely under-represents the papers published by authors who had NIH support. (Some types of literature were not represented, for example, retrospective clinical case series, presumably because they were not based on NIH-funded research.) There were initial concerns about charges of up to $3000 to be levied by publishers for submitting a paper to the database on behalf of the authors, but these fears were likely unwarranted, because investigators seem to be able to submit their published papers to PMC without permission or even assistance on the part of the journal. More information about open source publishing can be found at http://www.biomedcentral.com/openaccess/inquiry/myths/.

## NEUROLOGY PATIENTS AND THE INTERNET

Many neurologists are concerned about the type of information, or misinformation, that patients gather from the Internet. Data from the ALS Center at the University of Torino, together with related papers in other medical settings, shed light on the information-seeking behavior of patients with respect to online health information.

In the amyotrophic lateral sclerosis (ALS) study, Chio and colleagues,[1] interviewed 60 consecutive ALS patients and their caregivers regarding use of the Internet as a source of medical information. Only two-thirds of the study subjects felt that their physicians had provided enough relevant clinical information about ALS in the clinic setting; 55% of patients and 83% of caregivers expressed the need to learn more about the disease outside of the clinic setting. Similar numbers have been seen in other neurologic settings. The Internet was the most common source of information outside the clinic, even though only one-third of patients and two-thirds of caregivers actually derived information from online sources. The second most common source of medical information came from major media outlets, including newspapers and television.

The top goals for searching the Internet by the patient population were learning about outcome, disease-modifying therapies, and scientific research. By comparison, caregivers appeared to be more interested in experimental treatments and alternative therapies. Despite this level of use, patients were concerned about the reliability of the information they were reading on the Internet, and felt that data from medical meetings, television, and patient associations were more trustworthy.

Surprisingly, gender and age did not correlate with the likelihood of pursuing online health information. Some studies have shown higher rates of health-related use of the Internet with increasing educational level, whereas others have provided conflicting data on age, gender, and income. In unselected patients in a large primary care[2] and general population-based series,[3] 53% and 40%, respectively, of respondents used the Internet to obtain information about specific or general health issues.

The National Institute of Neurologic Disorders and Stroke (NINDS) Disorders Index (http://www.ninds.nih.gov/disorders/disorder_index.htm),     provides     moderately detailed information in nontechnical language about a large number of neurologic conditions and diseases, and is a useful source for neurologic patients and their providers. Links are provided to the Web sites of national, disease-specific, not-for-profit organizations from which patients can obtain additional information and assistance, and there is also a link to a preselected list of clinical trials registered with http://www.clinicaltrials.gov. The list of trials can be filtered by characteristics such as specific condition, study type, subject age, and location of study by state, allowing neurologists and patients to search for appropriate clinical trials. Viewers can also gain direct access to a prefiltered PubMed search of the medical literature on any disorder, and a link to Additional Resources from Medline Plus (http://medlineplus.gov/) leads to patient-oriented information provided by the US National Library of Medicine. These are outstanding resources to which neurologists can safely direct their patients.

## PERSONAL HEALTH RECORDS

Several online programs are available to help patients organize their personal medical information. These systems help patients manage their clinical records at a single online location that can be easily updated and then used to provide current medical records to their medical providers. Patient-controlled personal health records (PHRs) can reduce the likelihood of delays in making information available to providers, lessen the chance for miscommunication of key information, and may serve to keep individuals more engaged in their own health care.

Google Health (http://google.com/health) is the best organized and most user-friendly site among those described in this article. It serves as a central site for maintenance of medical records and has an interactive medication administration center. Free text functionality allows for annotation of most entries. There is ready access to a wide variety of useful proprietary tools ranging from assistance with converting paper medical records into electronic format to leveraging direct links from the Google Health record to medical groups. As an example, the Cleveland Clinic's MyConsult can provide second opinions for a wide variety of medical conditions. The Google Health site is supported by advertising and is free of charge to users.

Google Health has a simple function for extracting personal medication records from the computers of local pharmacies. Potential drug-drug interactions are automatically flagged from the lists of medications. A link to the pharmacy's online site (Walgreen's, in this case) allows the viewer to request prescription refills online. Once given access by the patient, doctors' offices also have the ability to see this data.

It is somewhat difficult to organize a printed summary of the record, but tools such as Lifestar offer free online services that allow patients to create views of their health history that can be printed or exported for sharing with health care providers, family, and caregivers. The security does not seem to be robust, compared with online banking sites, requiring only a username and password.

Several large companies are promoting the use of the PHR among their employees or customers. For instance, the 3 million members of Blue Cross Blue Shield of Massachusetts are able to securely populate their Google Health accounts with up to two years of health history. Similarly, the Dossia Founders Group (http://dossia.org) is a consortium of large employers who provide employees and their dependents with an independent, lifelong health record. The Dossia Founders Group includes AT&T, Applied Materials, BP America, Inc, Cardinal Health, Intel Corporation, Pitney Bowes, Sanofi-aventis and Wal-Mart. The site is only accessible for review by employees of these corporations.

Revolution Health (http://www.revolutionhealth.com), started by AOL founder Steve Case, allows users to store records, conduct research on health issues, take health-assessment tests, and gain easy access to health information and services. Editable categories include personal identification, emergency contacts, basic health information, family history, medical conditions, allergies, medications, immunizations, surgeries and procedures, doctors and care providers, hospitals and care facilities, and insurance. The page for each category opens with a large blank area that requires the user to scroll down to find the data field entry. The data fields are restrictive. For example, it is not possible to enter free text to annotate a particular entry with additional data. Medication interactions are not flagged. Microsoft HealthVault (http://www.healthvault.com) is an online shopping mall for health care, where companies can offer services, including a PHR.

Pinnacle (http://www.pinnaclecare.com) uses the online PHR to proactively manage medical care in the setting of concierge-type practice. Pinnacle charges $10,000 dollars or more to store and monitor medical records. Referrals to subspecialists are made on an as-needed basis, using a cohort of selected specialists around the country.

**NETWORKING**

Networking sites tailored to physicians soon followed the phenomenal success of the social networking site Facebook. Sermo (https://md.sermo.com/), one example of such a site, has more than 3000 licensed physicians who list neurology as their primary specialty. Membership is free, but to register, the user must first be verified by Sermo as a licensed physician. The core feature of the site is a posting, in which a member initiates an online conversation around a clinical case, a specific treatment, or any topic that might be of interest to fellow physicians. Most members choose unidentifiable usernames so that the postings are predominantly anonymous, and as a result the site is more like a chat room than a social network. Highly popular postings result in a financial reward (usually $500) to the originating physician. Sermo is sponsored by pharmaceutical companies, which are allowed to read, but not post, on the site, thereby presumably receiving insights into physicians' opinions about their products. The involvement of the pharmaceutical industry raises concerns about the lack of control of discussion of off-label use of drugs or devices, and potential conflicts of interest on the part of the participating physicians is not known. Pending federal legislation will require that those writing online product reviews will have to divulge the financial benefits they receive. It remains to be seen whether this regulatory activity will extend to sites such as Sermo.

A recently established online network called BioMedExperts (http://www.biomedexperts.com/) uses a novel approach to promote collaborations between biomedical scientists. The site has a prepopulated registry of more than 1.5 million authors who are listed in PubMed citations. Each scientist has been assigned a profile based on a list of concepts that are determined by the site and are extracted from each researcher's published abstracts. Concept categories include entries such as "Disorders," "Procedures," and "Phenomena." Registered members can search the database for individuals with specified research interests by entering key words, including concepts, investigator, or geographic location. Unique features include a list of new articles published by the user's previous co-authors. Members may enter additional information into their profile to improve the likelihood that they can be found by other scientists with similar interests.

## ADVOCACY

The ability of neurologists to act as advocates for their patients and for their profession is a critical, although underappreciated, aspect of modern practice. Several Web sites are well suited for this purpose.

The American Academy of Neurology (AAN) has been a leader in promoting awareness of legislative issues among its members, and more importantly, helping members become more involved in matters important to them and their patients. The advocacy Web page on the AAN's Web site (http://www.aan.com/go/advocacy) has up-to-date information about legislative developments of interest to neurologists at federal and state levels. The site contains AAN position statements and broader discussions of legislative issues. Vocus (http://www.aan.com/go/advocacy/active/vocus) allows the AAN to quickly notify its members about urgent legislative concerns, and in turn, have neurologists contact their legislators about these issues with just a few simple clicks of a mouse. Vocus provides information that is specific to the neurologist's legislative district, such as names and contact information for senators and congressmen. Legislators may be contacted using an individual letter or a form letter, making it easier for the busy practitioner to become involved in legislative issues.

Several advocacy organizations for neurologic patients use similar software to encourage their members to contact legislators about key issues. For instance, the National Multiple Sclerosis (MS) Society Web site (http://www.nationalmssociety.org/government-affairs-and-advocacy/index.aspx) educates the viewer about governmental issues relevant to MS and provides a simple conduit to contact relevant legislators by using a software program similar to Vocus (http://capwiz.com/nmss/issues/). The first-time visitor has to register online to enable these functionalities. Other neurologic patient advocacy organizations have varying degrees of expertise in exploiting the Internet for advocacy issues in this manner, but the model provides a powerful tool for helping neurologists become politically involved for the good of their specialty and their patients. (For access to specific disease-oriented sites, see the NINDS Disorders Index) (http://www.ninds.nih.gov/disorders/disorder_index.htm).

## SUMMARY

The Internet is a highly versatile tool for bringing information to physicians, and neurologists should seek the functions that best suit their individual styles of information gathering. Numerous barriers remain to achieving the Internet's potential. Scholarly publications can be difficult to access, although it seems that the publishing industry has recognized the inevitability of submission of many of their highest quality articles to PMC. More research is needed to understand the ways in which patients and their caregivers use the Internet. PHRs hold great promise, but vary greatly in mission, usability, and sophistication. The PHR is still in early stages of development, with many opportunities for improvement as electronic medical records come into widespread use by medical providers. Networking is still poorly developed within professional circles, but neurologists have begun to actively experiment with new sites as they come online. Several professional societies have highly developed Internet tools to leverage the effectiveness of those who seek to improve the lives of their patients through advocacy.

Fifteen years after its introduction into medicine, the Internet's value is still largely untapped. The neurologist's creativity and sense of curiosity will be crucial to the advancement of this tool in the service of acquiring knowledge and improving patient care.

## REFERENCES

1. Chio A, Montuschi A, Cammarosano S, et al. ALS patients and caregivers communication preferences and information seeking behaviour. Eur J Neurol 2008;15(1): 55–60.
2. Diaz JA, Griffith RA, Ng JJ, et al. Patients' use of the Internet for medical information. J Gen Intern Med 2002;17(3):180–5.
3. Baker L, Wagner TH, Singer S, et al. Use of the Internet and e-mail for health care information: results from a national survey. JAMA 2003;289(18):2400–6.

# Mobile Phones to Improve the Practice of Neurology

Neil Busis, MD[a,b,c],*

**KEYWORDS**

- Mobile phones • Smartphones • Information technology
- Neurology practice

## CASE STUDY: SOLVING A SPELL ON THE SCENE

*A young man feels funny and then loses consciousness. His friends record the event with the cameras on their cell phones, documenting left head and eye deviation with left arm posturing. A subsequent electroencephalogram demonstrates a temporal lobe seizure focus.[1]*

This case study only hints at the potential for smartphones to revolutionize medical care. As Zeiler and Kaplan,[1] the case authors, state, "One picture is worth a thousand guesses." Often patients cannot accurately describe their neurologic spells and neither can witnesses. Mobile voice and data interchange in the medical information domains of patient data, clinical decision support, and practice management bridges time and space, allowing near instantaneous diagnosis and treatment while at the same time redefining the meaning of "the point of care."[2–4]

This article addresses mobile health care via smartphones. The biggest advances may be expected to come about in developed countries, but this is not the case. A United Nations report describes mobile phones as having the greatest impact in developing countries.[5] Although many developing countries do not have widespread or even dependable broadband Internet access, much of their population has access to cell phones. These devices make it convenient to schedule appointments, receive medical results, and ensure timely alerts and reminders regarding upcoming tests, procedures, and medications.[6,7]

[a] Division of Neurology, Department of Medicine, UPMC Shadyside Hospital, Pittsburgh, PA 15232, USA
[b] Neurodiagnostic Laboratory, UPMC Shadyside Hospital, Pittsburgh, PA 15232, USA
[c] Pittsburgh Neurology Center, 532 South Aiken Avenue, Suite 507, Pittsburgh, PA 15232, USA
* Corresponding author. Division of Neurology, Department of Medicine, UPMC Shadyside Hospital, Pittsburgh, PA 15232.
*E-mail address:* nab@neuroguide.com

Neurol Clin 28 (2010) 395–410
doi:10.1016/j.ncl.2009.11.001
0733-8619/10/$ – see front matter

A disclaimer is in order. Technology articles are out of date as soon as they are written. The emphasis in this article, therefore, is on concepts and principles rather than specific hardware models and software versions.

## THE BIG PICTURE—SETTING THE STAGE
### Hardware/Network/Software Trends

Several interrelated developments will change how health care is accessed and provided.[8] Computing and communicating devices not only are getting smarter, smaller, faster, and cheaper but also are evolving from fixed to portable, non-networked to networked, wired to wireless, and location- and orientation-agnostic to location- and orientation-aware. We are moving to a world of health information technology literally at our fingertips, available at the point of care in clinical practice.

### Mobile Phones

Mobile phones are devices that transmit not only voice messages but also text and multimedia messages (messages composed of text, moving or still pictures, and sounds). Mobile phones can now acquire multimedia with built-in cameras and voice recorders. They are continually gaining computing power.

### Computer User Interfaces

Virtually all recent models of desktop and laptop computers employ a graphical user interface controlled by a mouse or some other pointing apparatus. In contrast, most of the successful smaller portable devices have adopted a touch-based interface. Users tap and choose icons, words, and so forth with a stylus or a finger. Recently introduced multitouch (or gesture) interfaces allow users to manipulate the objects on screen by touching two or more places on the screen at once, for example, touching a picture with two fingers and spreading them apart enlarges the picture.[9] This makes the interaction between users and portable devices more intuitive than through the use of a tiny trackball, pointing stick, stylus, and so forth to interact with a display.

### Networks

Advances in networks, most notably the ongoing transformation from wired to wireless, have accelerated the mobile computing revolution. Wireless networks can be narrower in range (a Bluetooth personal network, for example) or provide wider coverage (eg, the Internet) than many traditional local wired networks. Many mobile devices use several types and ranges of network interfaces, including satellite channels, cellular networks, Wi-Fi, and Bluetooth.

Cellular wireless networks depend on a series of cells—towers loaded with transmitters—which automatically transfer users' signals as they move from one tower's coverage area to another's. Each cell phone carrier uses proprietary network technology, which, with few exceptions, is incompatible with those of other carriers. It has recently been proposed that all cellular carriers begin sharing the same core network technology to allow devices acquired from one cellular carrier to be used on another carrier's network.

Wi-Fi is a local type of cellular network with a range of approximately 300 feet. Wireless access points broadcast a signal that users' devices pick up. The handoffs are usually not automatic when leaving one Wi-Fi coverage area and entering another; nevertheless, Wi-Fi transmission speeds are faster than on existing cellular networks.

Bluetooth personal networks allow the creation of a short-range personal area network of up to approximately 30 feet in range. For example, Bluetooth can connect a mobile phone to a wireless headset, a car's audio system, or a printer.

Voice over Internet Protocol may greatly increase access to long-distance telecommunications. Voice is translated into data that are transmitted over the Internet rather than through a cell phone carrier's proprietary networks. Users whose devices are equipped with Voice over Internet Protocol applications, such as Skype or Vonage, and who have broadband Internet connections can call similarly equipped devices anywhere in the world without paying cell phone charges.

### Global Positioning System and Accelerometers

The Global Positioning System (GPS) relies on location data computed from signals from satellites orbiting the Earth. GPS allows users of appropriately equipped mobile devices to detect their location (actually the location of their device) and broadcast it to others to find nearby attractions and resources (with reviews) and generate directions as a list or in real time, turn-by-turn. If the device is lost or stolen, GPS can help find it. GPS enhances social networking applications by pinpointing friends' locations. A built-in compass adds to the GPS functionality.

Accelerometers inform a device about its orientation in space. Appropriately equipped smartphones can automatically switch from portrait to landscape view when they are rotated. Accelerometers enhance user input options and can be used to control games or other devices. They can even act as an electronic carpenter's level.

### Cloud Computing

Cloud computing is an evolution of client-server computing. A client (a computer) is networked (wired or wirelessly) to a larger computer somewhere else (the cloud) in which most of the data and computing power resides.[10] This greatly enhances the information technology capabilities of small, relatively underpowered, computing devices, such as smartphones, because they are now able to offload large amounts of data storage and computations to more capacious and capable machines. The cloud can also be used to back up data on a mobile device. If a device is lost, the backup is simply retrieved from the cloud onto a replacement device. Moreover, the cloud allows synchronization of data among various devices. Users can ensure that desktop, laptop, and mobile devices contain the same contacts, calendar, Web browser bookmarks, and so forth, by synchronizing them with a server located in the cloud.

## ABOUT SMARTPHONES
### What are Smartphones?

Smartphones represent the convergence of mobile computers and cellular telephones.[11] Carrying around a communication device and a separate mobile computing device is no longer needed. Smartphones are the logical successors of traditional cell phones and personal digital assistants (PDAs), with more capabilities than both, separately or in combination. Just as it became inconceivable to buy a computer without Internet capability, one no longer thinks of buying a mobile computing device or a PDA without network potential. Mobile access to computing power, multimedia communications, the Internet, and individual physical location are in the palms of our hands. Phone numbers are now user-specific not location-specific.

### The Smartphone Market

Cell phones are replacing landlines as the preferred method of telephone communication.[12] The percentage of cell phones that are smartphones is relatively low in the world today, but the numbers are rising. In 2008, of the 1.19 billion mobile phones sold worldwide, 155 million (13%) were smartphones. Experts predict that in 2013, 280 million (20%) of the 1.4 billion phones sold will be smartphones.[13]

### Major Smartphone Platforms

Currently, the two major smartphone platforms in the United States[14] are the Apple iPhone (http://www.apple.com/iphone/) and various Research In Motion BlackBerry models (http://www.rim.com/). There are other smartphone platforms with smaller market shares. Palm makes smartphones (Pre and Pixi) based on its new operating system, webOS (http://www.palm.com/). They have phased out their older platform, the Palm OS, a previous market leader. Google provides its Android smartphone operating system for free and various manufacturers are developing devices based on this platform (http://www.android.com/). The Windows mobile platform (http://www.microsoft.com/windowsmobile/) has been around for years but is losing market share to these newer rivals. Nokia (http://www.nokia.com/) is the world leader in smartphones with its Symbian platform (http://www.symbian.org/) but has only a small market share in the United States. There are smartphones based on Linux (http://www.access-company.com/) and other proprietary technologies, although these constitute only a tiny portion of the market.

### The Smartphone Ecosystem

Each smartphone lies at the epicenter of its own ecosystem. A smartphone is connected via its cellular or Wi–Fi network to

1. An application store that contains software, which can be loaded on the smartphone
2. The Internet for e-mail and Web access
3. The cloud for synchronization, backup, and, in some cases, more intense data processing.

Smartphones have spawned a robust accessory market. The most popular accessories include wired and wireless headsets and speakers, cases, and wall and car chargers.

Because the different smartphone hardware operating systems are mutually incompatible (except that all are able to access the Web via browsers and e-mail), their ecosystems are all separate. The Apple iPhone ecosystem is the best developed (http://www.apple.com/iphone/apps-for-iphone/ and http://www.apple.com/mobileme/), and others are currently playing catch-up with their own application and accessory stores and with cloud computing systems.

### SMARTPHONE APPLICATIONS
#### Overview of Smartphone Functionality

Smartphones can think, sync, and link. They think by accessing references and databases that reside on smartphones themselves. They sync to other devices and to the cloud. They link to the Internet. Smartphone applications include those that are generally available to the public and those that are specific to a specialty, such as medicine.

There are three sources of applications—those built in by the manufacturer, those downloaded from third parties and then installed by a user, and those accessed via a mobile phone's Web browser.[15] Different manufacturers provide varying numbers and types of built-in applications. Third-party applications can be downloaded for some devices directly from the developers but in some smartphone ecosystems that can be done only via an intermediary. For example, iPhone applications can only be downloaded and installed (officially, at least) via the iTunes application store. Web-based applications are not installed on the device—they are accessed via an active Internet connection.

### Built-in Smartphone Applications

Most smartphones come with many built-in applications. They cover the core functions of smartphones—traditional functions, such as notes, and newer ones, such as GPS.

The primary function, of course, is the telephone. The software not only enables one-to-one voice communication but also allows easily setting up conference calls and voicemail for messages. Some of the newer smartphones feature visual voicemail, which streamlines the process of retrieving messages via the generation of a detailed list on smartphones themselves, thereby obviating calling and listening to a cumbersome audio menu. Messaging is a basic function of smartphones. This includes not only text messages but also multimedia messages, which incorporate still or moving pictures or sound.

In addition to information entered by a device owner, the contact management and calendar applications can include information provided by a user's organization. Some corporate contact and calendar databases reside on the cloud. For example, Microsoft Exchange uses ActiveSync to synchronize frequently updated data on a corporate server with a user's mobile device.

Web and e-mail access are now standard smartphone features. Mobile Web browsers enable users to search, browse, and interact with content formerly available only on desktop and laptop computers. E-mail applications can access individual or private accounts and organizational and corporate ones. With some e-mail protocols, the messages reside on a user's device, but with others, such as Microsoft Exchange, the device only views the mailbox contents—the actual messages are stored on a server somewhere in the cloud.

Notes and to-do lists are holdovers from original PDAs, such as the PalmPilot. Notes are small snippets of text used for references and reminders. To-do lists are useful as reminders of tasks recently assigned and yet to be completed. The more feature-rich smartphones allow notes and to-do lists to be synchronized to the cloud or to a user's desktop or laptop computer.

Multimedia capabilities are becoming incorporated into consumer and corporate smartphones. They allow users to access and acquire music and voice, photographs, and video. With voice recognition, users can say the name of a person or organization or the associated phone number, and the device processes the request and dials the correct number.

Newer smartphones have system-wide indexing and search. A single screen provides a gateway to relevant information in contacts, e-mail, calendars, notes, and so forth.

Location- and orientation-based applications are enabled by GPS and accelerometer capabilities, respectively. Some are built in, such as the map application and photo geotagging on an iPhone.

### Add-on Applications for Smartphones

Some add-on applications are useful to a wide variety of users and reside on the device. They can extend built-in functionality—for example, a barcode reader extends the functionality of a built-in camera—or they can add new functionality, such as an electronic wallet. Some applications act as a front end to Web-based services, including search engines, such as Google or Yahoo; social networking sites, such as Facebook or Twitter; news sites and RSS readers; Wikipedia and other references; and blogs and wikis.

Any Web site can be considered an add-on application because it can contribute functionality that is not built into smartphone software. Some Web sites are friendly to the limited feature set of mobile Web browsers, but some are not, so their utility varies by site and device.

### Health Care Applications for Smartphones

There is a rapidly expanding universe of specialized health care applications for users of all the major smartphone platforms. Applications for patients and providers are discussed.

### Applications for Patients

Lifestyle applications can help manage weight loss, diet and cooking, and exercise of brain and body. There are many applications for patient information and education, including general references such as Consumer Reports Health (http://www.consumerreports.org/health/) and the Mayo Clinic Health Letter (http://healthletter.mayoclinic.com/). Some are very specific, for example, a list for hikers of the most poisonous snakes. Applications may reside on a device or be accessed via the Web. A good example of the latter is the National Institute of Neurological Disorders and Stroke disease database with direct links to patient support groups (http://www.ninds.nih.gov/disorders/disorder_index.htm).

Smartphones allow patients to communicate with their health care providers by voice, text, and multimedia. In certain circumstances, patients are able to show their health care providers what is going on from a distance, as demonstrated in the case study discussed previously, in which a video of abnormal movements was shown or sent to the patient's neurologist. Communication can also be facilitated through foreign language translators. Patients can access and share personal medical information on smartphones. These include medication, allergy, and problem lists and can include comprehensive personal medical records. Medical social networks and communities, such as the BrainTalk Communities (http://brain.hastypastry.net/forums/), can be developed or accessed via mobile phones. For those patients with substantial neurologic impairments, such as limited mobility, access to virtual communities may greatly expand their horizons and sense of empowerment.[16]

Mobile phones have the potential to enhance the provision of health care around the world, wherever a cell phone infrastructure exists. Even in less developed areas, mobile phones can be used to send and receive test results, alerts, reminders, and advice. For example, text messages can remind patients to take their anti-HIV drugs. Mobile phones can be used for disease management, remote monitoring of symptoms and epidemics,[17] and questionnaires. They can even be used as prosthetics for sensory or cognitive impairments. For example, a smartphone application called Speak it! can transform text into speech.[18] It can give a voice to those who have been rendered voiceless, and can assist those who are sight impaired. Another smartphone application helps compensate for anterograde amnesia in memory-challenged patients.[19]

### Applications for Health Care Providers

There is a rich array of applications for health care providers. Some of the most compelling uses rely on built-in core smartphone functions. Many other applications are easily installed. Even more functionality is available if additional infrastructure – hardware or software on desktop or laptop computers–is also installed and utilized.

Physicians and other providers can use smartphones to easily communicate with offices, answering services, colleagues, and patients Pagers can be replaced by the two-way messaging capabilities.

Reference material and databases are plentiful. Some contain preclinical content, such as anatomic and radiographic atlases, and there are even audio collections with heart sounds. Clinical references cover diagnosis, treatment, practice guidelines, and practice parameters. Mobile versions, reformatted to best fit a mobile device's small screen, exist for several relevant Web sites, including the mobile version of the American Academy of Neurology's Web site (http://m.aan.com).

Users can search and retrieve full text of peer-reviewed medical literature via specially designed applications, such as PubMed On Tap for the iPhone, or via the smartphone's Web browser. Reference management tools are available. Papers for the iPhone, for example, for articles and abstracts saved in portable document format (PDF), has an interface similar to iTunes. There are instructions on how to perform medical procedures, incorporating sound and video. A series of instructional resources on how to perform electromyographic and nerve conduction studies by Dr Joseph Jabre is particularly useful (http://www.teleemg.com). Continuing medical education credits can be achieved over the Web on several free services.

Drug databases contain names of drugs, their indications, dosages, pharmacology, interactions, contraindications, cost, pill identifiers, and so forth. Drug-drug interactions calculated at the point of care are critically important. There are also databases for diagnostic tests that list indications, normal/abnormal values, and how to interpret certain laboratory results.

There are many multifunction clinical calculators, such as the free MedCalc,[20] and more specific ones, such as the National Institutes of Health (NIH) Stroke Scale calculator, for point-of-care stroke documentation and medical decision making. Practice management resources are also available for many smartphone platforms. These include reference materials, searchable databases, and calculators for proper diagnosis (*International Classification of Diseases, Ninth Revision-Clinical Modification [ICD-9-CM]*), evaluation and management, and procedure (*Current Procedural Terminology [CPT]*) coding.

Applications can assist in diagnostic testing. EyePhone, an application for the iPhone, is a visual acuity test optimized for the iPhone screen. Basic telemedicine can be achieved with smartphones by taking pictures or videos and sending them as multimedia messages between patients and providers.

More advanced telemedicine capabilities are possible with appropriate infrastructure.[21,22] A sophisticated camera and electronic medical record system at the point of care could transmit images and data to an offsite physician who is carrying only a smartphone. Access to imaging studies can be done via a smartphone if it is connected to a hospital or organization's digital radiology system. Mobile telephone microscopy is emerging in which the camera of a smartphone is connected to a microscope, and the images of the slides are sent for interpretation to an offsite pathologist. Remote patient monitoring is available for smartphones if they are connected to intensive care unit monitoring devices in a hospital.

Computer-assisted medical decision making is best done when a smartphone is connected to other computers. Patient alerts and reminders, electronic medical records, rounding lists, charge capture, and electronic prescribing are available as stand-alone applications, but functionality is greatly enhanced if a mobile device acts as a client for a hospital or organization's main electronic medical record system.

The same is true for physician quality measure reporting. Under the current model of the Physician Quality Reporting Initiative, providers submit numbers of patients with a particular diagnosis who received a certain type of treatment or advice. This works best if the patients' diagnoses and treatment have been stored in an electronic medical record. It would be difficult to do this from a smartphone operating in isolation.

The basis of continuous quality improvement is to model, measure, and manage. Another way to say this is plan, study, and act. By closing the feedback loop through the use of data collection at the point of care, smartphones will enable more valid continuous quality improvement projects in medicine.

Tying mobile phone data collection into a remote database permits epidemiologic studies to be performed even in developing countries. Clinical trials are also greatly extended using smartphone-based data collected by patients and providers. Location-specific capabilities enable patient tracking.[23]

Mobile phones are used as remote controls for games and for other electronic devices. It is probably not far off that simple robotic surgery will be controlled by an offsite surgeon using a mobile phone.

Patients often use the same applications that their providers use. Many patients use Epocrates, the National Institute of Neurological Disorders and Stroke Web site, and PubMed. It is useful to access these resources from time to time and try to see them from a patient's point of view (**Figs. 1** and **2**).

## SMARTPHONES AND PERSONAL DIGITAL ASSISTANTS IN MEDICINE—THE LITERATURE

Information technology can improve health care.[24] Case studies[25,26] and peer-reviewed medical literature[27] attest to the usefulness of smartphones and PDAs in medicine. In community hospitals and ambulatory clinics without wireless networks, real-time access to current medical literature may be achieved through applications on smartphones. Immediate availability of reliable and updated information obtained from authoritative sources on the Web makes evidence-based practice in community hospitals a reality.

An up-to-date bibliography is always available via a PubMed search (http://www.pubmed.gov) using the phrase, "Cellular Phone"[Mesh]. As of October 25, 2009, 1624 relevant articles were retrieved, 105 of them reviews. One recent study concluded, "enhancing standard care with reminders, disease monitoring and management, and education through cell phone voice and short message service can help improve health outcomes and care processes have implications for both patients and providers."[28]

## CHALLENGES AND SHORTCOMINGS

Although smartphones are promising devices and getting better almost every week, they have challenges and shortcomings. Interoperability is problematic for developers and end users. Platform-specific applications (those loaded directly onto a smartphone) are faster and may access more specific features of smartphones, but they require more resources and development time.[29] Small developers have to decide how many platforms they will support. The potential solution is to make well-designed, Web-based applications that are platform neutral. Their functionality is more limited, however, due to their inability to access some of the key built-in features of specific devices that make smartphones such a compelling platform. For example, network-based applications may be impeded by patchy, uncertain, or slow connectivity.

Data input is often clumsy and error prone.[30] Some smartphones have physical keyboards that are small and cramped, and typing on them is difficult. Some have virtual keyboards. Virtual keyboards can be reformatted for portrait and landscape modes and different keys can be available for different applications or different

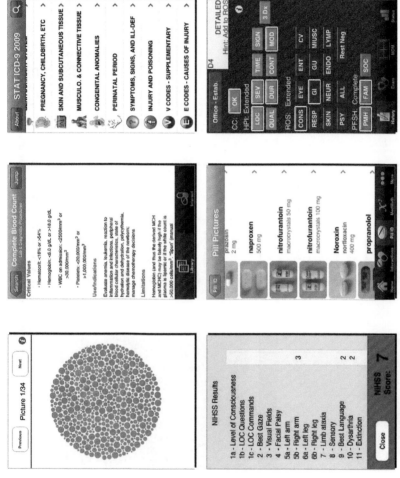

**Fig. 1.** Neurology applications for smartphones. (*Top row, left to right*) Test for color vision, database of laboratory tests, and *ICD-9-CM* (diagnosis codes) database. (*Bottom row, left to right*) NIH Stroke Scale calculator, drug database, and evaluation and management CPT code calculator. These examples are for the iPhone. Similar applications may be available for other smartphones.

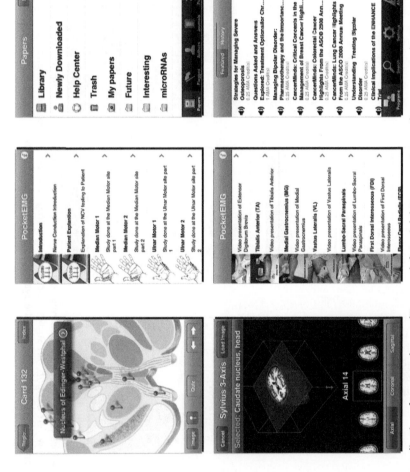

**Fig. 2.** More neurology applications for smartphones. (*Top row, left to right*) Neuroanatomy atlas, nerve conduction study instructions with illustrative videos, and reference manager (indexes and accesses PDF files of collected references). (*Bottom row, left to right*) Neuroradiology atlas, electromyographic instructions with illustrative videos, and free continuing medical education application. These examples are for the iPhone. Similar applications may be available for other smartphones.

languages, but there is no tactile feedback. Typing is slower on a virtual keyboard than on a physical keyboard, although many users do not mind or adjust to it within a short time.

Battery life can be limiting. Many smartphones have only a few hours of active battery life, barely enough to get through a full business day without recharging. Although battery life can be extended by turning off some of the features of the smartphone (for instance, GPS location, Wi–Fi, or Bluetooth), that partially defeats the intended purpose of smartphones.

Do smartphones actually access the real Web? The answer is sometimes yes and sometimes no. The small screen can be an impediment to users, because it is like looking at the Internet through a keyhole. Although almost all Web sites can be visited, to visualize many at a font size that is reasonable, a fair amount of horizontal and vertical scrolling is required, which may become tedious. One particularly troublesome development is the increasing use of plug-ins, such as Adobe Flash, for Web sites. Currently Flash solutions are absent or not completely satisfactory for smartphone platforms. Web sites without alternative non-Flash versions do not have full functionality on smartphones. The solution is to visit only Web sites optimized for mobile phone Web browsers, but the tradeoff is often a loss of functionality.

Privacy is concerning. Not only are there Health Insurance Portability and Accountability Act concerns about patient information on mobile devices, but also users of the devices may object to certain smartphone features. Carriers could monitor how devices are used on their networks and potentially intercept e-mail, Web transmissions, and so forth. Location-based services could monitor users' locations without their knowledge or approval.

Security remains a challenge with smartphones. What to do about loss or theft? Although Microsoft Exchange–based systems have Remote Wipe and Apple's MobileMe has introduced this functionality to their smartphones, there are ways to circumvent this safeguard.

Cloud computing has its downside. If all user data reside on remote servers and they fail without adequate backups, then important information can be irretrievably lost.[31]

What about viruses and worms (malware) for smartphones? These will probably become an increasing threat as more hackers devote their attention to these platforms. This is one instance in which the multiplicity of operating systems is actually a good thing. Because no smartphone maker controls the vast majority of devices (unlike the Windows-dominated personal computer [PC] world), it would be difficult for malware to inflict as great a negative impact on smartphones as it can on PCs. Antivirus software makers are starting to explore products for smartphones due to the anticipated threat.

## HEALTH PROBLEMS (POTENTIAL AND PROVED) AND UNINTENDED CONSEQUENCES

All technologic advances have negative aspects, and many cannot be predicted or anticipated. Edward Tenner terms this "the revenge of technology."[32] The potential adverse health consequences of cell phones are increasingly recognized.[33]

The biggest unsettled health-related question is whether or not cell phones cause cancer.[34–36] Although this has not been proved despite much investigation, absence of evidence is not evidence of absence. Some, but not all, authorities opine that further studies are needed.

Minor medical maladies are associated with overuse of smartphones. There is the so-called BlackBerry thumb, from overuse of the thumb-based keyboard.[37] There are scalp and ear dysesthesias reported from holding a cell phone too close to the ear during prolonged talking.[38]

More serious are the decreased attention and difficulties with multitasking inherent in having a conversation (voice or data) on a cell phone while doing something else important.[39,40] Talking or texting on cell phones while walking or driving leads to more accidents.[41] Hands-free conversations are shown no less distracting than holding a device to the ear.[42] State and federal lawmakers are beginning to prohibit certain cell phone uses while driving.[43]

Cell phones may cause stress when users are always available and on call. Users may become addicted to the Internet or to their devices (the so-called crackberry phenomenon).[44] Cell phones can sometimes serve as vectors of infection, just as neckties are.[45] Prolonged cell phone conversations can potentially have adverse electromagnetic[46] and thermal effects on central and peripheral nervous tissue.[47] Loud sounds through a receiver can cause hearing loss; this is more likely to occur from listening to music than from conversations.[48] Finally, there are concerns about sterility caused by cell phones, which is currently under investigation.[49]

There are potential problems with the software and hardware. The old adage, "garbage in–garbage out," applies to medical software and any other software. Users entering the wrong data leads to wrong decisions. More perniciously, medical software deficiencies or bugs may give erroneous results. A reported software bug caused a patient to get the wrong dose during radiation therapy with fatal consequences.[50]

Cell phones can cause electrical interference with other medical devices.[51,52] These can be in or on a patient (for example, a pacemaker or a ventriculoperitoneal shunt valve) or around or connected to a patient, such as a monitor, respirator, and so forth. The available literature demonstrates that different combinations of cell phones and devices have different degrees of electrical interference ranging from none to serious. As cell phones become more ubiquitous, manufacturers of cell phones and medical equipment will need to electrically isolate these devices from one another. When in doubt, ask the information technology personnel at a hospital or organization to test the devices to see if they are compatible before allowing them to be used together.

## WHAT DEVICE AND APPLICATIONS SHOULD YOU GET?

The answer depends on what problems you want to solve.[53,54] What do you want to sync and link to? What are your e-mail habits? What are your favorite applications? What carriers and networks work best in your area? What can you afford? What does your institution or organization mainly use? What does your institution or organization support? Are you willing to go it alone to use a device that is not supported by your information technology staff?

Currently, the iPhone and BlackBerry platforms are most popular among physicians.[55] The abundance of medical applications favors increasing popularity of the iPhone in the future.[56]

## WHERE DO WE GO FROM HERE?

Extrapolating from current trends, smartphones potentially can lead to pervasive computing, with these devices serving as the "remote control for your life."[57,58]

It is a safe bet that there will be smarter, smaller, faster, and cheaper devices and faster, more widespread networks that will allow seamless carrier conversions and carrier interoperability. As long as the applications are allowed, there may be liberation from the hegemony of the carriers by allowing users to avoid cellular networks with Voice over Internet Protocol.

More convergence lies ahead. Smartphones are becoming sufficiently capable that they can replace desktops and laptops for many applications. In some small businesses, networks of smartphones may replace landline telephones and PBX systems. There will be phone number convergence. Google Voice and related services will intercept messages from multiple phone numbers and assign them to a single new number. There should be better integration between the users' contacts and activities, especially by location-based services.

There should be better Internet-based applications; better ability to download, upload, and sync; and backup to and from the cloud. There should be better integration with social networking services, location-based services, other digital health care applications and platforms, and virtual communities. There should be smarter alerts and reminders via background patient-monitoring applications.

We hope for better battery life and better displays—some may be projected or some may be flexible and able to be rolled up or folded out. There may be better input with improved voice recognition and perhaps even keyboards projected onto larger spaces. There may be better accessibility for the visually and hearing impaired. There may be better security, including biometric logons (for example, using fingerprints).

We cannot predict future disruptive technologies or economic circumstances. As the saying goes, "the only guaranteed part of life is change." Anticipate the unanticipated—that one or more unexpected devices or applications will have a major impact on the world of mobile devices in the not-so-distant future.

## SUMMARY

Smartphones make mobile computing at the point of care practical. Smartphones can think, sync, and link. Built-in and user-installed applications facilitate communications between neurologists and their medical colleagues and patients and augment data acquisition and processing in the core medical information domains of patient data, clinical decision support, and practice management. Mobile telemedicine is becoming practical in certain scenarios. Smartphones can improve neurologic diagnosis and treatment, teaching, and research. Patients also can benefit from smartphone technology. In addition to enhanced communication, patient education, and social networking, these devices can promote healthy lifestyles, preventive medicine, and compliance and even serve as monitoring and prosthetic devices.

## REFERENCES

1. Zeiler SR, Kaplan PW. Our digital world: camera phones and the diagnosis of a seizure. Lancet 2009;373(9681):2136.
2. mHealth Initiative Vision. The mobilization of healthcare. Available at: http://mhealthinitiative.org/. Accessed September 20, 2009.
3. Bhanoo SN. New tool in the MD's bag: a smartphone 2009. The Washington Post. Available at: http://www.washingtonpost.com/wp-dyn/content/article/2009/05/18/AR2009051802234.html. Accessed September 20, 2009.
4. mHealth. Wikipedia. Available at: http://en.wikipedia.org/wiki/MHealth. Accessed September 20, 2009.
5. Vital Wave Consulting. mHealth for development: the opportunity of mobile technology for healthcare in the developing world. Washington, DC/Berkshire (UK): UN Foundation-Vodafone Foundation Partnership; 2009. Available at: http://www.unfoundation.org/press-center/publications/mhealth-for-development-mobile-technology-for-healthcare.html. Accessed September 20, 2009.

6. Vaitheeswaran V. Medicine goes digital—a special report on healthcare and technology. The Economist 2009. Available at: http://www.economist.com/specialReports/showsurvey.cfm?issue=20090418. Accessed September 20, 2009.

7. Denison DC. Using cellphones to change the world. Boston Globe 2009. Available at: http://www.boston.com/business/technology/articles/2009/10/14/mit_program_looks_at_ways_to_change_the_world_using_cellphones/. Accessed October 25, 2009.

8. Snyder S. The new world of wireless: how to compete in the 4g revolution. Upper Saddle River (NJ): Wharton School Publishing; 2009.

9. Ricknas M. Gestures set to shake up mobile user interfaces. Macworld (UK); 2009. Available at: http://www.macworld.co.uk/digitallifestyle/news/index.cfm?RSS&NewsID=27104. Accessed September 20, 2009.

10. Cloud computing in plain English. rPath. Available at: http://www.rpath.com/oorp/cloudinenglish. Accessed September 20, 2009.

11. Bertman J. Tech 101: a new generation of smartphones. MDNG Neurology 2009; 11(5):26.

12. America loses its landlines—cutting the cord. The Economist 2009;392(8644):55–6.

13. Hempel J. How blackberry does it. Fortune 2009;160(4):92–100.

14. AdMob Mobile Metrics. Metrics report 2009. Available at: http://metrics.admob.com/. Accessed September 20, 2009.

15. Fling B. Mobile design and development. Sebasopol (CA): O'Reilly Media, Inc; 2009.

16. Sarasohn-Kahn J. The wisdom of patients: health care meets online social media. California HealtHCare Foundation 2008. Available at: http://www.chcf.org/topics/chronicdisease/index.cfm?itemID=133631. Accessed September 20, 2009.

17. Golijan R. Healthmap app will tell you how diseased your neighborhood is. Gizmodo. Available at: http://gizmodo.com/5350585/healthmap-app-will-tell-you-how-diseased-your-neighborhood-is; 2009. Accessed September 20, 2009.

18. Vance A. Insurers fight speech-impairment remedy. The New York Times Online 2009. Available at: http://www.nytimes.com/2009/09/15/technology/15speech.html?scp=1&sq=speech-impaired&st=cse. Accessed September 20, 2009.

19. Svoboda E, Richards B. Compensating for anterograde amnesia: a new training method that capitalizes on emerging smartphone technologies. J Int Neuropsychol Soc 2009;15(4):629–38.

20. Tschopp M, Lovis C, Geissbuhler A. Understanding usage patterns of handheld computers in clinical practice. Proc AMIA Symp 2002;806–9.

21. Doty CA. Delivering care anytime, anywhere: telehealth alters the medical ecosystem. California HealtHCare Foundation; 2008. Available at: http://www.chcf.org/topics/view.cfm?itemID=133787. Accessed September 20, 2009.

22. Schwamm LH, Holloway RG, Amarenco P, et al. A review of the evidence for the use of telemedicine within stroke systems of care: a scientific statement from the American Heart Association/American Stroke Association. Stroke 2009;40(7):2616–34.

23. Kwok R. Personal technology: phoning in data. Nature 2009;458(7241):959–61.

24. Amarasingham R, Plantinga L, Diener-West M, et al. Clinical information technologies and inpatient outcomes: a multiple hospital study. Arch Intern Med 2009; 169(2):108–14.

25. BlackBerry Case Study. Hospital sees blackberry smartphones as a way to improve patient care and save lives. research in motion limited. Available at: http://na.blackberry.com/eng/newsroom/success/Trillium_HealthCentre.pdf. Accessed September 20, 2009.

26. BlackBerry. Revitalizing healthcare delivery with mobile communications. Research In Motion Limited; 2007. Available at: http://na.blackberry.com/ong/campaign/healthcarecampaign/smartphone_benefits.pdf. Accessed September 20, 2009.
27. Leon SA, Fontelo P, Green L, et al. Evidence-based medicine among internal medicine residents in a community hospital program using smart phones. BMC Med Inform Decis Mak 2007;7:5.
28. Krishna S, Boren SA, Balas EA. Healthcare via cell phones: a systematic review. Telemed J E Health 2009;15(3):231–40.
29. Krill P. Smartphones: a tower of babel for developers. Macworld; 2009. Available at: http://www.macworld.com/article/142576/2009/09/smartphone_development.html. Accessed September 20, 2009.
30. Haller G, Haller DM, Courvoisier DS, et al. Handheld vs. laptop computers for electronic data collection in clinical research: a crossover randomized trial. J Am Med Inform Assoc 2009;16(5):651–9.
31. Sarrel MD. The darker side of cloud computing. Available at: PCMag.com 2009; http://www.pcmag.com/article2/0,00.asp,2817,2330904. Accessed September 20, 2009.
32. Tenner E. Why things bite back: technology and the revenge of unintended consequences. New York (NY): Vintage Books; 1997.
33. Kharif O. Is cell-phone safety assured? or merely ignored? Bus Week 2009. Available at: http://www.businessweek.com/technology/content/sep2009/tc20090921_950531.htm. Accessed October 25, 2009.
34. Kundi M. The controversy about a possible relationship between mobile phone use and cancer. Environ Health Perspect 2009;117(3):316–24.
35. Lahkola A, Auvinen A, Raitanen J, et al. Mobile phone use and risk of glioma in 5 North European countries. Int J Cancer 2007;120(8):1769–75.
36. No link between mobile phone use and increased risk of glioma. Nat Clin Pract Neurol 2007;3:303.
37. Rx for BlackBerry thumb. Consum Rep 2009;74(1):12.
38. Westerman R, Hocking B. Diseases of modern living: neurological changes associated with mobile phones and radiofrequency radiation in humans. Neurosci Lett 2004;361(1–3):13–6.
39. Goodman MJ, Barker JA, Monk CA. A bibliography of research related to the use of wireless communications devices from vehicles. National highway traffic safety administration 2005. Available at: http://www.nhtsa.dot.gov/staticfiles/DOT/NHTSA/NRD/Multimedia/PDFs/Crash%20Avoidance/Driver%20Distraction/Wireless_Device_Biblio2k5.pdf. Accessed September 20, 2009.
40. Anderson J. Neurology study: brain too slow for cell phone use while driving. Ergonomics Today 2007. Available at: http://www.ergoweb.com/news/detail.cfm?id=1694. Accessed September 20, 2009.
41. Richtel M. U.S. withheld data on risks of distracted driving. New York Times Online 2009. Available at: http://www.nytimes.com/2009/07/21/technology/21distracted.html. Accessed September 20, 2009.
42. Ishigami Y, Klein RM. Is a hands-free phone safer than a handheld phone? J Safety Res 2009;40(2):157–64.
43. Hafner K. Texting may be taking a toll. New York Times Online 2009. Available at: http://www.nytimes.com/2009/05/26/health/26teen.html. Accessed September 20, 2009.
44. Carbonell X, Guardiola E, Beranuy M, et al. A bibliometric analysis of the scientific literature on Internet, video games, and cell phone addiction. J Med Libr Assoc 2009;97(2):102–7.

45. Brady RR, Verran J, Damani NN, et al. Review of mobile communication devices as potential reservoirs of nosocomial pathogens. J Hosp Infect 2009;71(4): 295–300.
46. Ferreri F, Curcio G, Pasqualetti P, et al. Mobile phone emissions and human brain excitability. Ann Neurol 2006;60(2):188–96.
47. Acar GO, Yener HM, Savrun FK, et al. Thermal effects of mobile phones on facial nerves and surrounding soft tissue. Laryngoscope 2009;119(3):559–62.
48. Kumar A, Mathew K, Alexander SA, et al. Output sound pressure levels of personal music systems and their effect on hearing. Noise Health 2009;11(44): 132–40.
49. Makker K, Varghese A, Desai NR, et al. Cell phones: modern man's nemesis? Reprod Biomed Online 2009;18(1):148–57.
50. Attalla EM, Lotayef MM, Khalil EM, et al. Overdose problem associated with treatment planning software for high energy photons in response of Panama's accident. J Egypt Natl Canc Inst 2007;19(2):114–20.
51. van Lieshout EJ, van der Veer SN, Hensbroek R, et al. Interference by new-generation mobile phones on critical care medical equipment. Crit Care 2007;11(5): R98.
52. Tri JL, Severson RP, Hyberger LK, et al. Use of cellular telephones in the hospital environment. Mayo Clin Proc 2007;82(3):282–5.
53. Helmreich D, Doriot P. CFI Group Smartphone Satisfaction Study 2009. CFI Group 2009. Available at: http://www.cfigroup.com/resources/whitepapers_register.asp?wp=41. Accessed October 25, 2009.
54. Halamka JD. The iPhone is what I want, the Blackberry is what I need. Life as a Healthcare CIO 2008. Available at: http://geekdoctor.blogspot.com/2008/08/iphone-is-what-i-want-blackberry-is.html. Accessed September 20, 2009.
55. Elmer-DeWitt P. Six out of 10 doctors prefer iPhones. CNNMoney.com 2009. Available at: http://brainstormtech.blogs.fortune.cnn.com/2009/08/04/six-out-of-10-doctors-prefer-iphones/. Accessed September 20, 2009.
56. Tharp T. Are iPhones or Blackberrys better for doctors and medical students? KevinMD.com 2009. Available at: http://www.kevinmd.com/blog/2009/09/iphones-blackberrys-doctors-medical-students.html. Accessed October 25, 2009.
57. Nadel B. Mobile tech 2010: trends to change our lives. InfoWorld 2009. Available at: http://www.infoworld.com/d/networking/mobile-tech-2010-trends-change-our-lives-691. Accessed September 20, 2009.
58. Rabinowitz E. When will healthcare go mobile? MDNG Neurology 2009;11(5): 16–8.

# Health Information Technology and Electronic Health Records in Neurologic Practice

Gregory J. Esper, MD, MBA[a],*, Oksana Drogan, MS[b],
William S. Henderson, MA[c], Amanda Becker, BA[b],
Orly Avitzur, MD, MBA[d], Daniel B. Hier, MD, MBA[e]

**KEYWORDS**

- Health information technology • Electronic health records
- Electronic medical records

Health information technology (HIT) reform is currently at the forefront of national health-care initiatives. Consensus opinion suggests that HIT and electronic health records (EHR) will improve the safety, quality, and efficiency of health care while supporting health-care delivery and facilitating the management of chronic conditions. However, despite prior endorsement of HIT by the Institute of Medicine,[1] the American Academy of Family Physicians,[2] and most recently President Barack Obama,[3] HIT implementation and use in the United States by physicians in general has been slow, with estimates ranging between 13% and 24%.[4–6] A recent study cited a figure as low as 4% as the actual adoption rate for fully functional EHR products, and adoption rates by non-primary care specialties have been reported to lag behind use by primary care specialties.[4]

Previously reported barriers to EHR implementation include reluctance to invest the money to purchase an EHR, lack of adequate funding and support by medical staff to

Funding support: The American Academy of Neurology Professional Association sponsored this study.

[a] Department of Neurology, Emory University School of Medicine, 1365 Clifton Road NE, Clinic A, Office 3445, Atlanta, GA 30322, USA

[b] American Academy of Neurology Professional Association, 1080 Montreal Avenue, St Paul, MN 55116, USA

[c] Upstate Neurology Consultants, Atrium Drive, Suite 200, Albany, NY 12205, USA

[d] Private Practice Neurology, 55 South Broadway, Tarrytown, NY 10591, USA

[e] Neuroscience Center University of Illinois at Chicago, 1801 West Taylor Street, 4F, Chicago, IL 60612, USA

* Corresponding author.

*E-mail address:* gesper@emory.edu (G.J. Esper).

Neurol Clin 28 (2010) 411–427

doi:10.1016/j.ncl.2009.11.014

neurologic.theclinics.com

implement EHR tools, inability to find an EHR product or components at an affordable cost, and doubts about return on investment. Additional obstacles for providers include lack of sophistication in evaluating EHR systems, poor interoperability amongst different technologies, lack of interoperability between systems, and the challenge of migrating from paper records to EHRs.[4,7,8] Physicians in smaller practices appear less likely to use EHRs than those in larger groups who are better able to realize economies of scale and who can justify a greater expense to provide care.[4,9]

Realizing the benefits and barriers to EHR implementation, the fact that governmental legislation will mandate the use of HIT in the future,[10–12] and the developing pay-for-performance guidelines established by the Centers for Medicare and Medicaid Services (CMS) that are heavily weighted toward use of HIT in general, physicians are becoming increasingly interested in efficient and effective ways to purchase, implement, and use to the fullest capability different HIT including EHRs. This article will define the various technologies that can be used for health care while focusing heavily on EHRs, governmental regulations, EHR functionality, implementation of EHRs in practices, and finances of EHRs, including cost/benefit analysis. Additionally, the authors will present survey data from the American Academy of Neurology Professional Association (the Academy) that highlights United States neurologists' experience with electronic health records.

## ELECTRONIC HEALTH RECORDS

An electronic health record is a computer-based program for documenting patient care.[13] The Institute of Medicine's EHR definition is

- The longitudinal collection of electronic health information for and about persons, where health information is defined as information pertaining to the health of an individual or health care provided to an individual
- The immediate electronic access to person- and population-level information by authorized, and only authorized, users
- The provision of knowledge and decision support that enhance the quality, safety, and efficiency of patient care
- The support of efficient processes for health-care delivery. Critical building blocks of an EHR system are the EHRs maintained by providers (eg, hospitals, nursing homes, ambulatory settings) and by individuals (ie, personal health records).

EHR core functionalities are the storage of health information and data; management of test results of all types; order entry and order management; evidence-based clinical decision support; electronic communication and connectivity; patient support; administrative processes, such as billing and coding; reporting clinical outcomes; and population health management.[14] Therefore, EHRs are intended to automate and streamline the clinician's workflow, make patient records increasingly available to health care providers, reduce medical errors, increase quality and safety of physician-patient interactions, reduce administrative burdens, and provide patients with access to their own health-care reports.

## ESTABLISHING THE FUNCTIONAL REQUIREMENTS OF AN ELECTRONIC HEALTH RECORD

As part of the selection process of an EHR, physicians and practices need to give careful consideration to functional requirements and may wish to list them so that prospective vendors can indicate presence or absence of such functionalities in their product.[15] EHRs differ considerably by look and feel. Practices will want to spend extensive time evaluating each product being considered for purchase to be sure that they like the method of data entry and ease of use. Although functionality is paramount, the EHR must be easily navigated to facilitate efficiency during patient visits.

Documentation of care is one of the most important features of an EHR. To facilitate use of the EHR, it is recommended that a computer be situated in each examination room. High-performing physicians prefer to document their care in real time while talking to patients. This documentation requires the physician to be at a computer while interviewing patients. If stationary, the computer often sits on a table in front of the physician, and patients face the physician alongside the table. The physician may need to regularly shift eye contact from the computer screen to the patients.[16] Some physicians like to tilt the screen slightly so that patients can follow along with the physician as the physician documents care. Similar adjustments need to be made if using a portable tablet personal computer. This adjustment helps to involve patients in the process by making patients active participants in care documentation. Documentation options include (1) writing notes and scanning them into the medical record; (2) dictating the note traditionally and scanning it into the record; (3) typing directly; (4) dictating using voice-recognition software, into either a word processing document that can be uploaded to the EHR or into EHR-based documentation templates that the vendor has created for the user; and (5) using point-click technology that allows data field entry that is searchable within the EHR database.[17] Documentation of patient care using EHR-only features is time consuming and slower than dictating. Most physicians benefit from using a combination of methods of entry in various parts of the charting process. Physicians adopting an EHR will need to think carefully about how they will document their care, primarily because it alters their workflow. Practices that rely upon traditional dictation will see little if any return on investment from an EHR.

Communications are essential to the efficient operation of a physician's office. The EHR functionality should support the ability of the physician to communicate with office staff, for office staff to communicate with each other, for physicians to communicate with outside physicians, and for the practice staff to communicate easily with patients. This communication may take place by letter, secure email, or secure fax.

All EHRs satisfying meaningful-use criteria must have the capability to electronically prescribe. Electronic prescribing should include decision support integrated with a medication list for reconciliation during patient visits. Electronic prescribing will form the basis for incentive payments to physicians groups for adoption of HIT. Electronic prescribing should allow two-way communication with pharmacies electronically through the Surescripts network. Surescripts certifies software used by prescribers, pharmacies, and payers/pharmacy benefit managers for access to the three core services: prescription benefit, history, and routing.

The EHR should allow an easy way to update allergies, medications, surgeries, and problem lists. These lists should be easily viewable throughout patient encounters and incorporable into patients' notes through a simple keystroke or macro function.

Decision support will become increasingly important as quality improvement initiatives grow. Decision support will prompt the physician to comply with evidence-based medicine guidelines, and it will identify potential opportunities to improve the care of patients. Examples include reminders ensuring that patients with a diagnosis of atrial fibrillation are taking Coumadin, that diabetic patients have had a recent hemoglobin A1C measurement, or that patients who have Alzheimer's dementia have a living will or power of attorney. The EHR vendor should also ensure that the evidence-based decision-support features are updated regularly.

Although EHRs have coding functionality, claims should still be vetted appropriately; most EHRs do not yet have the ability to send transactions by way of electronic data interfaces, so billing often needs to be done through another electronic program. As such, the EHR should be easily integrated with a practice management program that does the practice billing. International Classification of Disease (ICD)-9 and ICD-10 codes, Current Procedural Terminology (CPT) codes, CPT-II codes for the Physician Quality Reporting Initiative, and demographic information need to be shared between the EHR and the practice management program. Quality reporting capabilities are part of the meaningful-use criteria for incentive payments to physicians for use of health information technology, and the EHR should be able to readily generate needed reports documenting physician involvement in quality initiatives.

EHRs must have the capability to generate reports critical to practice management based on patient data; these reports can be integrated with reports from existing practice management software including already generated billing reports. For example, a practice may wish to extract data on finances, demographics, prescribing practices of its physicians, or frequency of a certain diagnosis. Report generation will be necessary to meet requirements for quality reporting initiatives.

A capable EHR should be able to interface with other health information technology. Such technologies could be procedural (eg, vital-signs apparatus, electroencephalography or electromyography systems, radiology viewing systems, and so forth); separate scheduling or practice management systems; or laboratory systems housing patient data that is repopulated into the electronic health record. Ultimately, EHR vendors will have to ensure system interfaces with personal health records such as Google Health or Microsoft HealthVault, among others.

The EHR should be able to interface with or provide a secure patient portal where patients can register for visits, update their medical records, communicate with their physicians, check laboratory results, and get appointments.

The EHR should have the capability to generate suitable materials for patient education, and these materials should be easily convertible into electronic or paper documents to be disseminated to patients.

## CERTIFICATION

Voluntary certification of EHRs is currently available through the Certification Commission for Health Information Technology (CCHIT), an independent nonprofit organization that certifies EHRs and other health information technologies as meeting certain minimum requirements in three areas: functionality, interconnectivity, and privacy. With a 3-year grant from the US Department of Health and Human Services,[18] CCHIT is currently the only federally recognized body that certifies ambulatory, inpatient, emergency room, and enterprise electronic health records; however, this may change in the near future if mandated by the Office of the National Coordinator for Health Information Technology (ONCHIT).

## ADOPTION AND IMPLEMENTATION OF ELECTRONIC HEALTH RECORDS

Because the cost of EHRs is considered to be one of the greatest roadblocks to implementation, the United States Government plans to invest $19 billion for HIT through the Health Information and Technology for Economic and Clinical Health (HITECH) Act, a part of the American Recovery and Reinvestment Act of 2009. This new law provides a financial incentive of up to $44,000 per physician under Medicare for meaningful-use of a certified electronic health record starting in 2011. Physicians reimbursed under Medicaid may receive up to $63,500. The precise cost of an EHR is difficult to judge. The total cost of ownership for a typical EHR is between $25,000 and $45,000 per physician, spread over a 3-year period.[16] This cost is divided between initial software-acquisition costs, implementation costs, training costs, interface costs, workstation costs, networking costs, server costs, and software updates and maintenance (**Table 1**).

A workgroup commissioned by ONCHIT presented initial criteria for meaningful-use on June 16, 2009.[19] However, these criteria are likely to change. The most up-to-date information on the incentive program and definitions for meaningful use can be found on the Web site of ONCHIT at http://healthit.hhs.gov/portal/server.pt. For more information, there is a specific tab on the ONCHIT Web site labeled "HEALTHIT/ RECOVERY" that has detailed information on the HITECH Act and the definition of meaningful use. Several of the initial objectives called for in 2011 are listed in **Box 1**.

Because participation in these core quality-improvement initiatives will likely be mandatory to receive the full payment for services under the CMS physician fee schedules, the ability to data mine and prove that core measures were fulfilled will likely require an electronic health record.

Although studies have shown that electronic health records, if implemented correctly, can decrease the opportunity for error, increase efficiency, and improve the quality of health care, extensive preparation for implementation is absolutely necessary. It is also imperative to consider return on investment when purchasing an EHR by understanding the present costs of delivering care, selecting the right system for the needs of the practice, preparing the group for the change to the new way of performing work, and defining group commitment to the entire process.[20]

Patient flow is supported by practice work processes, and for each one, the practice will want to assess how health information technology could be improved. Legacy scheduling systems may not interface with the new EHR, and scheduling operations may need to change. The practice manager should devise how patients will be scheduled, whether the old or new electronic scheduling system should be used, and what changes are necessary if used together. Automated reminders are beneficial, and the scheduling system should be integrated with an automated telephone reminding service such as Televox.

Some EHRs have the capacity to track room use and patient flow from waiting room to examination room to check out. They may also generate reports on time spent

**Table 1**
**Estimated expenses for implementation of electronic health records for a single-physician practice**

| Expense | Year 1 ($) | Year 2 ($) | Year 3 ($) | Total ($) |
|---|---|---|---|---|
| Software acquisition | 25,000 | — | — | 25,000 |
| Training costs | 1,000 | — | — | 1,000 |
| Implementation costs including lost productivity | 2,000 | — | — | 2,000 |
| Interfaces | 1,000 | — | — | 1,000 |
| Computers | 1,000 | — | — | 1,000 |
| Servers | 4,000 | — | — | 4,000 |
| Printers | 1,000 | — | — | 1,000 |
| Software maintenance | — | 2,500 | 2,500 | 5,000 |
| Total | 35,000 | 2,500 | 2,500 | 40,000 |

> **Box 1**
> **Initial guidelines for meaningful-use as put forth by the Office of the National Coordinator for Health Information Technology**
>
> - HIT should allow patients to access clinical information
> - HIT should comply with federal and state privacy standards
> - HIT must document patient progress and provide clinical summaries
> - HIT must provide for exchange of health information between providers
> - HIT must implement drug-interaction safeguards
> - HIT should send patients reminders about follow-up and preventive care
> - HIT should be able to submit immunization and laboratory data to relevant public health registries
> - HIT should support electronic prescribing

waiting and time spent with the physician that are useful in improving practice efficiency in a timely manner. Similarly, the practices of handling patient calls, prescription refills, and intra-office communication will be altered.

Implementation of an EHR is a complex process.[21,22] Its success depends upon a carefully executed plan, one that includes establishing a vision for how the organization will perform when the EHR is fully operational while simultaneously setting quantifiable goals.[23] Practice leaders who adhere to timelines, who are organized and detail oriented, and who are good communicators are needed to help the group set a management process that includes rules of participation and a mechanism for decision making. The leader has to be sure that key stakeholders are involved and that their input is heard. Physicians and staff must be prepared for the arrival of the EHR, and the implementation plan should be discussed before its initial use. Preparations, such as examination room technology readiness, must be addressed before the go-live date. A staged implementation of the EHR should be planned (ie, which functionalities will be used first and which can be added later). The full functionality of an EHR does not need to be realized within the first months or even year of operation. The practice will want a detailed implementation plan that sets forth milestones for vendor selection, contracting, delivery, setup, training, testing, and go-live date.

Vendor selection is a difficult task, and most practices will want to begin with a list of CCHIT-certified ambulatory EHRs. Other practices may wish to obtain help from a consultant in selecting an EHR, and independent evaluations are often helpful. The Academy maintains an entire section of the Web site devoted to the adoption of EHRs by neurologists (http://www.aan.com/go/practice/electronic). The Academy has produced annual reports on EHRs and health information technology since 2006 that document extensive assessments of multiple EHR products.

Purchase of an EHR begins with a request for proposal sent to multiple vendors. This request will allow the practice to compare the cost and features of several different EHRs before making a purchase. At the time of purchase, practices will want to carefully review the final contract which should delineate costs, features, support, training, and performance.[24] It should also delineate any penalties for failure of the EHR to meet agreed upon deadlines or performance measures. In addition, the contract needs to guarantee that patient data will be accessible to the practice even if the practice stops using the EHR.

Extensive training and frequent updates are the rule for ongoing use of the EHR. Practices need to have a plan to train their staff and physicians on use of the new EHR.[26] Before going live with the new EHR, make sure that it is tested extensively, and only after careful planning, training, and testing will the practice be ready. Many practices have found it useful to reduce their patient loads during the first days or weeks after going live with a new EHR. After going live, a period of reassessment is necessary. Ensure that enough technological equipment (eg, computers and printers) is present. Define whether the EHR is working as planned and whether more training is needed. Bring staff and physicians together to discuss problems and propose solutions.

## BENEFITS OF ADOPTING ELECTRONIC HEALTH RECORDS

In addition to adoption incentive payments under the HITECH Act, practices adopting EHRs can expect other financial benefits.[26–28] These financial benefits may include fewer chart pulls with reduced clerical costs, lower transcription costs, decreased malpractice premiums, reduced storage expenses, higher evaluation and management coding, reduced lost charges, and increased office efficiency requiring fewer employees (**Table 2**).

Not all of the benefits of an EHR are strictly financial.[26] Some of the non-financial benefits of EHRs include continuous access to patients' medical records by way of Internet connections, legible records, and compliance with medicolegal requirements (eg, date stamp, time stamp, and electronic signatures). EHRs provide practices an increased credibility with payers and patients, as surveys of the general public have shown widespread support for the adoption of EHRs.[28] EHRs can be the centerpiece of a strategy to do workflow re-engineering, stimulating practices to alter workflow to become leaner and more efficient. However, time-motion studies of practices have not shown changes in cycle time (door-to-door time for patient visits), physician contact time[26] (face-to-face time with the physician), or patient volumes with the implementation of an EHR. Specifically, EHRs have not been shown to cut wait times, increase practice volumes, or shorten physician time with patients.[28] Therefore, more research is needed to definitely show that EHRs accomplish intended benefits.

## NEUROLOGISTS' EXPERIENCE WITH ELECTRONIC HEALTH RECORDS: A SURVEY BY THE ACADEMY

Specific data regarding neurologist use of EHRs is sparse, as the majority of studies performed to date assess EHR use by primary care physicians. The Practice

**Table 2**
**Theoretical return on investment for electronic health records (without federal incentive payments)**

| Item | Base Amount ($) | Savings Rate (%) | Net Savings ($) |
| --- | --- | --- | --- |
| Transcription | 6,000 | 90 | 5,400 |
| Chart creation | 3,000 | 90 | 2,700 |
| Chart pulls | 6,000 | 90 | 5,400 |
| Rent for record storage | 4,000 | 90 | 3,600 |
| Reduction in lost charges | 4,000 | 2 | 8,000 |
| Reduction in billing Errors | 10,000 | 80 | 8,000 |
| Total | — | — | 33,100 |

Management and Technology Subcommittee (PMT) of the Academy embarked on a United States survey-based study designed to: (1) assess how many neurologists are using EHRs, (2) compare usage rate by practice setting, (3) determine what specific factors aid or limit neurologists in EHR implementation, (4) identify which EHR vendors were most used by neurologists and what costs were associated with implementation, and (5) understand how the Academy can further assist neurologists in selecting appropriate ambulatory EHR office solutions.

## Methods

The survey was sent to a random sample of 1200 Academy members. Selected participants received several reminders to complete the survey and could return it by faxing, mailing, or submitting responses online. Data collection lasted from January 31 until March 31, 2008.

## Response Rate

Forty-nine percent (585/1200) of neurologists responded to the survey. The margin of error for all respondents at a 95% confidence level was ± 3.8%. To check for non-response bias, the authors compared demographic profiles of respondents versus non-respondents (**Table 3**). There were no significant differences in gender or age distributions. However, significant differences were found between survey respondents and non-respondents in membership types. Slightly more neurologists who are more advanced in their professional careers (membership types Active and Fellow) answered the survey. Also, slightly fewer non-board certified neurologists (Associate type) and practice managers (Affiliate type) returned the survey.

## Reported Electronic Health Records Usage

Forty-seven percent of neurologists in the United States reported usage of an EHR. The majority of users in academic and private groups had been using EHRs for greater

**Table 3**
**Demographic characteristics of survey respondents and non-respondents**

| Demographic Characteristics | | Survey Respondents (N = 585) | Survey Non-respondents (N = 615) | p value |
|---|---|---|---|---|
| Age[a] (mean) | | 49.8. years (SD = 9.1) | 49.0 years (SD = 9.3) | 0.14 |
| Gender[b] (%) | Male | 70.5 | 70.2 | 0.91 |
| | Female | 29.5 | 29.8 | — |
| Academy membership type[c] (%) | Fellow | 13.3 | 7 | <0.001 |
| | Active | 67.7 | 64.2 | — |
| | Associate | 12.6 | 17.6 | — |
| | Affiliate | 6.8 | 11.2 | — |

[a] Data missing for nine members (1.5%) in the respondent sample and 20 members (3.3%) in the non-respondent sample.
[b] Data missing for two members (0.3%) in the respondent sample and four members (0.7%) in the non-respondent sample.
[c] Academy membership types descriptions: Fellow means certified in neurology, has been a member for at least 7 years and has demonstrated special achievement in the neurosciences; Active means trained and certified in neurology; Associate means fully trained in neurology but not yet certified; Affiliate means non-neurologist (business administrators in this survey's sample).

than 1 year at the time of the survey. Ambulatory academic practices far exceeded EHR use compared with ambulatory private practices (78% vs 37%). Furthermore, 34% of those in academic practices acknowledged having used an EHR for more than 5 years compared with 26% of those in private practice. Small private practices (with one to five neurologists) reported usage rates at 16%, consistent with national averages.

Neurologists' reasons for not using EHRs are reported in **Fig. 1** and varied depending on their practice settings. When asked to identify their top three reasons for not using EHR, private practice neurologists cited cost, doubts regarding return on investment, and lack of knowledge about which system to buy. Academic neurologists' top three reasons for not using EHR were "other," lack of knowledge about which system to buy, and concerns about the new EHR system slowing them down. Despite these concerns, 74% of academic practices and 51% of private practices currently not using an EHR will consider installing one within 3 years.

### Predicting Electronic Health Records Usage

The following demographic variables were used as covariates in a univariate logistic regression model to predict the use of EHRs: type of practice setting, person making information technology (IT) purchasing decisions for the practice, percentage of time spent in ambulatory clinical practice, age, and gender. All covariates, except for age, were categorical. A total of 505 cases were included in the model. The overall model was significant in predicting EHR use ($P<.001$) and its predictive accuracy was 76.2%, which was a substantial improvement over the 50.9% prediction rate of the baseline model without the predictor variables. **Table 4** shows all variables used in the equation. Two variables, type of practice and age, were significant in predicting EHR use. Compared to neurologists working in solo practice settings, the odds of using EHR increased if neurologists were employed in single-specialty groups with 5 to 10 neurologists, multispecialty groups, university groups, staff-model health maintenance organizations (HMO), government hospitals, or other public and private clinic settings. In addition, being older decreased one's odds of using EHR, with each additional year of age decreasing the odds of usage by a factor of 0.97.

### Electronic Health Records Vendors

Forty-six percent of academic practices use three commercially available EHRs from companies including Epic, Allscripts, and Cerner; government practitioners use VistA. Within private practices, the use of products marketed by other companies was more evenly distributed. Smaller private practices favored products from MediNotes, SOAPware, and eClinicalWorks. Thirty-seven percent of users in the academic and private practice groups use other EHRs, including combinations of local- or custom-designed EHRs, academic institution-designed EHRs (eg, Mayo), and other commercially marketed EHR systems.

### Electronic Health Records Cost and Implementation

Only 24% of all neurologists were aware of the cost of EHR implementation. As expected, the knowledge level varied greatly by practice type: 3% of academic neurologists, 45% of private practice neurologists, and 87% of small private groups were able to estimate the cost of full EHR implementation. Slightly less than half of all neurologists who could estimate the cost stated that the cost of implementation was more than $20,000 per provider. In both groups, at least 60% of practitioners stated that overhead costs were either reduced or unchanged.

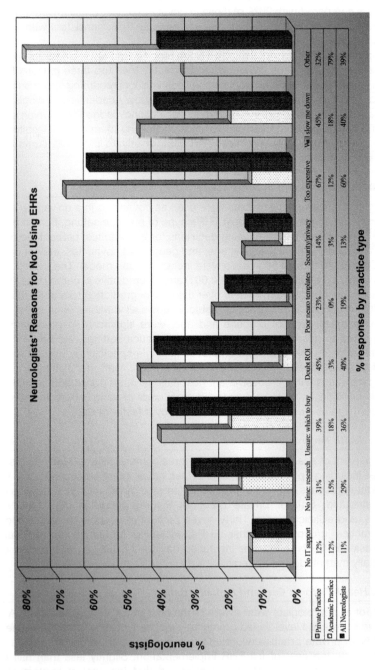

**Fig. 1.** United States neurologists' reasons for not using electronic health records.

**Table 4**
**Variables used in the univariate logistic regression to predict use of electronic health records**

| Variable | β | SE β | p | OR |
|---|---|---|---|---|
| Practice type | | | | |
| Solo practice | — | — | <0.001 | — |
| Single specialty (2–5) | 0.34 | 0.43 | 0.44 | 1.40 (0.6–3.3) |
| Single specialty (6–10) | 1.74 | 0.48 | <0.001 | 5.67 (2.2–14.5) |
| Single specialty (>10) | 1.85 | 0.51 | <0.001 | 6.33 (2.3–17.1) |
| Multispecialty private | 2.89 | 0.41 | <0.001 | 17.94 (8.0–40.1) |
| University based | 2.9 | 0.39 | <0.001 | 18.22 (8.4–39.3) |
| Staff-model HMO | 3.04 | 0.87 | <0.001 | 20.86 (3.8–114.0) |
| Government hospital/clinic | 4.1 | 0.81 | <0.001 | 59.71 (12.1–294.4) |
| Other public or private | 2.67 | 0.51 | <0.001 | 14.39 (5.3–39.2) |
| No clinical practice | 1.32 | 1.31 | 0.32 | 3.73 (0.3–48.6) |
| Person making IT decisions | | | | |
| Office manager | — | — | 0.1 | — |
| Senior partner | 1.11 | 0.64 | 0.08 | 3.04 (0.9–10.7) |
| All physicians | 0.17 | 0.53 | 0.75 | 1.19 (0.4–3.4) |
| Office manager and physicians | 0.33 | 0.46 | 0.48 | 1.38 (0.6–3.4) |
| Other | 0.84 | 0.45 | 0.06 | 2.31 (1.0–5.5) |
| Time in clinical practice <10% | — | — | 0.22 | — |
| 10%–30% | 0.2 | 0.65 | 0.75 | 1.22 (0.3–4.3) |
| 31%–60% | 0.01 | 0.59 | 0.98 | 1.01 (0.3–3.2) |
| 61%–90% | 0.75 | 0.59 | 1.63 | 0.20 (0.7–6.6) |
| >90% | 0.4 | 0.59 | 0.49 | 1.50 (0.5–4.7) |
| Age | −0.03 | 0.01 | 0.01 | 0.97 (0.9–0.99) |
| Gender: male | 0.18 | 0.95 | 0.2 | 0.29 (0.73–2.0) |

*Abbreviations:* β, beta weight; HMO, health maintenance organization; OR, odds ratio with 95% confidence interval; SE, standard error.

When asked whether there was a decrease in their practices' productivity over the first 6 months that could be directly attributed to implementing EHR, 45% of all neurologists answered in the affirmative. In the first six months of EHR usage, approximately two thirds of all neurologists reported spending one or more additional hours each day on work activities.

### Electronic Health Records Functional Use

Percent of neurologists using various functions typically found in EHRs is shown in **Table 5**. By far, the most common feature used within EHRs was clinical documentation. Academic neurologists and private-practice neurologists were similar in their use of laboratory-result functions, medication prescription generation, medication lists, and other features. Academicians did use EHRs for imaging results 82% of the time, compared with 68% of private-practice neurologists. Safety features, such as drug formulary compliance, drug-drug interaction checks, education materials for patients, Health Insurance Portability and Accountability Act (HIPAA) protected intra-office communication through the EHR, and decision-support capability (evidence-based medicine confirmation of practice decision) all appeared to be

**Table 5**
**Percent of neurologists using various functions of electronic health records[a]**

| Function | Private Practice (%) | Academic Practice (%) |
|---|---|---|
| Allergy checks | 57 | 57 |
| Clinical note documentation | 93 | 94 |
| Decision support capability | 17 | 17 |
| Diagnoses | 61 | 56 |
| Drug-drug interaction checks | 45 | 42 |
| Drug formulary compliance | 20 | 25 |
| Education materials (eg, prescription handout) | 32 | 24 |
| Imaging results | 68 | 82 |
| Intra-office HIPAA protected communication about patients | 49 | 44 |
| Lab results | 85 | 94 |
| Medication lists | 85 | 82 |
| Medication prescription generation | 67 | 65 |
| Patient scheduling | 77 | 62 |
| Preventive service reminders and physician quality reporting initiative | 18 | 14 |
| Problem lists | 58 | 57 |
| Other | 14 | 5 |

[a] Participants could choose as many responses as applicable.

used by less than half of neurologists. Few practitioners (<20%) had begun physician-quality reporting initiative documentation at the time of the survey.

### Electronic Health Records Satisfaction and Impact on Care and Reimbursement

Overall, of neurologists who have already implemented EHRs into their practice, 69% of academic neurologists and 80% of private-practice neurologists were somewhat or very satisfied that they had done so. The majority of neurologists reported that EHR improved quality of care (69%) and patient safety (68%) within their practices. Almost all physicians (90%) indicated that the EHR improved access to relevant information within patients' medical records.

Academic and private groups differed on the question of whether EHR use improved reimbursement; 36% of private neurologists compared with 20% of academic neurologists agreed that EHR use increased reimbursement. However, at least half of respondents in each group neither agreed nor disagreed with the statement about impact on reimbursement.

### Academy Role in Assisting with Electronic Health Records Adoption

When asked how neurologists would prefer to receive updates about EHR from the Academy, the top three choices were (1) through the Academy Web site (48%), (2) through printed news (48%), and (3) through annual meeting courses (30%). The top three needed types of data were information about the most reliable or popular systems (62%), tools to maximize EHR functionality (57%), and information on reduced costs by way of vendor alliances with the Academy (41%).

## SURVEY CONCLUSIONS
### *Usage Rate of Electronic Health Records*

This survey demonstrates that EHR adoption by United States' neurologists, with the exception of small groups, exceeds the previously reported national averages for primary and specialty care.[4–6,9,29–33] This finding is unexpected, as the authors had suspected that usage rates for neurologists would be similar to those defined for other specialties by prior studies. Study methodology conforms to recently published criteria of high-quality EHR usage studies by Jha and colleagues,[6] and this survey addresses their recommendations for future measurement of HIT usage by conforming to American Association for Public Opinion Research standards and by clearly defining EHR use in the survey instrument. Survey respondents were also representative of United States neurologist demographics based on group size and location of practice.

Identification of such a high EHR usage rate was aided by the study's response rate, which was comparable to that of some studies[4,30,31,33–35] and greater than obtained in others.[5,9,29,36] Most of these studies that assessed specialists' usage of EHRs derived lower usage rates, but none of those studies directly focused on neurologists. In comparison with a similarly conducted survey by the American Academy of Ophthalmology of its members, response rate using Internet-based and telephone-based questionnaires was 15.6%, and EHR usage rate was approximately 18%.[29]

The study conforms to the findings of multiple prior surveys that document greater use of HIT in larger practices. In the authors' study, odds ratios for using EHRs were high for large organizations including multispecialty private practices, university settings, staff-model HMOs, and government hospitals/clinics. Though the driving factor for HIT implementation in these large organizations is economies of scale, the authors were not surprised to see age as a significant indicator of HIT usage, as younger neurologists are more likely not only to be more computer proficient but also to have had greater exposure to computer use in health care during their training.

### *Survey Limitations*

The statistically significant difference in survey responders compared with non-responders may have had an effect on the usage-rate measurement. Because respondents tended to be more advanced in their professional careers and also tended to be board-certified, this could have skewed the usage rate upward, as these neurologists may have had more time to establish practices and thus evaluate and implement EHRs in the office setting. The total effect, however, could not be measured by this study.

### *Use of Electronic Health Records Safety Functionalities*

Despite the high EHR usage rate, neurologists underutilized most safety features that EHRs possess including drug-drug interaction checks, drug formulary compliance, and decision-support capability. This underutilization may be caused by early rollout of EHRs before safety features were comprehensively included or updated. Alternatively, lack of familiarity with all functions of an EHR because of inexperience with a system may have contributed to these results; this would not be functionally different than a user employing a basic EHR rather than a fully functional EHR.

If safety features are to be effectively used, office-visit workflow may need to be re-engineered, and products must be easier to use. Safety functionalities, such as medication reconciliation and drug-drug interactions, are difficult to achieve without HIT. Other features, such as laboratory monitoring, have important implications for use in neurologic conditions including stroke, epilepsy, neuromuscular disorders, multiple sclerosis, and autoimmune disease. As evidence-based decision-support tools are incorporated into EHRs, they will theoretically assist physicians in patient-specific or diagnosis-based medical decision making. However, this has been difficult to prove based on the results of two recent studies.[30,37]

### Barriers to Usage

EHR usage barriers encountered in this study were similar to those cited in prior studies, but principally for private-practice neurologists, who mainly cited high cost and dubious return on investment.[36] The majority of neurologists surveyed who stated that they knew the costs of implementation estimated an expense under $20,000. Recent data from the Medical Group Management Association documents that EHR capital cost per full-time equivalent physician is greater than $15,000 75% of the time, EHR operating cost is higher than $250 per month over 50% of the time, and over $1000 per month almost 20% of the time.[38] To further facilitate EHR adoption, however, all stakeholders should consider providing financial incentives for adoption, payment for use of an EHR, and protection of physicians from liability for record tampering by external parties.[4] Neurologists expecting to implement EHR systems in the coming years should keep in mind the tangible and intangible returns on investment.[20] Detailed cost data for the systems inquired about in this survey were not available, as prices varied according to factors including, but not limited to, number of physicians in a practice, number of sites of implementation, geographic area, time to installation, and EHR functions desired.

Neither productivity gains nor reductions were definitively demonstrated in the study. This survey did not take into account whether provider schedules were adjusted during the period of implementation. Also, the authors do not know if practitioners who spent more than 1 hour in excess of traditional work time did so with the same schedule or an adjusted workflow. Ultimately, given the recent CMS initiatives addressing pay for performance, the continual threat of government-enacted cuts in physician reimbursement, and the new mandates for HIT within practices by 2016 according to the American Recovery and Reinvestment Act, productivity and reimbursement will likely be contingent on efficient HIT implementation.

### Educational Initiatives

The PMT undertook this survey to develop a baseline against which progress in HIT adoption by neurologists could be measured. Better performing practices have been shown to use EHRs; this correlation bodes well for those neurologists who have implemented EHRs and for those who are considering doing so.[39] The purchase and implementation of an EHR system is a significant initial expense for a practice and carries with it ongoing financial and regulatory implications. Neurologists and all other physicians will face increasing pressure to use HIT to be reimbursed for their services and to comply with governmental, payer, and legal policies. According to these survey results, all specialty medical societies should consider developing educational materials in multiple forms of media, including podcasts and print news, to assist their members in this decision process. Dissemination of information by way of society Web sites should also be considered so that these societies can better support their members in the selection and implementation of an EHR system.

## FUTURE TRENDS IN ELECTRONIC HEALTH RECORDS

The Office of the National Coordinator for Health Information Technology is committed to establishing an electronic health network, to be known as the Nationwide Health Information Network, that will allow health information to be exchanged between providers and hospitals throughout the country; the goal would be to facilitate integration, interoperability, and connectivity among all electronic systems.[40] Future EHRs will be configured to exchange information with personal health records so that patients will be able to download information from EHRs or upload information to EHRs, thereby facilitating access by providers to updated, medically relevant information. The Continuity of Care Document and the Continuity of Care Record are two standards for summarizing health information in an EHR and allowing exchange of information between two EHRs. These documents are likely to aid substantially in supporting data interchange in the coming years. Furthermore, EHRs of the future are expected to play an increasing role in bio-surveillance, including the detection of new pandemics or bioterrorism attacks.[41]

## SUMMARY

The tipping point for EHRs has been reached and universal adoption in the United States is now inevitable. Neurologists will want to choose their electronic health record prudently. Careful selection, contracting, planning, and training are essential to successful implementation. Neurologists need to examine their workflow carefully and make adjustments to ensure that efficiency is increased. Neurologists will want to achieve a significant return on investment and qualify for all applicable financial incentives from payers, including CMS. EHRs are not just record-keeping tools but play an important role in quality improvement, evidence-based medicine, pay for performance, patient education, bio-surveillance, data warehousing, and data exchange.

## ACKNOWLEDGMENTS

The authors would like to thank the Practice Management and Technology Subcommittee of the Academy for their assistance in preparation of the survey and comments on the manuscript.

## REFERENCES

1. Institute of Medicine Committee on Quality of Health Care in America. Crossing the quality chasm: a new health system for the 21st century. Washington, DC: National Academy Press; 2001.
2. Martin J, Avant R, Bowman M, et al. The future of family medicine: a collaborative project of the family medicine community. Ann Fam Med 2004;2(Suppl):S3–32.
3. Obama B. Remarks of President Barack Obama: address to Joint Session of Congress. Available at: http://www.whitehouse.gov/the_press_office/remarks-of-president-barack-obama-address-to-joint-session-of-congress/. Accessed August 30, 2009.
4. DesRoches CM, Campbell EG, Rao SR, et al. Electronic health records in ambulatory care – a national survey of physicians. N Engl J Med 2008;359(1): 50–60.
5. Gans D, Kralewski J, Hammons T, et al. Medical groups' adoption of electronic health records and information systems. Health Aff (Millwood) 2005;24(5): 1323–33.

6. Jha AK, Ferris TG, Donelan K, et al. How common are electronic health records in the United States? A summary of the evidence. Health Aff (Millwood) 2006;25(6): w496–507.

7. Kleaveland B. Making it to the EHR promised land. How to solve common EHR adoption problems. MGMA Connex 2008;8(5):42–5.

8. Thakkar M, Davis DC. Risks, barriers, and benefits of EHR systems: a comparative study based on size of hospital. Perspect Health Inf Manag 2006;3:5.

9. Menachemi N, Perkins RM, van Durme DJ, et al. Examining the adoption of electronic health records and personal digital assistants by family physicians in Florida. Inform Prim Care 2006;14(1):1–9.

10. Department of Health and Human Services. 42 CFR Part 411 Centers for Medicare & Medicaid Services (CMS), HHS. Medicare Program; Physicians' referrals to health care entities with which they have financial relationships; exceptions for certain electronic prescribing and electronic health records arrangements; final rule. Fed Regist 2006;71(152):45139–71.

11. Department of Health and Human Services. 42 CFR Part 423 Centers for Medicare & Medicaid Services (CMS), HHS. Medicare program; standards for e-prescribing under Medicare Part D and identification of backward compatible version of adopted standard for e-prescribing and the medicare prescription drug program (version 8.1). Fed Regist 2008;73(67):18917–42.

12. Department of Health and Human Services, Office of the National Coordinator for Health Information Technology. The O.N.C. Coordinated Federal Health I.T. Strategic Plan: 2008–2012, Objective 1.32008, Washington, DC, published on June 3, 2008.

13. National Institutes of Health National Center for Research Resources. Electronic health records overview. McLean (VA): Mitre Corporation; 2006.

14. Committee on Data Standards for Patient Safety, Board on Health Care Services. Key capabilities of an electronic health record system. Washington, DC: National Academy of Sciences; 2003.

15. Adler KG, Edsall RL. Electronic health records: the 2007 FPM user-satisfaction survey. Fam Pract Manag 2007;14(4):27–30.

16. Ventres W, Kooienga S, Vuckovic N, et al. Physicians, patients, and the electronic health record: an ethnographic analysis. Ann Fam Med 2006;4(2): 124–31.

17. Esper GJ. Electronic health record (EHR) documentation options: why do they matter? (as part of course 2AC.005: making sure your electronic health record system is a success). American Academy of Neurology Annual Meeting. Chicago (IL), April 13, 2008.

18. Certification Commission for Health Information Technology. Physician guide to certification for 08 EHRs. Chicago: Certification Commission for Healthcare Information Technology; 2008.

19. Panel offers initial criteria for defining 'Meaningful Use'. Available at: http://www.ihealthbeat.org/Articles/2009/6/16/Panel-Offers-Initial-Criteria-for-Defining-Meaningful-Use.aspx. Accessed August 19, 2009.

20. Aita S. Implementing an E.H.R. with R.O.I. in mind. J Med Pract Manage 2008; 23(4):244–6.

21. Miller RH, Sim I, Newman J. Electronic medical records: lessons from small physician practices. San Francisco: California HealthCare Foundation; 2003.

22. Yoon-Flannery K, Zandieh SO, Kuperman GJ, et al. A qualitative analysis of an electronic health record (EHR) implementation in an academic ambulatory setting. Inform Prim Care 2008;16(4):277–84.

23. Kaufman J. How can I ensure successful implementation of my EHR? (as part of course 2AC.005: making sure your electronic health record system is a success). Seattle (WA): American Academy of Neurology; 2009.

24. Rowden-Racette K. Negotiating deals with tech vendors. Physician practice technology guide. 2009; 24–9.

25. Nelson R. Marathon-like training is a way to prepare for EHR implementation. Mod Med 2009. Available at: http://www.physicianspractice.com/index.cfm?fuseaction=articles.details&articleID=1370. Accessed August 19, 2009.

26. Gottschalk A, Flocke SA. Time spent in face-to-face patient care and work outside the examination room. Ann Fam Med 2005;3(6):488–93.

27. Menachemi N, Brooks RG. Exploring the ROI associated with health IT: a report to the state of Florida. Tallahassee: Florida State University; 2005.

28. Poissant L, Pereira J, Tamblyn R, et al. The impact of electronic health records on time efficiency of physicians and nurses: a systematic review. J Am Med Inform Assoc 2005;12(5):505–16.

29. Chiang MF, Boland MV, Margolis JW, et al. Adoption and perceptions of electronic health record systems by ophthalmologists: an American Academy of Ophthalmology Survey. Ophthalmology 2008;115:1591–7.

30. Linder JA, Ma J, Bates DW, et al. Electronic health record use and the quality of ambulatory care in the United States. Arch Intern Med 2007;167(13):1400–5.

31. Shields AE, Shin P, Leu MG, et al. Adoption of health information technology in community health centers: results of a national survey. Health Aff (Millwood) 2007;26(5):1373–83.

32. Simon JS, Rundall TG, Shortell SM. Adoption of order entry with decision support for chronic care by physician organizations. J Am Med Inform Assoc 2007;14(4):432–9.

33. Simon SR, Kaushal R, Cleary PD, et al. Physicians and electronic health records: a statewide survey. Arch Intern Med 2007;167(5):507–12.

34. Audet AM, Doty MM, Peugh J, et al. Information technologies: when will they make it into physicians' black bags? Med Gen Med 2004;6(4):2.

35. Simon SR, McCarthy ML, Kaushal R, et al. Electronic health records: which practices have them, and how are clinicians using them? J Eval Clin Pract 2008;14(1):43–7.

36. Menachemi N. Barriers to ambulatory EHR: who are 'imminent adopters' and how do they differ from other physicians? Inform Prim Care 2006;14(2):101–8.

37. Zhou L, Soran CS, Jenter CA, et al. The relationship between electronic health record use and quality of care over time. J Am Med Inform Assoc 2009;16:457–64.

38. MGMA. 2007 Digest: what counts in group practice. MGMA Connex 2007;7(3):12–4 16, 18 passim.

39. Shortell SM, Schmittdiel J, Wang MC, et al. An empirical assessment of high-performing medical groups: results from a national study. Med Care Res Rev 2005;62(4):407–34.

40. Nationwide Health Information Network. Available at: http://www.nhinwatch.com/. Accessed September 12, 2009.

41. Greenspan H, Cothren R. Achieving effective bio-surveillance. Available at: http://www.healthmgttech.com. Accessed September 12, 2009.

# Hot Topics in Risk Management in Neurologic Practice

David E. Thiess, JD[a], Justin A. Sattin, MD[b],
Daniel G. Larriviere, MD, JD[c],*

**KEYWORDS**

- Civil law • Informed consent • Patient autonomy
- Physician liability

Physicians practice medicine within a legal environment. Generally speaking, when judging the actions of physicians, the law uses the customs and values of the medical profession as reference points. Nevertheless, caring for patients with neurologic disease requires an understanding of certain aspects of civil law. This is especially true in selected types of interaction between physicians and neurologic patients, including obtaining informed consent, treatment of acute stroke with tissue plasminogen activator (tPA), reporting drivers with dementia, reporting drivers with epilepsy, and assessing the capacity to vote for those with dementia. This article provides a brief survey of these areas. In each instance, the neurologist is encouraged to become familiar with the laws in his or her own state.

## INFORMED CONSENT

The concept of informed consent developed out of courts' respect for the principle of patient autonomy and the right to be free from nonconsensual interference with one's body.[1] The physician's duty to obtain informed consent notably extends beyond the acquisition of a patient's signature on a consent document. Physicians instead meet the terms of informed consent by ensuring that patients receive the appropriate amount of information before agreeing to treatment.

[a] American Health Lawyers Association, 1025 Connecticut Avenue NW, Suite 600, Washington, DC 20036-5405, USA
[b] Department of Neurology, Clinical Science Center H6/546, University of Wisconsin, 600 Highland Avenue, Box 5230, Madison, WI 53792-5230, USA
[c] Department of Neurology, University of Virginia School of Medicine, PO Box 800394, Charlottesville, VA 22908-0394, USA
* Corresponding author. Department of Neurology, University of Virginia School of Medicine, University of Virginia, PO Box 800394, Charlottesville, VA 22908-0394.
E-mail address: dgl6t@virginia.edu (D.G. Larriviere).

Neurol Clin 28 (2010) 429–439
doi:10.1016/j.ncl.2009.11.005
0733-8619/10/$ – see front matter

neurologic.theclinics.com

In the United States, courts have historically used two standards to determine whether a physician has conveyed enough information to the patient for the consent to be informed. Under a physician-based standard, a court will seek to determine the information a similarly-situated physician would usually find necessary to convey to a patient in order for the patient to fully understand the issues in the decision at hand. Courts in other states measure informed consent against a reasonable patient standard by asking what information a similarly situated patient would want to know before treatment.[1]

The physician-based standard resembles the malpractice standard, asking what a similarly situated, reasonable practitioner would do. Under this standard, trial counsel will introduce expert testimony from other physicians (expert witnesses) to demonstrate the amount and kind of information reasonable physicians feel would be necessary before a patient could make a particular medical decision.

In contrast, the reasonable patient standard maintains that a patient's need for disclosure of information material to treatment should take precedence over medical expediency[2] and is a logical extension of the desire to protect patient autonomy. The reasonable patient standard asks physicians to take account of a patient's particular circumstances in assessing the information material to treatment, rather than deferring to standards set by the medical profession.[3] Not surprisingly, courts are moving away from the physician-based standard in favor of the reasonable patient standard.[1] Currently, approximately half of states endorse the reasonable patient standard.[1]

### Elements of Informed Consent

Whereas two standards measure the adequacy of information conveyed for informed consent, courts across jurisdictions consider some types of information essential. In general, physicians should fully communicate the relevant diagnosis with each patient. If an evaluation is required before a diagnosis is rendered, physicians should discuss the tests they recommend, along with their associated risks.[1] Additionally, physicians should always discuss the nature and purpose of the treatment they propose, along with the possible risks and outcomes. Whether physicians must mention a possible outcome varies with its severity and probability of occurrence. That is, while physicians probably do not need to mention a 5% chance of treatable infection, they should certainly warn of a 1% chance of paralysis.[1] Physicians should further fully disclose alternatives to treatment, prognosis if treatment is accepted versus declined, and any existing conflicts of interest. Courts have not typically required physicians to provide their particular success rates with the proposed treatment or procedure, but physicians are required to answer patients truthfully if asked.[1]

### Liability for the Failure to Inform

There are considerable legal ramifications for the failure to provide satisfactory information to a patient before treatment. In addition to malpractice lawsuits brought by the patient, some courts have allowed third parties to bring suit against physicians when a patient has harmed the third party as a result of insufficient information. For example, in *Coombes v Florio*,[4] Dr Florio did not inform his patient, Sacca, that the medications he prescribed might cause drowsiness, dizziness, fainting, or altered consciousness. Sacca therefore did not have reason to refrain from driving. While on medications prescribed by Dr Florio, Sacca drove over a sidewalk, killing Coombes' son and Coombes sued Dr Florio for failing to warn Sacca about driving while on the medications. The Massachusetts Supreme Court allowed Coombes to sue Dr Florio for negligently failing to provide appropriate information to Sacca about driving while taking the prescribed medications. The Court noted that the doctor's duty of reasonable care, owed to a patient, includes the duty to provide appropriate warnings about side effects so a patient may make an informed decision about taking the prescribed medication and what activities to avoid when doing so. The Court then reasoned that because the foreseeable risk of injury is not limited to the patient, affected third parties may bring suit against the physician.[4]

The Coombes decision does not change informed consent requirements for physicians, but does broaden the scope of who might be able to sue the physician for foreseeable injuries that result from a failure to inform a patient about the possible side effects of treatments or medications in the state of Massachusetts. At least two other states with cases on point have reached a similar conclusion.[5,6] It is too soon to say whether other states will adopt the rationale used in Coombes. No matter to whom the duty of informed consent extends, physicians should discuss the risks, benefits, and side effects of recommended treatments with their patients. The physician should provide the patient with adequate time to ask questions and document the discussion in the medical record.

## LIABILITY FOR TPA DECISIONS IN ACUTE STROKE

In light of mixed opinions regarding the risks and benefits of intravenous thrombolysis with recombinant human tPA, many physicians have expressed concern that tPA use or non-use may expose them to legal liability.[7–9] The following presents two important elements of malpractice law that arise in tPA cases, standard of care and causation, and discusses how courts have analyzed those elements to reach a decision on physician liability for tPA decisions.

### Standard of Care and Causation with Respect to tPA

In medical malpractice cases, the injured plaintiff has the burden of proving that the defendant physician's conduct violated the applicable standard of care. The standard of care in medical malpractice cases is generally thought to mean what most similarly situated physicians, practicing in the same specialty or subspecialty, would have done in similar circumstances.[10]

There are two clinical practice guidelines concerning tPA that may be used by expert witnesses to define the standard of care when they testify in malpractice cases. The American Academy of Neurology (AAN) Practice Advisory on Thrombolytic Therapy for Acute Ischemic Stroke[11] and the American Heart Association (AHA) Guidelines for the Early Management of Adults with Ischemic Stroke[12] support the use of intravenous tPA for acute ischemic stroke, with certain inclusion and exclusion criteria. However, the North American Emergency Medicine Physician organizations have issued position statements concluding that tPA should not be considered standard of care,[13] suggesting its use be restricted to medical centers with a specific stroke therapy infrastructure.[14]

If the guidelines can be used as evidence of the applicable standard of care in these cases, it seems reasonable to conclude that a neurologist would be expected to use the drug in the appropriate circumstances and that an emergency medicine physician would not be expected to use the drug—all things being equal. Thus, a plaintiff who is suing an emergency medicine physician for failing to use tPA might have a more difficult time proving that the doctor violated the standard of care than would a plaintiff who was suing a neurologist for the same reason.

This is not to say that a neurologist who does not give tPA to an otherwise qualified patient must be considered to have breached the standard of care. If that neurologist could show that a significant minority of neurologists would not have given tPA in the same or similar circumstances, then his actions may be considered to have met the standard of care. This follows what is known as the respectable minority rule.[15] To prove this case, a neurologist would have to establish that there is reason to doubt the validity of the underlying data supporting the use of intravenous-tPA in acute stroke. This is becoming more difficult in light of a recent randomized, controlled trial confirming the drug's safety and efficacy[16] and population-based studies showing that the drug is as beneficial in community practice as it is in the research setting.[17,18]

The other pivotal element of malpractice claims regarding the administration of tPA is causation. If a jury were to find that a physician breached the standard of care by not offering tPA to the patient or plaintiff, the plaintiff must still prove that the failure to give tPA was the cause of the injuries.

In medical malpractice cases, a plaintiff traditionally demonstrates legal causation by showing that there is a greater than 50% chance that defendant's conduct was a substantial factor in producing the injury in question.[19] However, 20% to 38% of stroke patients will be asymptomatic, or almost so, at 3 months if they receive no treatment.[20] With treatment, 31% to 50% of patients will be asymptomatic, or almost so, at 3 months. Because there is a less than 51% chance of recovery with or without treatment, it would be very difficult in an individual case to say that the defendant's conduct caused the plaintiff's ultimate condition.

However, some jurisdictions do not employ the traditional method of assessing causation that requires a greater than 50% chance the physician substantially contributed to the outcome. Some jurisdictions have allowed a plaintiff to recover for the lost opportunity to achieve a better outcome. Under this loss-of-chance theory of causation, a plaintiff may recover for the reduction in his or her chances of achieving a better outcome, rather than for the outcome itself.[21]

Whether a plaintiff whose chances of a better outcome are slim will be able to recover for the lost opportunity occasioned by a defendant's negligent conduct is dependent in large part (but not exclusively) on whether that case arises in a jurisdiction that follows the traditional causation analysis or if it is brought in a jurisdiction that will allow the plaintiff to present evidence of, and recover for, the lost opportunity. In general, over half the states allow evidence of lost opportunity to be presented, while a smaller minority hews to the traditional causation analysis.[22]

### Analysis of Trials and Appeals

A search of all state and federal court cases involving the use or non-use of tPA for acute ischemic stroke reveals 20 cases at the trial court level and 6 appellate cases that involved malpractice suits for failing to use tPA in stroke. No cases were found in which physicians were sued for injury allegedly caused by giving tPA.

Of the 20 trial court verdicts, 5 were for the plaintiff, 14 were for the defendant, and one case did not reach the verdict stage at the trial level. Three trials involved a neurologist; juries found for the neurologist in all three. Plaintiffs found the most success when they named the hospital as a defendant, with courts finding for the plaintiff in 5 of 12 such cases. State-level trial courts do not typically issue written opinions, meaning that it is difficult to discern how the analysis proceeded in each of the trial verdicts.

One appellate case from Texas, *Young v Memorial Hermann Hospital System*, exemplifies how causation traditionally plays out in tPA cases.[23] In that case, a 37-year-old male suffering from altered mental status was brought to the emergency room at 21:15 hours but was not diagnosed with stroke until 02:30 hours. The plaintiff sued, alleging the failure to timely diagnose his stroke precluded him from receiving tPA and experiencing a better outcome.[1] The court required the plaintiff to show a 51% or greater chance of avoiding injury if tPA were administered in a timely manner.[1] In analyzing the plaintiff's evidence, the federal court noted that the absolute benefit of tPA in the National Institute of Neurological Disorders and Stroke trial was 11% to 13% and that a 1997 subgroup analysis found a 17% benefit of tPA in younger patients with lower National Institutes of Health stroke scale scores (in which group plaintiff would have been included). Because the plaintiff could not show that he had a better than 51% chance of avoiding his current condition with timely treatment, the defendants were entitled to a summary judgment in their favor (which precludes a jury from deciding the matter, among other consequences).[1] Of six total appellate tPA cases, three additional cases analyzed the causation requirement in a similar manner and held for the defendants.[24–26]

An appellate case from Kentucky illustrates one approach courts may take that increases the chances physicians will be found liable for failure to administer tPA. In *Lake Cumberland LLC v Dishman*, the plaintiff's expert witness testified that the plaintiff fell in a subgroup of persons that "within a reasonable degree of medical certainty" would have had a significantly better outcome had she been given tPA.[3,27] In effect, the expert witness performed an individualized assessment of the plaintiff's likelihood of improvement in relation to the published data in acute stroke cases to create a more-likely-than-not possibility that the plaintiff would have been better off with treatment. The plaintiff had undergone cerebral angiography for the complaint of worsening dizzy spells. She suffered a postprocedural stroke, which went undetected by the hospital staff for an undetermined length of time and for which tPA was not administered. At the outset, the appellate court noted that Kentucky follows the traditional view of causation. Thus, the issue on appeal was whether the jury could have reasonably concluded that there was a greater than 50% chance that the hospital's failure to administer tPA to the plaintiff was a substantial factor in causing her injuries. The appellate court viewed the expert witness' subgroup analysis as satisfying Kentucky's causation requirement. As a result, the Court held that a jury could have reasonably concluded that the plaintiff's injuries were caused by the defendant's negligence.[3]

Litigation regarding use of tPA highlights two intriguing issues in the law of medical malpractice: divergent practices in different medical specialties and the puzzle of deciding whether the physician's error caused harm in situations where a bad outcome would still have been the most likely result even if the physician had adhered to the standard of care. With respect to standard of care, at trial, neurologists may cite the AAN clinical guidelines in support of tPA as the standard of care in acute stroke. Neurologists who do not give tPA to a qualified patient, however, will need to establish a reason to question the validity of the underlying data supporting the use of tPA in acute stroke. It is noteworthy that our search returned no appellate cases in which a defendant neurologist or emergency medicine physician was sued for administering tPA.

Less commonly appreciated by physicians concerned about liability exposure is that the law accommodates differing views on what constitutes a sufficient link between a defendant's conduct and a plaintiff's injuries to warrant recovery. The traditional causation analysis would limit recovery in most cases involving stroke patients because the a priori probability of a better outcome with appropriate treatment is less than 51%. However, in some cases the loss-of-chance theory of causation allows plaintiffs to recover for the lost opportunity of a better outcome attributable to the defendant's negligence. A cogent approach to the quantification of lost chance in these cases is necessary to ensure that justice is served and that physicians are treated fairly.

Even in a jurisdiction using the traditional view of causation, a stroke patient may recover damages if the expert witness is able to credibly classify a particular plaintiff in a small group of similarly situated patients who would have benefited from tPA treatment, as was done in *Lake Cumberland LLC v Dishman*. The basis for the expert's assessment in that case is not mentioned in the court's opinion. However, whether based on personal experience or the published results of a subgroup analysis, such individualized assessments would be subject to vigorous exploration and critique by the defense attorney on the ground that the estimated probabilities lack a sufficient scientific foundation. Should the witness prove unable to substantiate his or her assessment, he or she would run a very real risk of losing credibility with the jury if the case were tried. Further, many courts have been unwilling to allow juries to speculate about whether a plaintiff fits into a group of people who may benefit from tPA treatment. However, the willingness of an expert witness to state that the failure to use tPA "more likely than not" prevented the plaintiff's recovery from the stroke would probably prevent a court from granting summary judgment for the defendant before the trial reached the jury, thereby making a favorable settlement for the plaintiff more likely.

## DRIVERS WITH DEMENTIA

Some patients with dementia who operate a motor vehicle pose a significant risk to themselves and others. Physicians are frequently in a position to observe symptoms that indicate the danger a patient poses before an accident occurs. The resulting conundrum for physicians is how to mitigate the danger by effectively ensuring the patient does not continue to drive or drive more often than appropriate while respecting the confidentiality of the physician-patient relationship. A loss of driving ability can have considerable impact on a person's autonomy and personal liberty, especially among elderly patients. Physicians confronted with this dilemma must balance the need for public safety with the real likelihood that the patient may not seek medical care or reveal the full extent of her or his symptoms knowing the physician will share that information with state authorities. In addition, a decision by the state to suspend the patient's driving privileges may have a significant impact on the patient's health. Studies have shown that driving cessation is a strong predictor of increased depressive symptoms.[28] In most states, the physician has the option to report the patient to the state authorities. In other states, physicians are required to do so. The American Medical Association has compiled a brief summary of state reporting laws.[29]

### Reporting is Governed by State Law

Most states have laws governing driving-related reports of patients with dementia. These laws vary widely. When faced with the issue for the first time, physicians should consult an attorney or their risk management department regarding the laws of their state.

In general, a physician reports his or her concerns to a state department of motor vehicles (DMV). An official with the DMV will then contact the patient to arrange a formal evaluation of the patient's driving ability to determine if they may retain their license to drive. In most cases, the state, not the physician, determines whether a patient can operate a vehicle safely enough to retain the right to drive.

In a majority of states, physician reporting to the DMV is optional. Optional reporting provides the physician and the patient with the most flexibility in terms of resolving conflicts about driving and the greatest chance of preserving their relationship in those instances in which the patient is not safe to drive. In these states, physicians may encourage a patient to voluntarily stop driving or self-report to the DMV when the patient's cognitive function makes driving dangerous. Optional reporting also takes advantage of the physician's unique position to observe the danger a patient poses on the road, and the ability to weigh the danger to the public against the individual circumstances of a particular case. Thus, where a patient has little family or external support, and the danger on the road is low, a physician may decide that the patient should retain the mobility associated with the ability to drive and choose not to report that patient to the DMV.

In a handful of states, it is critical to note, a physician has the legal duty to report a patient to the DMV for retesting and possible termination of driving privilege. Thus, even in a case in which a patient obeys a physician's direction to stop driving, the physician may still be obliged to report the patient.

State legislation often describes the conditions for which a physician should report a patient. For example, Pennsylvania law allows physicians the discretion to report based on a host of conditions and symptoms, including seizure disorders, unstable diabetes or hypoglycemia, periodic loss of consciousness, mental or emotional disorders, or any other condition that, in the opinion of the physician, could interfere with the ability to control and safely operate a motor vehicle.[30] In comparison, Montana law provides only that a physician may voluntarily report a person whose medical condition will significantly impair a person's ability to safely operate a motor vehicle.[31]

Physicians face potential liability in the reporting process. First, where physicians are not permitted or mandated to report, they may face lawsuits or professional penalties for violating physician-patient confidentiality.[32] For example, in Hawaii, generally doctors may not disclose to any person any information pertaining to a patient's diagnosis, treatment, or health,[33] and doing so may result in fine or license revocation.[34,35] Despite the fact that courts have been reluctant in imposing liability on physicians for failure to report,[36] a handful of states in which physicians help assess driving safety permit liability to be imposed on physicians for their assessments.[29] However, most states with discretionary reporting also provide physicians specific legal protections for doing so. These states generally immunize physicians against lawsuits arising out of the physician's decision to report. Some states also prohibit the DMV from disclosing the name of the reporting physician to the patient.[36]

Though the federal Health Insurance Portability and Accountability Act (HIPAA) regulates disclosing patient information, HIPAA's regulations have provisions recognizing the requirements of state law and the need to manage risks to public safety. HIPAA allows physicians to report patients to the DMV when required by state law and discretionarily when the patient poses a serious threat to public safety behind the wheel.[37] However, where state law does not allow physicians to report, HIPAA does not absolve them of the liability or professional consequences of reporting created by state law.

### Physician Guidelines Regarding Reporting

The American Medical Association and AAN encourage reporting patients who pose a safety risk to themselves and the public.[32,38] Both organizations favor reporting only when a patient has not self-reported to the DMV or if the patient has ignored the physician's advice to discontinue driving. Until state laws are changed, physicians who practice in states without immunity for reporting will have to choose between their obligation to protect the health of their patients and the public, on the one hand, with the potential legal liability associated with the ethically questionable act of violating physician-patient confidentiality on the other. In these circumstances, neurologists can avoid the ethical dilemma if the patient freely agrees not to drive. Neurologists should create an environment within the physician-patient relationship wherein the patients can make such a choice by engaging in honest and repeated discussions with the patient and the caregivers about risks that the patient poses to himself and others by continuing to drive.

## DRIVERS WITH EPILEPSY

Epileptic seizures are the most common cause of accidents associated with acute driver incapacity.[39] Approximately 700,000 of 180 million licensed drivers in America have epilepsy.[40] Generally, state laws governing the physician's ability or requirement to report drivers with dementia also apply to reporting drivers with epilepsy. For physicians, the similar rights, obligations, liabilities, and legal protections are implicated when reporting those with epilepsy as reporting those with dementia. A minority of states mandate physician reporting, but it is voluntary in the majority of states.[40] However, unlike state laws governing driving and dementia, states laws governing driving and epilepsy reflect the fact that epilepsy may result in only intermittent impairment of driving ability. Rather than prohibiting driving completely for patients with seizures, a slight majority of states require patients with epilepsy to be free of seizures for a fixed period of time before they may resume driving. As of 2001, the median restriction among state laws was 6 months, with a range between 3 and 12 months.[40] On the other hand, a substantial number of states employ more flexible approaches to driving restriction. These flexible approaches commonly employ individual clinical factors to assess when an epileptic patient may resume driving.[40] For example, some state laws outline that driving can resume in a shorter period if the seizure occurred during a physician-directed reduction of antiepileptic medication.[40] Conversely, repetitive seizures in a short time frame after a certain seizure-free period can mean the patient will need to wait a longer time before resuming driving.

## VOTING WITH DEMENTIA

In an environment where political groups battle over the validity of each and every vote by counting chads and dimples, one issue drawing national concern in recent years has been voting by persons with cognitive disabilities. Although federal law protects the right to vote generally, whether cognitively impaired individuals may be disenfranchised based on their condition is determined by state law and there is considerable disparity among states with regard to this issue. Often, state standards for capacity to vote are only vaguely defined, with little case law to provide clarity. If any generalization can be made, though, it is that many states prohibit voting by persons declared incompetent by a court.

### Laws Addressing the Right to Vote

Only nine states currently focus their standard specifically on the person's capacity to vote: Connecticut, Florida, Ohio, Massachusetts, Iowa, New Mexico, Wisconsin, Delaware, and Oregon; and none of them provide a standard to assess that capacity.[41] About two thirds of states and the District of Columbia have laws which prevent persons from registering to vote on the basis of certain legal classifications not specifically related to the capacity to vote.[41] For example, states may disenfranchise someone if that person has been judged insane, if he or she is under the care of a court-appointed guardian, or if a court has found him or her generally incompetent. This approach treats mental capacity as an all-or-nothing matter: diminished capacity as to some matters is treated as having diminished capacity for all matters and is clearly incompatible with current principles of mental health law. However, this may be changing. In states where legal classifications determine voting rights, some courts are beginning to take measures that restore voting rights to those with cognitive disorders. For example, guardianship courts are beginning to tailor their judgments to specific matters, meaning individuals may retain the right to vote where they previously would not.[42] In an escalating number of states, guardianship orders are now required to specify which rights a person retains.[42]

### Assessment of Voting Capacity

In general, a court must determine whether an individual has the capacity to vote, if such an assessment is to be made.[41] With the exception of Wisconsin, voting registration officials may not assess the capacity to vote. Wisconsin is the only state that has a formal judicial procedure whereby an election official may challenge someone's capacity to vote. The final determination is still made by a court.[43]

Federal courts have rarely spoken about the appropriate standard for capacity in voting. However, in 2001, a federal District Court in Maine offered some clarification for the capacity to vote. In *Doe v Roe*, three persons challenged the Maine constitution which disenfranchised those "under guardianship for reasons of mental illness."[44] The District Court found that a person has the capacity to vote if he or she understands the nature and effect of voting and has the capacity to choose among the candidates and questions on the ballot.[44] Because it is a trial-level decision, the *Doe v Roe* standard does not have the force of law across the country. However, it is highly relevant as a beginning point for understanding the fundamental aspects of the capacity to vote in the United States, and as the beginning of potential reforms to come.

### Executing the Right to Vote

There are several points at which individuals with dementia might face barriers to voting.[40] First, registration forms may ask if a person has a legal guardian or has been declared incompetent by a court. These questions are appropriate and anticipated, assuming the particular state law defines capacity to vote using such classifications. Second, voter registration staff may suspect a person is not competent to vote and refuse to give out an application for registration. As mentioned, Wisconsin is the only state in which registration officials may question the capacity of a potential voter. Third, there is a paucity of voting technologies tailored to individuals with cognitive impairment.

Finally, family or long-term care staff might not believe an individual competent to vote and as a result may not assist him or her in the process of voting. In practice, the decision of whether an individual is competent to vote often falls to family and long-term care staff who are in daily contact with the cognitively-impaired person. Although they serve an important screening role in voting[40]—because some cognitively impaired patients who clearly lack capacity to vote end up casting ballots—there is a risk that they may make unwarranted assumptions about an individual's capacity to vote and, as a consequence, fail to help the individual exercise the right to the franchise. If the patient does not express an independent desire to go to the polls, his or her ability to vote often goes unutilized as caregivers may simply fail to broach the subject with the patient.

Neurologists may play a meaningful role in this process by raising the subject of voting in discussions with their cognitively impaired patients and their caregivers to ascertain the patient's interest in voting and to uncover any tacit assumptions being made by those taking care of the patient. If the patient expresses a desire to vote, the neurologist should consider performing an evaluation to determine whether the patient understands the nature and effect of voting and has the capacity to choose among the candidates and questions on the ballot.

## REFERENCES

1. Furrow BR, Greaney TL, Johnson SH, et al. Health law. at 310. 2nd edition. St. Paul (MN): West Group; 2000. p. 313–4.
2. Wheeldon v Madison, 374 N.W.2d 367, 375 (S.D.1985).
3. Larriviere DG, Beresford HR. Professionalism in neurology: the role of law. Neurology 2008;71:1283–8.
4. 877 N.E.2d 567 (Mass. 2007).
5. Joy v Eastern Maine Med Ctr, 529 A.2d 1364 (Me. 1987).
6. McKenzie v Hawaii Permanente Medical Group, Inc, 47 P.3d 1209 (Haw. 2002).
7. Bambauer KZ, Johnston SC, Bambauer DE, et al. Reasons why few patients with acute stroke receive tissue plasminogen activator. Arch Neurol 2006;63:661–4.
8. Weintraub MI. Thrombolysis (tissue plasminogen activator) in stroke: a medico-legal quagmire. Stroke 2006;37:1917–22.
9. Schneider SM. Goldstein LB. Adams JG. et al. Improving the chain of recovery for acute stroke in your community: task force report. 2002. Incentives for enhancing stroke care. Available at: http://www.ninds.nih.gov/news_and_events/proceedings/stroke_2002/acute_stroke_incentives.htm. Accessed September 1, 2009.
10. Bryan v Burt, 486 S.E.2d 536, 539 (Va. 1997).
11. Report of the Quality Standards Subcommitte of the American Academy of Neurology. Practice advisory: thrombolytic therapy for acute ischemic stroke. Neurology 1996;47:835–9.
12. Adams HP, del Zoppo G, Alberts MJ, et al. Guidelines for the early management of adults with ischemic stroke. Stroke 2007;38:1655–711.
13. AAEM Work Group on Thrombolytic Therapy in Stroke. Position statement of the American Academy Of Emergency Medicine on the use of intravenous thrombolytic therapy in the treatment of stroke. 2002. Available at: http://www.aaem.org/positionstatements/thrombolytictherapy.php. Accessed September 1, 2009.
14. Canadian Association of Emergency Physicians Committee on Thrombolytic Therapy for Acute Ischemic Stroke. Thrombolytic therapy for acute ischemic stroke. CJEM 2001;3:8–12.
15. Hood v Phillips, 537 S.W.2d 291 (Tex.Civ.App. 1976).
16. Hacke W, Kaste M, Bluhmki E, et al. Thrombolysis with alteplase 3 to 4.5 hours after acute ischemic stroke. N Engl J Med 2008;359:1317–29.
17. Wahlgren N, Ahmed N, Davalos A, et al. Thrombolysis with alteplase for acute ischaemic stroke in the Safe Implementation of Thrombolysis in Stroke-Monitoring Study (SITS-MOST): an observational study. Lancet 2007;369:275–82.
18. Hill MD, Buchan AM, Canadian Alteplase for Stroke Effectiveness Study (CASES) Investigators. Thrombolysis for acute ischemic stroke: results of the Canadian Alteplase for Stroke Effectiveness Study. CMAJ 2005;172:1307–12.
19. Herskovits v Group Health Co-op. of Puget Sound, 664 P.2d 474 (Wash. 1983).
20. Tissue plasminogen activator for acute ischemic stroke. The National Institute of Neurological Disorders and Stroke rt-PA Stroke Study Group. N Engl J Med 1995; 333:1581–7.
21. Hodson JD. Medical malpractice: loss of chance causality. 54 ALR 4th 10, §. 2[a] (2007).
22. Saroyan Z. The current injustice of the loss of chance doctrine: an argument for a new approach to damages. 33 Cumb. L. Rev. 15, note 99–100. (2002).

23. 2006 WL 1984613 (S.D.Tex. 2006) (slip copy).
24. Ensink v Mecosta County General Hospital, 687 N.W.2d 143 (Mich.App. 2004).
25. Joshi v Providence Health System of Oregon Corp, 149 P.3d 1164 (Or. 2006).
26. Potter v Ingham Regional Medical Center, 2003 W.L. 356360 (Mich.App. 2003).
27. 2007 WL 1229432 (Ky.App. 2007).
28. Marottoli RA, Mendes de Leon CF, Glass TA, et al. Driving cessation and increased depressive symptoms: prospective evidence from the New Haven EPESE. Established Populations for Epidemiologic Studies of the Elderly. J Am Geriatr Soc 1997;45(2):202–6.
29. American Medical Association. State licensing requirements and reporting laws. Available at: http://www.ama-assn.org/ama1/pub/upload/mm/433/chapter8.pdf. Accessed January 9, 2009.
30. Sullivan J. Physicians as gatekeepers for society: confidentiality of protected health information versus duty to disclose at-risk drivers. 16 Health Law. 20 (2003).
31. M.C.A. § 37-2-311.
32. Bacon D, Fisher RS, Morris JC, et al. American Academy Of Neurology position statement on physician reporting of medical conditions that may affect driving competence. Neurology 2007;68:1174–7.
33. Haw. Rev. Stat. § 432D-21.
34. Haw. Rev. Stat. § 436B-7(3), Haw. Rev. Stat. § 436B-16(b).
35. Kane KM. Driving into the sunset: a proposal for mandatory reporting to the DMV by physicians treating unsafe elderly drivers. 25 U. Haw. L. Rev. 59, 60 (2002).
36. Stone DH. You take my space, I take your air: an empirical study of disabled parking and motor vehicle laws for persons with disabilities. 33 Ohio N.U.L. Rev. 665 (2007).
37. 45 C.F.R. § 164.512(a); 45 C.F.R. § 164.512(j).
38. Opinion 2.24 Impaired Drivers and Their Physicians. Code of medical ethics. Chicago: American Medical Association; 2006. Available at: http://www.ama-assn.org/ama/pub/physician-resources/medical-ethics/code-medical-ethics/opinion224.shtml. Accessed January 9, 2009.
39. Chadwick DW. Driving restrictions and people with epilepsy. Neurology 2001;57:1749–50.
40. Krauss GL, Ampaw L, Krumholz A, et al. Individual state driving restrictions for people with epilepsy in the US. Neurology 2001;57:1780–5.
41. Karlawish JH, Bonnie RB, Applebaum PA, et al. Addressing the ethical, legal, and social issues raised by voting with persons with dementia. JAMA 2004;292:1345–50.
42. Hurme SB, Applebaum PS. Defining and assessing capacity to vote: the effect of mental impairment on the rights of voters. 38 McGeorge L. Rev. 931 (2007).
43. Wis. Stat. Ann.§ 54.25(2) (c)1.g (West Supp. 2006).
44. 156 F.Supp. 2d 35 (D.Me. 2001).

# Neurological Malpractice and Nonmalpractice Liability

James C. Johnston, MD, JD, FCLM, FACLM[a,b,*]

**KEYWORDS**

• Medical malpractice • Neurologic misadventures
• Neurological liability • Forensic neurology

This article provides an overview of the liability issues affecting neurologists. It focuses on current trends in malpractice law, with illustrative management strategies for several common recurring claims involving selected neurologic conditions. Nonmalpractice liability issues are discussed with particular attention to the unique risks engendered by the expert witness.

## MALPRACTICE TRENDS

The overall medical malpractice claims frequency (number of claims filed) in the United States is at a historic low; payouts in constant dollars have plummeted, down 45% since 2000.[1,2] The result, however, is a paradoxically adverse impact on the specialty of neurology. The cumulative data from an insurance consortium review of 3812 neurology claims between 1985 and 2008 paints a disturbing picture[3]: the absolute number of paid neurology claims significantly increased over the past 5 years; the extraordinarily high payment ratio (percentage of paid claims to claims closed) more than doubled in the past 5 years (39.58% in 2007); neurology continues to have the highest average indemnity payment of all specialties including neurosurgery and obstetrics ($614,577 in 2007); and neurology claims, compared with every other specialty group, are the most costly to defend.

Several unique factors inherent to the specialty of neurology may explain these alarming statistics, which are at odds with general malpractice trends. First, the unprecedented growth of sophisticated neurodiagnostic tests, the proliferation of powerful neuropharmacologic agents, and the advent of more invasive procedures

[a] 321 High School Road NE, Suite D3–750, Bainbridge Island, Seattle, WA 98110, USA
[b] Barrister Sole, 323-100A Ponsonby Road, Auckland 1011, New Zealand
* 321 High School Road NE, Suite D3–750, Bainbridge Island, Seattle, WA 98110.
*E-mail address:* johnstonMDJD@aol.com

Neurol Clin 28 (2010) 441–458
doi:10.1016/j.ncl.2009.11.008
0733-8619/10/$ – see front matter
**neurologic.theclinics.com**

raise the standard of care, increasing the level of accountability and hence likelihood of suit. Second, neurologists, more so than other specialists, confront a diverse array of legal issues beyond the scope of traditional practice involving brain death, genetic testing, competency issues, neurotoxic insults, and evaluation of the neurologically impaired child. These varied conditions, governed by expanding legal doctrines, evolving regulatory control, and political whims, expose the neurologist to a variety of often novel claims. Third, neurologic liability extends beyond the physician-patient relationship to include a host of third parties. For example, there is tort liability for negligence to a patient that also injures a fetus, child, or spouse. In addition to the duty to warn of imminently dangerous patients, there is now a duty to warn third parties of communicable diseases. Neurologists have a duty to warn patients of medical conditions that may impair driving (epilepsy, sleep disorders, stroke); they may also be required to warn others directly, either by statute or an imposed tort duty to warn of foreseeable harm. The result is an everexpanding pool of potential claimants. Fourth, the very nature of neurologic disease or injury spells a grave outcome for many patients, which is undoubtedly reflected in the indemnity payments. The confluence of these factors may herald a fundamental shift transforming neurology from a low-risk specialty to one plagued by malpractice claims.

## NEUROLOGIC MISADVENTURES

Medical misadventure refers to personal injury from either a negligent act or omission, or an adverse outcome of properly rendered care. The most prevalent neurologic misadventure is unquestionably diagnostic error, occurring in one third of all claims and in 45% of paid claims over the past two decades.[4] These errors commonly stem from the failure to perform an adequate history and examination, which is the most prevalent procedure resulting in claims against neurologists.[5] The most frequent incorrectly diagnosed conditions are malignant neoplasm of the brain, followed by headache (HA), intracranial and intraspinal abscess, nontraumatic subarachnoid hemorrhage (SAH), and vertebral fracture.[6] Other prevalent misadventures, in decreasing order of frequency, include improperly performed procedure, failure to supervise or monitor a case, medication errors, failure to recognize a complication of treatment, delay in performance, procedure performed when not indicated or contraindicated, procedure not performed, and failure to instruct or communicate with the patient.[7]

## CLAIMS AGAINST NEUROLOGISTS
### General Remarks

The provision of medical care meeting or even exceeding the prevailing standard may not effectively shield the neurologist from a lawsuit. A solid physician-patient relationship, valid consent, and proper medical record documentation are essential for successful risk management and malpractice defense.

The root of a malpractice claim is injury or perceived injury; however, most suits are actually triggered by a breakdown in the physician-patient relationship caused by poor communication. A thorough understanding of the relationship is crucial; meeting patient expectations through effective communication significantly reduces the risk of suit.

Informed consent issues are a frequent source of malpractice suits, wholly unrelated to negligence claims. The legal theories of consent detailed in the literature are equally applicable to all specialties, and discussed elsewhere in this issue.

Poor documentation is the leading factor in the forced settlement of most malpractice claims. The literature is replete with recommendations for ensuring that records are clear, accurate, complete, legible, and timely without alterations or other evidence of spoliation. It is redundant to reiterate good record-keeping principles in this article; however, one legal maxim must be emphasized: "If it is not in the record, it never happened."

### Specific Claims

The extraordinarily broad scope of neurologic malpractice liability precludes a compendium of potential claims. Even limiting the claims to diagnostic errors is overwhelming. Moreover, such a listing is quickly outdated because emerging diagnostic and therapeutic options open the door for new claims. A more instructive approach is to consider the most prevalent patient conditions generating suits against neurologists. These include, in decreasing order of frequency, back disorders, cerebrovascular accident, convulsions, displacement of intervertebral disk, HA, epilepsy, occlusion and stenosis of cerebral arteries, migraines, nontraumatic SAH, and malignant neoplasm of the brain.[8]

Back disorders and intervertebral disk displacement are not discussed because these claims are generally attributable to straightforward diagnostic errors, few result in an indemnity payment, and the total indemnity is a small percentage of that paid for all neurology claims.[9] This article outlines several management strategies pertaining to the remaining conditions, arbitrarily grouped together as stroke, epilepsy, and HA, the latter subsuming migraine, brain tumor, and SAH. Lack of space precludes discussion of the myriad disparate claims involving these conditions. Several key topics were selected because they affect a large segment of the general population, are frequently seen by neurologists and nonneurologists alike, generate recurring claims, and have the potential for exceptionally high indemnity payments or judgments.

The discussion of each condition is written from a legal perspective, focusing on the origin of frequently encountered malpractice claims as opposed to discussing arcane details of sometimes obscure legal principles. This format requires oversimplification of the medical points, which necessitates omitting many conditions, truncating differential diagnoses, and ignoring various diagnostic and therapeutic options. It focuses solely on malpractice issues, and is not a substitute for conventional medical writings. Nor is it a treatise of neurologic malpractice; indeed, an impossible feat for a single article or even a single volume. This article is simply designed to provide the neurologist with a rudimentary understanding of how lawsuits arise, and generate some discussion on adapting practice patterns to improve patient care and minimize liability risk. References are kept to a minimum and, as much as possible, selected to provide the reader with additional background material for specific topics.

### HEADACHE
### General Considerations

HAs are ubiquitous, arguably the most common disorder encountered by the practicing physician, and the most common presenting symptom in malpractice claims against neurologists.[10] HA may be of little clinical significance or, paradoxically, herald potentially catastrophic illnesses, such as brain tumor, SAH, or meningitis. A complete and accurate diagnosis of the patient with HA requires a detailed history coupled with a full neurologic and general medical examination, as well as diagnostic testing and neuroimaging in selected cases. The single most important step in the evaluation is to classify the type of HA and ascertain whether it is acute, long-standing, or with recent change. This practical approach allows the neurologist to determine the need for any diagnostic testing and initiate a proper treatment plan, all with the appropriate degree of urgency. Too often, the inexperienced, poorly trained, or hurried neurologist distorts a patient's history or fails to perform an adequate examination, resulting in the wrong diagnosis. Most malpractice suits stem from the failure to elicit an accurate history. The art of history taking cannot be taught in this article or in any other book; it includes an innate ability to establish a rapport, and instill confidence and trust. The author suggests the following methodology for the sole purpose of demonstrating several pitfalls that may lead to misdiagnosis, and recommends that neurologists formulate their own techniques, which will evolve with time, experience, and continuing education (**Box 1**).

### Specific Approach

Evaluating the patient with HA requires a systematic approach to exclude more serious conditions, diagnose the primary HA, and formulate a treatment plan. There are particular aspects of each step that seem to generate recurring claims. This overview is limited to nontraumatic HAs in the adult population, with particular attention to the more common diagnostic and treatment errors.

The first step is to exclude serious conditions causing secondary HAs, which may share many of the same clinical features as a primary HA. The differential diagnosis of HA is exceedingly long, and indications for diagnostic testing must be made on an individual basis. The neurologist performing a history and examination should direct particular attention to warning signs or "red flags" suggesting a secondary HA, and proceed with appropriate diagnostic and therapeutic intervention. The author proposes the mnemonic "SIGNAL" to account for the most commonly misdiagnosed secondary HAs (**Box 2**).

The second step, after excluding secondary HAs, is to diagnose the primary HA in accordance with International Headache Society criteria.[20] It is beyond the scope of this article to review the various HA syndromes; however, the importance of correctly

---

**Box 1**
**History taking methodology in HA**

- Allow ample time for the consultation. Introduce yourself and invite the patient to sit for an interview before changing into a gown. Advise the patient that you have read the referral letter, but never accept either the patient's or referring physician's diagnosis.

- "Tell me about your HAs." Allow the patient to speak uninterruptedly before asking questions. Then begin open-ended queries to determine the quality, severity, location, duration, and time course of events, as well as precipitating, exacerbating, and relieving factors. It is helpful to ask the patient to describe a particular attack. Determine whether the patient has more than one type of HA. It is essential to separately evaluate each HA type, which may not be possible during the initial consultation because of time constraints. Subsequent appointments should be arranged accordingly.

- Communication skills are critical. Knowing which clues to follow and when to interrupt the patient are fundamental to an accurate history. Failure to understand the patient's terminology often leads to a misdiagnosis. The word "throbbing," for example, may be incorrectly translated into a migraine. The HA specialist must avoid distorting the history to fit a preconceived diagnostic category.

- The scope of the history must be sufficiently broad to address systemic diseases that may be relevant to the HA. Past, family, and social histories provide valuable information about the patient's condition. Before concluding the history, it is often enlightening to solicit the patient's opinion regarding the cause of the HA.

**Box 2**
**Warning signs of secondary HA**

1. Sudden onset (thunderclap) HA. The sudden onset of severe HA mandates immediate and thorough evaluation for potential etiologies, such as SAH, intracerebral hemorrhage, venous or sinus thrombosis, intracranial or extracranial arterial dissection, aneurysmal expansion, pituitary apoplexy, or less common conditions.[11] Of these, SAH warrants further discussion. Aneurysmal hemorrhage accounts for 85% of nontraumatic cases and is the focus of this discussion.[12] It is among the most frequently missed serious causes of HA, and has a mortality rate of 50%.[13] More than half of patients presenting to the emergency room with a sentinel HA and SAH are misdiagnosed.[14] The failure to diagnose SAH consistently results in the highest percentage of paid claims (61.6%), and the highest average and highest total indemnity for all claims involving diagnostic error.[15] The sine qua non of SAH is a sudden HA classically described as the "first" or "worst HA of my life," often associated with nausea or vomiting, and followed by signs of meningeal irritation. Perhaps a better description is that the HA presents with maximal severity at onset. There may be cognitive impairment; focal deficits; or, in up to one half of cases, a history of premonitory symptoms suggestive of a sentinel bleed or aneurysmal expansion.[16] The known migraineur presenting with a sentinel HA may be misdiagnosed as having breakthrough symptoms; a thorough history is essential, because most patients recognize that the HA is different from a typical migraine.[17] The patient with thunderclap HA must have immediate CT of the brain and, if negative, a lumbar puncture to include spectrophotometric evaluation for xanthochromia.[18] The failure to perform a CT is the most common error; further evaluation based on the clinical presentation, and CT and lumbar puncture results, may warrant four-vessel cerebral angiography and neurosurgical consultation for definitive intervention.[19]

2. Increasing or worsening HA. The patient's HA pattern must be interpreted in light of the overall history. Recent-onset HAs with progression may indicate a tumor, subdural hematoma, or other mass lesion, and focal deficits may be present. A slow-growing mass, however, may not be associated with any neurologic deficits. Chronic primary HAs with progression may represent the development of a new, superimposed HA disorder (primary or secondary), or transformation of the primary disorder. It may be impossible to clinically distinguish the transformed migraine, often precipitated by medication overuse, from a new HA disorder. The presentation of an escalating HA, whether acute or chronic, warrants investigation.

3. Generalized disease with HA. There are a plethora of systemic diseases presenting with acute HA including intracranial (eg, meningitis, encephalitis, sphenoid sinusitis) and generalized (eg, Lyme disease) infections; neoplasm (including paraneoplastic disease and leptomeningeal metastases); vascular conditions; autoimmune disorders; metabolic diseases; and toxic exposures. The diagnosis requires proficient examination with attention to systemic signs serving to guide diagnostic intervention. For example, the older patient with HA and visual symptoms may require temporal artery biopsy for giant cell arteritis.

4. Neurological or focal signs with HA. A HA associated with transient or permanent focal deficits other than a typical aura requires further evaluation.

5. Activity, exertion or cough HA. These HAs are frequently associated with posterior fossa structural abnormalities and warrant MRI to provide a definitive diagnosis.

6. Labor, pregnancy or postpartum HA. The new onset of HAs or progression of known primary HAs during pregnancy or postpartum raises the concern of sinus thrombosis, cerebral infarction, carotid dissection, pituitary apoplexy, and preeclampsia. These disorders most commonly occur during the third trimester or postpartum, present with HA, and may be associated with focal signs or seizures.

diagnosing the patient cannot be overstated. It is commonplace for the neurologist to label a patient with a particular HA type during the initial consultation and, despite a poor response to treatment, never consider revisiting the diagnosis. These patients are branded with the wrong diagnosis, and resultant therapy is ineffective as well as potentially harmful. It creates a breeding ground for malpractice claims.

The third step is to treat the primary HA with a comprehensive multimodality approach incorporating pharmacologic intervention predicated on evidence-based guidelines.[21] This approach is frequently ignored by the neurologist content with simply prescribing a medication. Management strategies for acute and chronic HA are detailed in the neurologic literature, and each therapeutic modality is subject to a unique array of claims.[22,23] A significant number of these suits, however, allege medication errors, such as failure to manage rebound phenomena; inappropriate use of medications (triptan prescribed in coronary artery disease), failure to properly monitor medication (liver failure on valproic acid); and failure to recognize side effects (β-blockers aggravating Raynaud phenomena).

The majority of patients with refractory HA have been misdiagnosed or improperly treated because of one of the following errors: incomplete or incorrect diagnosis (undiagnosed secondary HA, misdiagnosed primary HA, or failure to recognize multiple HA types); improper imaging studies ("normal" CT overlooking posterior fossa lesion); ignoring exacerbating factors or triggers (failure to provide dietary instructions); poor pharmacotherapeutic management (subtherapeutic dosage); and neglecting rebound phenomena, which leads to persistent HAs.

### Neuroimaging in the HA Patient

The role of neuroimaging in the adult patient with HA and a normal neurologic examination remains a controversial topic.[24] The American Academy of Neurology (AAN) Practice Guidelines state that "neuroimaging is not usually warranted in patients with migraine and a normal neurologic examination," but should be considered in patients with an abnormal neurologic examination or "patients with atypical headache features or headaches that do not fulfill the strict definition of migraine or other primary headache disorder."[25] These parameters presuppose an accurate diagnosis of the patient's HA, which is frequently not the case. The most common diagnostic error in neurology is to label a patient with migraine or other HA disorder in the absence of neuroimaging, only to find that subsequent evaluation uncovers a brain tumor.[26] Arguments that earlier diagnosis would not have materially affected the outcome are generally unsuccessful. There may be absolutely no relationship between the HA and brain tumor, but the trier-of-fact will likely find otherwise if the neurologist failed to order a timely imaging study. The decision to forego neuroimaging in a patient with HAs requires a great deal of experience and clinical acumen. For many neurologists, it is simply prudent to perform an imaging study on every HA patient early in the evaluation. There is no point in repeating a test if it was already performed, assuming no change in the patient's condition. There are no evidence-based recommendations in the United States regarding the relative sensitivity of MRI compared with CT in nonacute HA disorders, although a European Task Force recommends MRI.[27] Most experts agree MRI is the superior choice because of its sensitivity to venous thrombosis, extracranial hematomas, neoplasms, and meningeal disease; and ability to visualize the posterior fossa, cervicomedullary junction, and pituitary region. Unfortunately, neurologists may be deterred from ordering these studies because of onerous preauthorization requests or concerns over deselection, and failure to diagnose brain tumor will likely remain one of the most common malpractice claims.

## CEREBROVASCULAR DISEASE

Globally, almost 6 million people die from stroke each year; it is the third leading cause of death in the United States with almost 800,000 strokes annually.[28] Stroke therapy has changed dramatically over the past decade with the development of specific treatment options (thrombolysis, endovascular therapy) and refinement of prevention strategies (anticoagulation, carotid endarterectomy [CEA]). These recent advances, along with improved diagnostic modalities, create a heightened expectation of proper stroke management and, combined with the catastrophic impact of stroke, portend increasing litigation in this area.

### Thrombolytic Therapy

Tissue plasminogen activator (tPA) thrombolysis arguably represents the neurologic standard of care for acute ischemic stroke, despite the fact that an extremely low percentage of eligible patients receive the drug at this time. Intravenous administration of tPA within 3 hours of ischemic stroke significantly improves functional outcome in selected patients.[29-34] Recent data suggest modest but significant clinical improvement in patients treated 3 to 4.5 hours after onset of stroke symptoms, resulting in a science advisory for this population.[35,36] The therapeutic window is narrow, and strict adherence to the approved protocol inclusion and exclusion criteria is imperative.[37,38] The hospital, emergency department, radiology team, and neurology and neurosurgery consultants should establish a dedicated stroke center capable of responding to every acute ischemic stroke patient in a timely fashion and, if indicated, administering tPA.[39] Alternatively, tPA-eligible patients must be promptly transferred to another institution for definitive treatment if it can be accomplished within a suitable time frame. Failure of the hospital to provide appropriate facilities and personnel (streamlined emergency room intake, CT technicians continuously available) may create liability for all parties including the neurologist.

The failure to recommend or administer tPA to an eligible patient may constitute negligence, unless it can be proved that tPA would not have made a material difference in the patient's outcome. The neurologist deciding not to use tPA in an acute ischemic stroke should clearly document the reasons for that decision in the medical records. It is equally important for the neurologist to resist pressure from the emergency physician or family to use tPA unless the patient meets all inclusion and exclusion criteria. Modification of the criteria, especially the time constraint, decreases the benefit of tPA and increases the risk of intracerebral hemorrhage.[40] Determination of the time of stroke onset is crucial. It is a common error to label the onset as the time symptoms were first observed rather than the last time the patient was known to be well. For example, if the patient awakens with deficits, then the onset time must be considered the last time the patient was known to be well (usually the night before), not when the symptoms were first noticed on wakening. The same holds true for patients unable to communicate these details. Likewise, patients with stroke-related neglect syndromes cannot reliably observe the onset time. Another frequent error is the administration of anticoagulants or antiplatelet agents during the first 24 hours after tPA administration, which greatly increases the risk of intracerebral hemorrhage. Again, it is imperative to follow the guidelines.[41] There are cases, however, where the neurologist may consider all of the risks and benefits, and decide it is in the patient's best interest to deviate from the protocol. This decision should be discussed with the patient or legal representative and family, and thoroughly documented in the records.

The failure to obtain valid informed consent may precipitate a malpractice action separate from negligence.[42] Informed consent mandates a frank discussion regarding the benefits and risks of tPA, including the potential for hemorrhage, coma, and death.[43] The acute stroke patient may not be able to fully participate in the process because of communication deficits or cognitive impairment. Options should then be discussed with a close family member and documented, but only a legal representative (guardian or person with written power of attorney) can give consent. If the patient is unable to give consent and no legal representative is available, the neurologist may proceed with tPA when it is the most reasonable option. Courts recognize an implied consent; there is an assumption that a competent individual would have agreed to the procedure.[44]

### Anticoagulation Therapy

The use of heparin to prevent an impending stroke remains controversial despite the absence of supporting evidence, and immediate anticoagulation is occasionally recommended for fluctuating basilar artery thrombosis, extracranial arterial dissection, and imminent carotid artery occlusion, as well as certain cases of cardioembolic and noncardioembolic cerebral infarction. It is increasingly difficult to defend any complications in these circumstances because the weight of the evidence is against anticoagulation.[45]

Warfarin may be beneficial in the first few months after an ischemic event, but there is no definitive evidence that the benefits of long-term anticoagulation for thrombosis or embolism outweigh the potential risks except in patients with nonvalvular atrial fibrillation, prosthetic heart valves, and acute myocardial infarction.[46] Nonvalvular atrial fibrillation affects 2.5 million Americans and the prevalence increases with age; it increases the risk of stroke fourfold to sixfold across all age groups.[47,48] The annual rate of ischemic stroke in untreated nonvalvular atrial fibrillation patients increases with high-risk factors, such as hypertension, left ventricular dysfunction, transient ischemic attack (TIA), or prior stroke.[49] Anticoagulation with warfarin significantly reduces this risk of stroke, and represents the generally accepted standard of care for stroke prevention in these patients.[50] Multiple separate guidelines and over two dozen randomized trials in the past two decades consistently advocate anticoagulation for nonvalvular atrial fibrillation patients with additional risk factors conferring high risk of stroke.[51] These guidelines differ in the classification of risk criteria; however, every statement labels prior stroke or TIA high risk, and recommends anticoagulation. If warfarin is contraindicated, or the patient is at low risk of stroke, then antiplatelet therapy is the appropriate treatment.

Neurologists may be reluctant to use warfarin because of the required follow-up and monitoring, or they may inappropriately minimize the medication dosage out of undue concern about bleeding. This is a frequent subject of litigation, with the claim that a major stroke would have been prevented if the patient had been properly anticoagulated. It is, therefore, imperative to identify patients at risk for stroke in accordance with established clinical guidelines. Accurate diagnosis is essential, including appropriate neuroimaging before initiating therapy. The reasons for or against anticoagulating a patient at risk should be documented in the medical records. For example, if the increased risk of bleeding caused by gait instability outweighs the potential benefits of anticoagulation, then careful documentation may protect against litigation if the patient suffers a massive embolus. Patient and family education concerning the management of anticoagulation is crucial, and should be clearly documented. Certain medications must be avoided or used with extreme caution because of the increased risk of hemorrhage when combined with warfarin (aspirin, barbiturates, cephalosporins, sulfa drugs, high-dose penicillin). Establish and follow written procedures for monitoring patients on warfarin, or enlist one of the anticoagulant management services.

## CEA and Angioplasty

Over one quarter of recently symptomatic patients with a high-grade carotid stenosis (70%–99% diameter reduction) suffer an ipsilateral stroke within 2 years, despite appropriate management of risk factors and antiplatelet therapy.[52] CEA significantly reduces the incidence of cerebral infarction in these patients and may be considered to represent the standard of care; it is moderately useful for symptomatic patients with 50% to 69% stenosis, not indicated for symptomatic patients with less than 50% stenosis, and individualized decisions are required for the smaller benefit in asymptomatic patients with 60% to 99% stenosis.[53] There must be careful patient selection (ie, attention to patients with a high-grade tandem lesion in the ipsilateral intracranial arteries, or asymptomatic patients with severe contralateral carotid artery stenosis or occlusion), and skill of the surgical team is paramount. The most common malpractice claims are failure to diagnose TIA or minor stroke, and failure to perform an evaluation for carotid stenosis, allowing the patient to suffer a recurrent or massive stroke. Every patient with a TIA or stroke should have appropriate neuroimaging unless surgery is plainly contraindicated. Patients with symptomatic carotid artery stenosis greater than 70% should be offered CEA or carotid angioplasty. Other degrees of stenosis require individualized considerations, which must be well documented. Delay in referring a TIA patient with high-grade stenosis for definitive treatment may also constitute negligence, since a high percentage of strokes occur within 48 hours of the TIA.[54] Surgery should be offered as soon as possible after a TIA or nondisabling stroke, preferably within 2 weeks of the last symptomatic event.[55] Premature surgical intervention following a moderate to severe stroke creates a liability risk for extension or hemorrhagic conversion of the infarction; however, there is insufficient evidence to support or refute delaying CEA for 4 to 6 weeks.[56] Carotid angioplasty is a more recent procedure, and its indications are still evolving. Informed consent issues are critical, and all decisions should be thoroughly documented in the medical records.

## EPILEPSY

There are over 2 million epileptics in the United States.[57] Approximately 150,000 adults present annually with a first seizure, with almost half recurring to be classified as epilepsy; the lifetime cumulative risk of a seizure ranges from 8% to 10%, with a 3% chance of developing epilepsy.[58] These disorders present formidable legal challenges because of the variable clinical symptoms, diverse etiopathogenetic mechanisms, and diagnostic and therapeutic complexity in patients who commonly harbor intellectual impairment, cognitive dysfunction, and psychiatric symptoms.[59,60]

## Driving

Every state restricts issuance of a driver's license to individuals who have suffered loss of consciousness. The laws differ among the states, but generally require that an individual be seizure free for a period of time before obtaining a license. This seizure-free interval is variable within individual state jurisdictions, ranging from no fixed duration to 1 year. A physician's evaluation must be submitted to the state before a license is issued. Neurologists are rightfully concerned about their potential liability when certifying that a patient with epilepsy is capable of driving. Some states grant immunity to the physician, although the level of immunity varies among the jurisdictions, ranging from "good faith" immunity to immunity from suit. In other states, physicians are not granted statutory immunity from liability for the information they provide to the state or for damages arising out of a seizure-related accident. In states without physician immunity laws, courts may still refuse to impose liability on the neurologist who exercised reasonable care and good faith in reporting to the state.

Six states (California, Delaware, Nevada, New Jersey, Oregon, and Pennsylvania) have express mandatory reporting statutes requiring physicians to report patients with epilepsy (or other disorders associated with a loss of consciousness or impaired ability to drive) to the state.[61] All other states have voluntary reporting statutes. The neurologic standard of care for reporting the epileptic patient varies according to the laws and regulations of each state. It is incumbent on neurologists to know the relevant statutes in their jurisdiction, and have an understanding of the common law trends for any ambiguous issues. The neurologist has a duty to advise patients of the legislation in their particular state, and emphasize the importance of complying with the law. If the state has an explicit self-reporting requirement, patients should be advised in writing to comply, retaining a copy of the letter in the medical records. The discussion of driving restrictions and restrictions on other activities, the effect of discontinuing or reducing dosage of a drug, and possible side effects of medications in relation to driving should be clearly documented in the records. These issues should be reiterated and documented on any change in medication because of the increased risk of breakthrough seizures.

If an epileptic patient continues to drive because the neurologist failed to report where reporting is mandatory, or failed to instruct the patient in a voluntary reporting state, then a seizure-related accident may trigger a malpractice suit by the patient or the patient's estate. It is imperative that the neurologist clearly document patient instructions in the medical records, and keep a copy of any notification sent to the state. It is also advisable to record any factors that may mitigate liability for not filing a report. The patient who drives against medical advice is a special concern for every neurologist, especially in voluntary reporting states. *Tarasoff* reasoning may be applied to the neurologist who advises a patient not to drive, learns the patient continues driving, and fails to take any further action.[62] In this situation, the neurologist should inform the patient in writing about the potential consequences of driving, and consider filing a voluntary report with the appropriate state agency. There may be statutory protection for a voluntary report that is made in good faith and consistent with the prevailing standard of care. The level of protection varies among jurisdictions, however, and it is advisable to consult legal counsel.

Neurologists may be liable to third parties for failing to report a patient or certifying a patient to drive. This is an emerging area of liability, and most decisions turn on whether the neurologist owes a duty to the third party. Courts have ruled in both directions, and the issue remains far from settled.[63] Neurologists should adapt practice patterns to comport with the relevant legal trends in their jurisdiction, but even third-party liability is minimized by effective patient discussions, proper reporting, and thorough documentation, as outlined previously.

### Teratogenesis

There are over 0.5 million women with epilepsy of childbearing age in the United States; 3 to 5 births per 1000 are to epileptic women.[64] Epilepsy is the most common neurologic disorder in pregnancy, and it raises a host of legal and medical issues. The most serious concern, however, is the potential for congenital malformations in the offspring of mothers taking antiepileptic drugs (AEDs). These mothers have an up to 7% risk of bearing a child with congenital malformations, threefold higher than nonepileptic mothers.[65] This higher risk is probably multifactorial with genetic and social components, but AEDs are clearly implicated as human teratogens.[66] All conventional AEDs (phenytoin, phenobarbital, carbamazepine, and valproic acid [VPA]) taken during the first trimester share an increased risk of malformations, which commonly include orofacial clefts, congenital heart disease, neural tube defects, and urogenital malformations.[67] It is not clear if the increased risk is imparted from one or some AEDs; however, VPA harbors a greater risk of major fetal malformations and should be avoided in women who may become pregnant.[68] The teratogenic potential of the newer AEDs remains unknown, and these drugs should be avoided during pregnancy.

Malpractice suits for AED-induced fetal malformations have the potential for extraordinarily large settlements or judgments, and tolling of the statute of limitations is commonplace. The neurologist must address a variety of complex issues in epileptic women who take AEDs during their reproductive years to minimize liability for these claims. The recent guidelines are not particularly helpful because of a paucity of evidence limiting the strength of many findings and recommendations.[69,70] The following suggestions are provided to focus on some of the clinical points that seem more commonly raised in lawsuits. Detailed counseling early in the reproductive years should include a discussion of the increased risk of seizures during pregnancy, importance of medication compliance, necessity of regular follow-up with AED levels, risk of malformations, folic acid and vitamin K supplementation, and the importance of avoiding coteratogens. Before pregnancy, it is important to determine whether AEDs are necessary; for example, if the patient is receiving an anticonvulsant for migraine, depression, or some other disorder, it may be possible to discontinue the drug. Additionally, if the patient with a single type of seizure has been in remission for 2 to 5 years, and has a normal neurologic examination with no EEG abnormalities, then it may be reasonable to gradually withdraw the drug. The taper must be performed slowly over months, and completed 6 months before conception, because seizure recurrence is most likely during this time. If treatment is indicated, every effort should be made to place the patient on monotherapy with the lowest effective dose of the most suitable AED. Frequent daily dosing avoids high peak levels, possibly reducing the potential for teratogenesis. The free (non–protein-bound) AED levels should be monitored at least preconception, at the beginning of each trimester, the last month of pregnancy, and 2 months postpartum. Pregnancy screening should include serum alpha fetoprotein at 16 to 18 weeks and a level II ultrasound at 18 to 20 weeks. If indicated, amniocentesis may be offered at 18 to 20 weeks. The patient should be properly counseled if there is a serious malformation, and provided with the option to terminate the pregnancy. The administration of folic acid in the early stages of pregnancy probably decreases the incidence of neural tube defects and, despite the limited guideline recommendations, should be given to all women of childbearing potential. Optimal dosage for epileptics remains controversial, and data must be extrapolated from nonepileptic women; it is a matter of clinical judgment but should be between 0.4 and 4 mg/d.

It is not uncommon for women with epilepsy to present to the neurologist after becoming pregnant. In general, the risk of uncontrolled epilepsy is greater than the risk of AED-induced teratogenesis, and drug treatment must be continued throughout pregnancy. For several reasons, it is a serious albeit common error to change medications for the sole purpose of reducing teratogenic risk. First, there is a risk of precipitating seizures that may reduce placental blood flow and impair fetal oxygenation. Second, the critical period of organogenesis has usually passed, and discontinuing an AED does not lower the risk of congenital malformations. Third, exposing the fetus to a second agent during the crossover period is akin to polytherapy and increases the teratogenic risk. If an epileptic woman presents after conception on effective mono-therapy, the AED, even if VPA, should generally not be changed. Lastly, hemorrhagic disease of the newborn may occur in neonates exposed to hepatic enzyme inducing AEDs, and requires special attention including maternal administration of oral vitamin K during the last month of pregnancy.

## NONMALPRACTICE LIABILITY

Neurologists must be cognizant of the morass of laws and regulations affecting their practice, raising the specter of adverse licensing sanctions, civil penalties, and crim-inal prosecution. This nonmalpractice liability penumbra generically includes creden-tialing disputes (professional licensure, hospital privileges, professional organization membership); reimbursement issues (fee disputes, program exclusion, denial of managed care contracts); and myriad ad personam (assault, manslaughter, homicide), economic (antikickback, self-referral, and antitrust violations; false claims), and regu-latory (violations of Americans with Disabilities Act, Health Insurance Portability and Accountability Act, Emergency Medical Treatment and Labor Act) crimes.[71] The rele-vant legal principles governing these diverse areas are substantially the same for all specialties and do not warrant review in this article.[72–78]

## FORENSIC NEUROLOGY LIABILITY

Many neurologists have addressed managed care constraints by expanding their practices to incorporate medical record reviews, independent medical examinations, and expert witness services. These lucrative activities generally do not invoke a physi-cian-patient relationship (thereby precluding a malpractice claim), but may lead to administrative penalties, civil lawsuits, and criminal prosecution. In particular, expert witness activities engender unique risks warranting further discussion.[79–81]

Anecdotal reports of neurologists advancing specious complaints are legion.[82] One review of expert witness testimony involving neurologists demonstrated improper testimony and erroneous conclusions regarding malpractice in 37% of cases.[83] It is "alarmingly common for accomplished neurologists to hire themselves out for [one-sided testimony]."[84] These partisan experts have flourished behind the common law expert witness immunity shield and lack of professional oversight. Today, there is a trend toward accountability with increased expert witness liability.[85] Friendly expert lawsuits (retaining party sues the expert) are increasing.[86] The traditional immunity is not absolute, and most states ruling on this issue have carved out exceptions to hold the expert liable for professional negligence.[87,88] One state Supreme Court explained that an "absence of immunity will... protect the litigant from the negligence of an incompetent professional."[89] This may represent an effective means of stemming the proliferation of negligent experts. Courts have also upheld suits against opposing and independent experts. Some jurisdictions continue to favor immunity for testimony, but that does not necessarily extend to nontestimonial expert activity (discovery of facts, literature search).[90] Nor does it protect the expert from criminal prosecution for improper testimony or misrepresentation of a degree or license.[91] The expert neurologist may also be liable for defamatory communications, and face administra-tive, civil, or criminal charges for negligent or intentional spoliation of evidence.[92]

Expert testimony and related activities are subject to increasing scrutiny by state licensing boards and professional organizations. The American Medical Association considers testimony to be the practice of medicine and subject to peer review, and supports state licensing boards in disciplining physicians who provide fraudulent testimony or false credentials.[93] Some boards have expanded the definition of medical practice to include testimony, allowing disciplinary action if warranted.[94] The AAN adopted *Qualifications and Guidelines for the Physician Expert Witness*, promulgated a code of professional conduct for legal expert testimony, and established a formal disciplinary procedure for errant neurologists with potential sanctions ranging from censure to expulsion.[95–98] AAN disciplinary actions may trigger the American Board of Psychiatry and Neurology to revoke certification.[99] The Seventh Circuit Court of Appeals validated these forms of discipline, stating in dicta that the American Academy of Neurologic Surgeons had a duty to discipline a neurosurgeon for irresponsible testimony.[100]

This complex, evolving area of law will create a more perilous liability climate for the future expert. The standard of care for expert services varies with the particular facts of each case, but salient guidelines applicable to all circumstances include the following: fulfill the AAN qualifications before accepting a case; review all relevant medical information; review the standard of care for the time of occurrence; perform adequate discovery of facts; review and understand the relevant literature; properly assemble and present the case; avoid losing or destroying any evidence; provide accurate, impartial, and truthful testimony; avoid conflicts of interest; do not discuss the case outside the course of litigation; and ensure compensation is reasonable, not contingent on outcome. It is important to remember that all deposition and trial testimony constitutes a permanent public record, which may be accessed from various national repositories. Some professional organizations maintain copies of depositions and court testimony (eg, the Defense Research Institute, in Chicago; Association of Trial Lawyers of America, in Washington; Collaborative Defense Network for Expert Witness Research; and various medical groups, such as the American Association of Neurological Surgeons).

## REFERENCES

1. Hunter J, Cassell-Stiga G, Doroshow J. True risk: medical liability, malpractice insurance and health care. Americans for Insurance Reform (a project of the Center for Justice and Democracy). Available at: http://www.insurance-reform. org. Accessed August 15, 2009.
2. Baker T. The medical malpractice myth. Chicago: Univ of Chicago Press; 2005.
3. Risk management review (Neurology). Rockville (MD): Physicians Insurers Association of America; 2008.
4. Id. at Exhibit 5.
5. Id at Exhibit 7.
6. Supra note 3 at Exhibit 5–2.
7. Supra note 3 at V and Exhibit 5.
8. Supra note 3 at Exhibit 6.
9. Supra note 3 at V.
10. Supra note 3 at Exhibit 6 for claims closed in 2007.
11. Evans R. Secondary headache disorders. Neurol Clin 2004;22:1–260.
12. Greer D. Management of subarachnoid hemorrhage, unruptured cerebral aneurysms, and arteriovenous malformations. In: Fisher M, editor. Stroke III: investigation and management, Handbook of clinical neurology, vol. 94, series 3. Amsterdam, Netherlands: Elsevier; 2009. p. 1239–49.
13. van Gijn J, Kerr RS, Rinkel GJ. Subarachnoid hemorrhage. Lancet 2007; 369(9558):306–18.
14. Rothrock J. Headaches due to vascular disorders. Neurol Clin 2004;22:21–37.
15. Supra note 3 at V and Exhibits 5-3, 8–9.

16. Mayer PL, Awad IA, Todor R, et al. Misdiagnosis of symptomatic cerebral aneurysm: prevalence and correlation with outcome at four institutions. Stroke 1996; 27:1558–63.

17. Available at: http://www.medlink.com. Accessed August 13, 2009.

18. Kelly ME, Dodd R, Steinberg GK. Subarachnoid hemorrhage. In: Fisher M, editor. Stroke part II: clinical manifestations and pathogenesis, Handbook of clinical neurology, vol. 93, series 3. Amsterdam, Netherlands: Elsevier; 2009. p. 791–808.

19. Bederson JB, Connolly ES, Batjer H, et al. Guidelines for the management of aneurysmal subarachnoid hemorrhage: a statement for healthcare professionals from a special writing group for the Stroke Council, American Heart Association: The American Academy of Neurology affirms the value of this statement as an educational tool for neurologists. Stroke 2009;40:994–1025.

20. Headache Classification Subcommittee of the International Headache Society. The international classification of headache disorders. 2nd edition. Cephalalgia 2004;24(Suppl 1):1–160.

21. American Academy of Neurology. Report of the quality standards subcommittee: practice parameter: evidence-based guidelines for migraine headache (an evidence-based review). Neurology 2000;26(55):754–62.

22. American Academy of Neurology 61st Annual Meeting. Headaches in adults, 2FC.001; acute treatment of migraine headache, 7TP.002. Seattle (WA), April 25 to May 2, 2009 (access via Marathon Multimedia Syllabi2view).

23. Silberstein S, Lipton R, Dodick D, editors. Wolff's headache and other pain. 8th edition. New York: Oxford University Press; 2008.

24. Evans RW. Diagnostic testing for migraine and other primary headaches. In: Evans RW, editor. Migraine and other primary headaches. Philadelphia (PA): WB Saunders Company. Neurol Clin 2009;27(2):393–415.

25. Frishberg B, Rosenberg J, Matchar D, et al. Evidence-based guidelines in the primary care setting: neuroimaging in patients with nonacute headache. US Headache Consortium, Available at: http://www.aan.com/professionals/practice/pdfs/g10088.pdf. Accessed December 3, 2009.

26. Richter v Northwest Memorial Hospital, 532 N.E. 2d 269 (Ill. App. 1988).

27. Sandrini G, Friberg L, Janig W, et al. Neuropsychological tests and neuroimaging procedures in nonacute headache: guidelines and recommendations. Eur J Neurol 2004;11(4):217–24.

28. Available at: http://www.cdc.gov. Accessed August 10, 2009.

29. The National Institute of Neurological Disorders and Stroke rt-PA Stroke Study Group. Tissue plasminogen activator for acute ischemic stroke. N Engl J Med 1995;333:1581–7.

30. Hacke W, Kaste M, Fieschi C, et al. Intravenous thrombolysis with recombinant tissue plasminogen activator for acute hemispheric stroke: the European Cooperative Acute Stroke Study (ECASS). JAMA 1995;274:1017–25.

31. Hacke W, Kaste M, Fieschi C, et al. Randomized double-blind placebo-controlled trial of thrombolytic therapy with intravenous altepase in acute ischemic stroke (ECASS II). Lancet 1998;352:1245–51.

32. Marler JR, Tilley BC, Lu M, et al. Early stroke treatment associated with better outcome: the NINDS rt-PA Stroke Study. Neurology 2000;55:1649–55.

33. Clark WM, Wissman S, Albers GW, et al. Recombinant tissue-type plasminogen activator (altepase) for ischemic stroke 3 to 5 hours after symptom onset. The ATLANTIS study: a randomized controlled trial. JAMA 1999;282:2019–26.

34. Hacke W, Donnan G, Fieschi C, et al. Association of outcome with early stroke treatment: pooled analysis of ATLANTIS, ECASS, and NINDS rt-PA stroke trials. Lancet 2004;363:768–74.
35. Hacke W, Kaste M, Bluhmki E, et al. Thrombolysis with alteplase 3 to 4.5 hours after acute ischemic stroke. N Engl J Med 2008;359:1317–29.
36. del Zoppo GJ, Saver JL, Jauch EC, et al. American Heart Association Stroke Council. Expansion of the time window for treatment of acute ischemic stroke with intravenous tissue plasminogen activator: a science advisory from the American Heart Association/American Stroke Association. Stroke 2009;40:2945–8.
37. American Academy of Neurology. Report of the quality standards subcommittee: practice advisory: thrombolytic therapy for acute ischemic stroke (summary statement). 1996 (Reaffirmed February 18, 2003).
38. Adams HP, del Zoppo GJ, Alberts MJ, et al. Guidelines for the early management of adults with ischemic stroke: a guideline from the American Heart Association/American Stroke Association Stroke Council, Clinical Cardiology Council, Cardiovascular Radiology and Intervention Council, and the Atherosclerotic Peripheral Vascular Disease and Quality of Care Outcomes in Research Interdisciplinary Working Groups: The American Academy of Neurology affirms the value of this guideline as an education tool for neurologists. Stroke 2007;38:1655–711 [Erratum: Stroke 2007;38(6):e38, 2007;38(9):e96].
39. Levine SR, Adamowicz D, Johnston KC. Primary stroke center certification. Continuum 2008;14(6):98–116.
40. Adams, Harold P, Brott T, et al. Guidelines for the early management of patients with ischemic stroke: a scientific statement from the Stroke Council of the American Stroke Association. Stroke 2003;34:1056–83.
41. Schellinger P, Kohrmann M, Hacke W. Thrombolytic therapy for acute stroke. In: Fisher M, editor. Stroke III: investigation and management, Handbook of clinical neurology, vol. 94, series 3. Amsterdam, Netherlands: Elsevier; 2009. p. 1155–93.
42. Backlund v University of Washington, 975 P.2d 950 (1999).
43. American Academy of Neurology. Consent issues in the management of cerebrovascular diseases: a position paper of the American Academy of Neurology Ethics and Humanities Subcommittee. Neurology 1999;53:9–11.
44. Canterbury v Spence, 464 F.2d 772 (D.C. Cir. 1972), cert. denied, 408 U.S. 1064 (1974).
45. Coull BM, Williams LS, Goldstein LB, et al. Anticoagulants and antiplatelet agents in acute ischemic stroke: report of the Joint Stroke Guideline Development Committee of the American Academy of Neurology and the American Stroke Association (a Division of the American Heart Association). Neurology 2002;59:13–22 (Reaffirmed August 2, 2008).
46. Schwartz NE, Diener H, Albers GW. Antithrombotic agents for stroke prevention. In: Fisher M, editor. Stroke III: investigation and management, Handbook of clinical neurology, vol. 94, series 3. Amsterdam, Netherlands: Elsevier; 2009. p. 1277–94.
47. English J, Smith W. Cardio-embolic stroke. In: Fisher M, editor. Stroke II: clinical manifestations and pathogenesis, Handbook of clinical neurology, vol. 93, series 3. Amsterdam, Netherlands: Elsevier; 2009. p. 719–49.
48. Sloan MA. Use of anticoagulant agents for stroke prevention. Continuum 2005;11(4):97–127.
49. Freeman WD, Aguilar MI. Stroke prevention in atrial fibrillation and other major cardiac sources of embolism. Neurol Clin 2008;26:1129–60.

50. American Academy of Neurology. Report of the quality standards subcommittee: practice parameter: stroke prevention in patients with nonvalvular atrial fibrillation. Neurology 1998;51:671–3.

51. American Academy of Neurology 61st Annual Meeting. Neurology update i: stroke, 3FC.002. Seattle (WA), April 25 to May 2, 2009.

52. Rothwell P. Carotid endarterectomy, stenting, and other prophylactic interventions. In: Fischer M, editor. Stroke III: investigation and management, Handbook of clinical neurology, vol. 94, series 3. Amsterdam, Netherlands: Elsevier; 2009. p. 1295–325.

53. Chaturvedi S, Bruno A, Feasby T, et al. Carotid endarterectomy: an evidence based review: report of the therapeutics and technology assessment subcommittee of the American Academy of Neurology. Neurology 2005;65:794–801 (Reaffirmed February 9, 2000).

54. Easton D, Saver J, Albers G, et al. Definition and evaluation of transient ischemic attack: a scientific statement for healthcare professionals from the American Heart Association/American Stroke Association Stroke Council; Council on Cardiovascular Surgery and Anesthesia; Council on Cardiovascular Radiology and Intervention; Council on Cardiovascular Nursing; and the Interdisciplinary Council on Peripheral Vascular Disease: The American Academy of Neurology affirms the value of this statement as an educational tool for neurologists. Stroke 2009;40:2276–93.

55. Fairhead J, Mehta Z, Rothwell P. Population-based study of delays in carotid imaging and surgery and the risk of recurrent stroke. Neurology 2005;65(3): 371–5.

56. American Academy of Neurology 61st Annual Meeting. Update on endovascular treatment of cerebrovascular diseases, 7AC.005. Seattle (WA), April 25 to May 2, 2009.

57. Browne R, Holmes G. Epilepsy. N Engl J Med 2001;344:1145–51.

58. Engel J, Pedley T, editors. Epilepsy: a comprehensive textbook. 2nd edition. Philadelphia: Lippincott-Raven Publishers; 2008.

59. Bortz J. Neuropsychiatric and memory issues in epilepsy. Mayo Clin Proc 2003; 78:781–7.

60. Krumholz A, Wiebe S, Gronseth G, et al. Practice parameter: evaluating an apparent unprovoked first seizure in adults (an evidence based review): report of the Quality Standards Subcommittee of the American Academy of Neurology and the American Epilepsy Society. Neurology 2007;69:1996–2007.

61. Available at: http://www.efa.org. Accessed August 11, 2009.

62. Tarasoff v Regents of the University of California, 551 P.32d 334 (Cal. 1976).

63. Harden v Dalrymple 883 F.Supp. 963 (D Del. 1995). Cf. Praesel v. Johnson 41 Tex. Super. Ct. J. 630 (1998).

64. Hirtz D, Thurman D, Gwinn-Hardy K, et al. How common are the common neurological disorders? Neurology 2007;68:326–37.

65. Morrow J, Russell A, Guthrie E, et al. Malformations risks of antiepileptic drugs in pregnancy: a prospective study from the UK epilepsy and pregnancy register. J Neurol Neurosurg Psychiatr 2006;77:193–8.

66. Holmes L, Harvey E, Coull B, et al. The teratogenicity of anticonvulsant drugs. N Engl J Med 2001;344(15):1132–8.

67. American Academy of Neurology. Practice parameter update: management issues for women with epilepsy: focus on pregnancy (an evidence based review): teratogenesis and perinatal outcomes. Report of the Quality Standards Subcommittee and Therapeutics and Technology Assessment Subcommittee of

the American Academy of Neurology and American Epilepsy Society. Neurology 2009;73:133–41.

68. Wyszynski D, Nambisan M, Survet T, et al. Increased rate of major malformations in offspring exposed to valproate during pregnancy. Neurology 2005;64:961–5.

69. American Academy of Neurology. Practice parameter update: management issues for women with epilepsy – focus on pregnancy (an evidence based review): obstetrical complications and change in seizure frequency. Report of the Quality Standards Subcommittee and Therapeutics and Technology Assessment Subcommittee of the American Academy of Neurology and American Epilepsy Society. Neurology 2009;73:126–32.

70. American Academy of Neurology. Practice parameter update: management issues for women with epilepsy: focus on pregnancy (an evidence based review): vitamin K, folic acid, blood levels, and breastfeeding. Report of the Quality Standards Subcommittee and Therapeutics and Technology Assessment Subcommittee of the American Academy of Neurology and American Epilepsy Society. Neurology 2009;73:142–9.

71. Beresford HR. Neurology and the law: private litigation and public policy. Philadelphia: F.A. Davis Co; 1998.

72. Miles J. Health care and antitrust law: principles and practice. Eagan (MN): West Publishing; 2009.

73. American Bar Association, health law section. 7th National institute on civil false claims act and qui tam enforcement, 2008.

74. American Health Lawyers Association. Health law practice guide. 2nd edition. Eagan (MN): West Publishing; 2009.

75. Boumil M, Sharpe D. Boumil and Sharpe's liability in medicine and public health (American Casebook Series). Eagan (MN): West Publishing; 2004.

76. Rozovsky F, Giles C, Kadzielski M. Health care credentialing: a guide to innovative practices. New York: Wolters Kluwer: Aspen Publishers; 2009.

77. Rozovsky F. Consent to treatment: a practical guide. 4th edition. New York: Wolters Kluwer: Aspen Publishers; 2008.

78. Boyle L. HIPAA: a guide to health care privacy and security law. New York: Wolters Kluwer: Aspen Publishers; 2008.

79. Shandell R, Smith P. Securing the medical expert. In: Shandell R, Smith P, editors. The preparation and trial of medical malpractice cases. New York: Law Journal Press; 2008. 7–1 to 7–24.

80. Freemon F. The origin of the medical expert witness. J Legal Med 2001;22:349–73.

81. Matson J, Daou S, Soper J. Effective expert witnessing: practices for the 21st century. 4th edition. New York: CRC Press; 2004.

82. McAbee G. Improper expert witness testimony: existing and proposed mechanisms of oversight. J Leg Med 1998;19:257–72.

83. Safran A, Skydell B, Ropper S. Expert witness testimony in neurology: Massachusetts experience 1980–1990. Neurol Chronicle 1992;44:2477–84.

84. Holtz S. The neurologist as an expert witness. AAN Education Program Syllabus 7DS.003 (2002).

85. Hanson R. Witness immunity under attack: disarming hired guns. Wake Forest Law Rev 1996;31:497.

86. Aufrichtig v Lowell, 650 N.E.2d 401 (N.Y. 1995).

87. Butz v Economou, 438 U.S. 478 (1978).

88. Restatement (Second) of Torts §588.

89. Marrogi v Howard, 805 So.2d 1118 (La. 2002).

90. Gustafson v Mazer, 54 P.3d 743 (2002).

91. Brennan M, Dilenschneider D, Levin M, et al. Finding and researching experts and their testimony. Available at: http://www.expertwitnesswhitepaper.com. Accessed August 13, 2009.

92. Hite C, Taylor R. Spoliation of evidence in state and federal courts in Virginia. J of Civil Litigation 2007;XIX:391–405.

93. Weintraub M. Expert witness testimony. Neurol Clin 1999;17:363–9.

94. Cohen F. The expert medical witness in legal perspective. J Legal Med 2004;25: 185–209.

95. Williams M, Mackin G, Beresford H, et al. American Academy of Neurology qualifications and guidelines for the physician expert witness. Neurology 2006;66:13–4.

96. §6.4 Code of Professional Conduct, American Academy of Neurology Professional Association 2008.

97. Available at: http://www.aan.com/go/diooiplinary. Accessed August 12, 2009.

98. Williams M, Nelson S. Impeccable or impeachable? Guidance for physician expert witnesses. AAN Education Program Syllabus 5PC.002 (2009).

99. American Board of Psychiatry and Neurology: General information and board policies, §B.4. revocation of certificates, 2009.

100. Austin v American Association of Neurological Surgeons, 253 F.3d 967 (7th Cir. 2001).

# Consent Issues in Neurology

Emily B. Rubin, JD, MD[a],*, James L. Bernat, MD[b,c]

## KEYWORDS

- Informed consent • Valid consent, Shared decision making
- Emergency exception • tPA • Surrogate
- Do-not-resuscitate • Carotid endarterectomy

The requirement that doctors obtain valid consent from patients before providing medical treatment has long been ingrained in both legal doctrine and medical ethics. As Gert and Culver[1] state:

*It is an ideal outcome of the consent process for patients to make treatment decisions which are based solely on their own stable ranking of the harms and benefits involved, as these rankings are applied to the treatment choices at hand.*

Although valid consent to treatment should underpin all relationships between clinicians and patients, practitioners often treat consent instead as simply the requirement to obtain a patient's signature on a form before an invasive procedure. Studies have shown that failure of clinicians to provide sufficient information about patients' conditions and treatment options is the most common source of patient dissatisfaction.[2]

This article summarizes the foundations of the informed consent doctrine, discusses the recent evolution in thinking about consent and medical decision making, and addresses common situations in neurologic practice that pose challenges in obtaining valid consent.

## FOUNDATIONS OF THE INFORMED-CONSENT DOCTRINE

The doctrine of informed consent has foundations in both law and ethics. The legal doctrine, developed in a series of legal cases between the early and mid–twentieth century, is based on two core principles: (1) A physician has a fiduciary duty to his patient based on the trust and confidence that the patient places in him or her, and

[a] Departments of Internal Medicine and Pediatrics, Massachusetts General Hospital, 55 Fruit Street, Boston, MA 02114, USA
[b] Dartmouth Medical School, 1 Rope Ferry Road, Hanover, NH 03755, USA
[c] Department of Neurology, Dartmouth-Hitchcock Medical Center, 1 Medical Center Drive, Lebanon, NH 03756, USA
* Corresponding author. Departments of Internal Medicine and Pediatrics, Massachusetts General Hospital, 55 Fruit Street, Boston, MA 02114.
*E-mail address:* emmyrubin@gmail.com (E.B. Rubin).

Neurol Clin 28 (2010) 459–473
doi:10.1016/j.ncl.2009.11.007
0733-8619/10/$ – see front matter © 2010 Elsevier Inc. All rights reserved.

**neurologic.theclinics.com**

it is a breach of faith for the physician not to provide adequate information to the patient; and (2) individuals have the right to self-determination, which requires that they be allowed to make decisions regarding what will be done with their own bodies.[3]

Legal claims by patients that a clinician failed to elicit informed consent before providing medical treatment were originally treated as battery, and patients treated without proper consent were considered to have been unlawfully touched in violation of laws against battery.[3] As Justice Cardozo[4] famously stated in the 1914 case *Schloendorff v Society of New York Hospital*:

> *Every human being of adult years and sound mind has a right to determine what shall be done with his own body and a surgeon who performs an operation without his patient's consent commits an assault for which he is liable in damages.*

The case law ultimately evolved so that a complaint that a claim of treatment without appropriate consent is now treated as negligence rather than battery. A doctor who fails to solicit proper consent to treatment is considered to have violated the professional duty to provide a patient with sufficient information to make a medical decision and is liable for malpractice.[3] Patients generally must prove that the physician did not provide adequate information about the treatment and that the patient would not have consented to assume the risk had it been disclosed.[5]

The ethical doctrine of informed consent is based on the concept of respect for personal autonomy, which is in turn derived from moral rules not to deprive an individual of freedom and not to disable.[6] The focus on autonomy in medical decision making, which was a departure from the traditional paternalistic model that previously dominated medical practice, strengthened in the mid–twentieth century in response to the evolving legal landscape and concern about civil liberties in the wake of Nazi atrocities and the Tuskegee Syphilis Study.[7] Although there is disagreement between moral philosophers and ethicists about the most appropriate way to frame the analysis of autonomy (some describe it as a principle and others as a concept derived from moral rules), it is commonly understood that patients should have the right to make medical decisions based on their own priorities and values.

## ELEMENTS OF VALID CONSENT

Informed consent has three basic elements. First, the patient must have the capacity to consent to or refuse the proposed medical intervention. Second, the physician must present adequate information to the patient about the proposed medical intervention. Third, the patient's decision must be made freely and without coercion by a clinician or any third party.[6]

Many ethicists and other observers prefer the term *valid consent* or *effective consent* to *informed consent*. The term *informed consent* implies that the only relevant factor in determining whether consent is adequate is whether the patient has received sufficient information, essentially disregarding the additional requirements of patient capacity and lack of coercion.[8,9] The authors therefore use the term *valid consent* in the remainder of this article to indicate consent that satisfies the three elements described above.

Although this article discusses consent as it relates to certain specific medical interventions, valid consent is best conceptualized as a process and not an event. Ideally, clinicians and patients should be engaged in an ongoing process of sharing information sharing and making decisions throughout a patient's course of treatment. In this process, the clinicians provide information and expertise to help patients make decisions consistent with their own values.

### Capacity to Consent to Treatment

A patient has capacity to make medical decisions for himself when he or she

*possesses the mental capacity to understand the relevant medical information, to appreciate the medical situation and the possible consequences of treatment decisions, and to manipulate this information rationally to reach a decision.*[8]

This article uses the word *competent* to describe a patient who has the capacity to make medical decisions. This ethical construct should not be confused with the legal determination of competence, which is a separate issue.

In situations involving neurologic impairment, assessing capacity can be particularly difficult. Aphasia or other types of cognitive impairment, however, do not necessarily render a patient incompetent to make his or her own medical decisions. Specific instruments should be used to help clinicians assess competency in patients with Alzheimer dementia, aphasia, or other cognitive impairments.[8] In assessing a patient's capacity, particularly in a neurologic emergency, clinicians should inform the patient clearly that he or she is being asked to make a treatment decision and ask the patient directly whether he or she feels able to make a decision.[9]

Although there is consensus among ethicists about the criteria for assessing capacity, there is disagreement about how to define capacity in a patient who under-stands and appreciates the information received, but proposes to make a decision about treatment that most people would consider irrational. Gert and Culver[6] provide examples, including that of a severely depressed woman who understands that elec-troconvulsive treatment (ECT) likely would prevent her death, but refuses it because she is afraid of ECT. She technically understands and appreciates the information conveyed to her, but has what they consider an irrational fear of ECT.

Observers who believe that patients in this category should be treated against their expressed wishes either (1) define competence in a way that excludes these patients, or (2) define these patients as competent but assert that the exercise of paternalism is justified when a patient who is competent to make medical decisions proposes to make a decision that most would consider irrational. In the first category, Gert and colleagues[6] suggest that the best definition of competence is the "ability to make a rational decision." They assert that no one voluntarily makes an irrational decision and that anyone proposing to make an irrational decision must be under the influence of a condition that destroys the person's ability to do so (eg, a cognitive or volitional disability or phobia). They would classify a patient who proposes to make a treatment decision that the vast majority of people would view as irrational under the circum-stances as incompetent to make that particular medical decision.

Other observers treat competence and irrationality as distinct concepts, noting that a patient who is competent to make treatment decisions can nevertheless make what seems to the physician to be an irrational decision—that is, a decision that is likely to cause harm to the patient without adequate justification or counterbalancing benefit. Whether one views irrationality as a marker of incompetence or as a potential rationale for exercising paternalism, the fundamental question remains the same: Is it ever permissible for a physician to impose treatment on a patient who understands and appreciates the information given but proposes to make a decision that seems to the physician to be irrational? The authors discuss this question briefly in the section on paternalism below.

### Adequate Information

The second criterion for valid consent is the provision of adequate information about the risks and benefits of the proposed intervention and its alternatives. The key question is: What type and amount of information constitutes "adequate information" in a given situation? It is well accepted that physicians have an ethical obligation to give patients, at a minimum, the following information as a prerequisite to valid consent: (1) the significant risks and benefits associated with the proposed intervention, (2) any alternatives to the proposed intervention and their accompanying risks and benefits, and (3) the nature of the patient's condition and the likely course of that condition without any intervention.

The difficulty lies in determining how much specificity and breadth are appropriate or, in fact, morally required. Physicians are not required to outline every risk associated with a given medical treatment. The importance of disclosure of a given risk is generally considered to be a function of two factors: (1) the likelihood of the event and (2) the severity of the outcome if the event should occur. Very likely events, regardless of severity (eg, pain following abdominal surgery), and rare but very severe events (eg, death during abdominal surgery) are generally considered to be part of the required disclosure.

Although physicians ultimately should be guided by ethical considerations in determining how to communicate with patients, the legal standards related to informed consent are nevertheless instructive in thinking about what degree of disclosure is appropriate. There are two different legal standards for assessing whether the information given to a patient is adequate: (1) the physician-based standard and (2) the patient-based standard. Roughly half of states follow the physician-based standard and the other half use the patient-based standard. Under the physician-based standard, a patient bringing a claim for breach of informed consent must show (1) that a reasonably prudent practitioner would have provided the information and (2) that the patient would not have undergone the procedure had that information been given.[3] Under the patient-based standard, a physician must disclose all "material risks." That is, if a physician believes that a reasonable person in the patient's position "would be likely to attach significance to the risk or cluster of risks in deciding whether or not to forego the proposed therapy," the physician must disclose the risk.[10]

The type of information that a reasonable physician should disclose or that a reasonable patient would want to know is evolving as medical practice becomes more complex, as the delivery of medical care becomes increasingly fragmented, and as the data about harms and benefits associated with particular treatments become more detailed and accessible. Physicians should be as specific as possible in describing potential risks and benefits to maximize the accuracy of the information and the utility of the information to the patient. Wherever possible, quantitative outcomes information, such as volume-outcome studies (eg, data about the outcomes of different procedures at high-volume vs low-volume centers), numbers needed to treat, and numbers needed to harm should be discussed with patients. Where a treatment is intended to minimize the risk of a certain outcome (eg, warfarin therapy to prevent stroke in atrial fibrillation), clinicians should couch risk information in terms of absolute risk reduction rather than relative risk reduction to maximize the patient's understanding of the true benefits of the proposed intervention.[10]

Finally, several studies have shown significant variation in the preferences of patients regarding medical information sharing and decision making. Mazur and colleagues[11] found in one study that 22.5% of patients preferred physician-based decision making regarding invasive medical procedures and that greater than 40% of the patients found the doctor's opinion most important for making their decision. In a separate study, they found that 21.4% of patients preferred physician-based decision making and that 43% preferred disclosure of risks to be done in qualitative terms only without quantitative information.[12] Given the wide variation in patient preference, it is appropriate for physicians to take into account a given patient's preferences for information sharing. In the absence of explicit instructions to the contrary, however, physicians should err on the side of full disclosure of significant risks in as quantitative terms as possible.

### Absence of Coercion

The third and final element of valid consent is the absence of coercion from any source. Gert and colleagues[13] define coercion as:

> the use of such powerful negative incentives (for example, threats of severe pain or significant deprivation of freedom) that it would be unreasonable to expect a patient to resist them.

It is not coercive for a physician to strongly recommend treatment if the physician believes that the treatment would be the best course of action. It is, in fact, the physician's responsibility to do so. The physician does, however, have a professional and ethical responsibility to present all alternative treatment options and to explain clearly the reasoning for recommending one course over another. As Gert and colleagues[13] observe:

> One of the most difficult tasks is to present all the relevant information in a manner that genuinely allows patients to make free, informed decisions based on their values or beliefs, but yet to present it forcefully enough that patients are most likely to make what doctors believe to be rationally acceptable decisions.

Clinicians must understand that the way in which they frame the discussion of a proposed intervention can have a profound impact on how a patient makes decisions and can, at the extreme, exert a coercive effect on patients. Studies have shown, for example, that the majority of patients choosing between two treatment options with similar benefits will choose the one couched in terms of relative risk reduction rather than the one couched in terms of absolute risk reduction because the relative risk numbers tend to magnify the benefit.[10] Tversky and Kahneman[14] demonstrated that choices framed in terms of gains (eg, the chance of saving lives) tend to be risk averse, whereas choices framed in terms of losses (eg, the risk of death) are generally more risk-taking. Murphy[15] studied decision making in cardiopulmonary resuscitation (CPR) and found that a patient's decision on resuscitation depends largely on how the question is framed and whether likely outcomes are specifically addressed This article discusses this effect further in the section on do-not-resuscitate (DNR) orders.

Although clinicians usually should offer an opinion regarding the optimal course of action for a given patient, they should make every effort to present factual information as objectively as possible and then offer an opinion, making the line separating information and opinion very clear.

## WRITTEN DOCUMENTATION OF CONSENT

There is much more to the process of valid consent than obtaining a signed consent form. It is generally understood, however, that certain medical interventions should not be undertaken without first documenting in writing the provision of valid consent. There are no explicit standards delineating which specific interventions should be preceded by written consent and hospitals differ in their requirements regarding written consent forms. One 2003 survey of intensivists and general internists showed that there was little uniformity regarding the use of written consent forms for commonly performed invasive medical procedures. Written consent forms were routinely obtained for gastrointestinal endoscopy, bronchoscopy, and medical research, but generally not for Foley catheterization and nasogastric intubation. Practice was mixed regarding written consent forms for central venous catheterization and diagnostic procedures, such as thoracentesis and paracentesis.[16] Some hospitals ask patients to sign "blanket" consent forms on admission, which are then interpreted to signify consent to various diagnostic and therapeutic procedures during the admission. As a general principle, the more invasive a medical intervention is and the higher the accompanying risks, the more important it is to document the consent process through a written form before a specific procedure or intervention.

## TREATMENT WITHOUT VALID CONSENT

Medical treatment in the absence of valid consent is appropriate only when (1) a surrogate consents on behalf of the patient, (2) the emergency exception to valid consent applies, or (3) paternalism can be rigorously justified.

### Surrogate Decision Making

When a patient is deemed incompetent to make medical decisions for himself, a surrogate decision-maker should be identified to provide consent for medical interventions. Ideally, through a durable power of attorney or other document appointing a health care proxy, a patient will have legally authorized a specific individual to act on his or her behalf. In the absence of such clarity, clinicians should first turn to the nuclear family for surrogate decision-making under the well-accepted (though not always accurate) assumption that nuclear family members are likely to be most concerned for the patient's welfare, and are in the best position to know the patient's values and wishes concerning health care.

The overarching goal of surrogate decision-making is to make a decision on behalf of the patient that is consistent with what the patient would decide if he or she were capable of making that decision. Family members or other surrogates are therefore ethically bound to attempt to make decisions that the patient would make if he or she were competent to do so. If a patient has made explicit, relevant statements related to his or her wishes regarding health care (either in a living will or in an informal setting), the surrogates are bound to follow those wishes. In the absence of expressed wishes, the surrogate has a moral duty to consider the patient's overall values and life goals and make health care decisions consistent with those values and goals. Finally, if little is known about the patient's specific values, the surrogate must attempt to make decisions in the "best interests" of the patient, taking into account all of the benefits and burdens of treatment or test.[8]

### Emergency Exception

Consent is presumed in true medical emergencies where it is not possible to secure valid consent from the patient or a surrogate. As Fleck and Hayes[17] describe, the moral legitimacy of claiming this exemption depends on the following conditions being met:

*(1) There is widely accepted and incontrovertible evidence that this emergent therapy is likely to have a positive therapeutic result, (2) delay in therapy will almost certainly have adverse or irreversible consequences, (3) there are no alternative therapies available that would be nearly as safe and effective, and (4) treating physicians are confident that reasonable persons who, given this possible circumstance to consider in advance, would agree to the therapeutic intervention and agree to forego explicit informed consent.*

Generally, presumed consent applies to only the standard accepted treatment for any given condition.

### Paternalism

A detailed discussion of paternalism in medicine is beyond the scope of this article. In nearly all instances, paternalism cannot be justified. In the rare (and largely theoretical) case in which a patient proposes to make a medical decision that is seriously irrational and the proposed treatment will clearly avoid death or severe disability while causing significantly less harm than it prevents, a physician may be justified in treating the patient against his or her will. An example would be a young woman with acute appendicitis who refuses surgery because she does not want to have a scar.[8]

One difficulty with acting in violation of a patient's wishes is determining that the decision of the patient is truly irrational (ie, that the reasons given for the decision are inadequate or that the patient is accepting harm with no discernible benefit in return). This is inherently a subjective determination and any clinician proposing to overrule refusal of treatment by a patient should take great lengths to ensure that no religious justification or legitimate value judgment underlies the patient's refusal. In addition, the clinician should explain to the patient why the clinician believes the patient's decision is irrational and make every attempt to convince the patient to accept treatment, with the help of family and friends if necessary. Treatment should be forced on a patient only as a last resort and only if the harms inflicted by forcible treatment are reasonably considered to be outweighed by the harms of doing nothing.[8]

### THE EVOLUTION OF SHARED DECISION MAKING

Perhaps because of its history as a legal doctrine, many clinicians view informed consent as obtaining a signature on a form before an invasive procedure to avoid legal liability. But valid consent is more properly viewed as a process of communication that proceeds continuously throughout the course of medical treatment. It is a dynamic process between physician and patient that enables the patient to decide whether the overall course of treatment is consistent with his or her values and priorities.

The model of medical decision making that has emerged over the last decade in recognition of the importance of ongoing collaboration between physicians and patients is called *shared decision making*. Ezekiel and Linda Emanuel[18] defined a model of medical decision making called *the deliberative model*, under which:

> clinicians help patients define their best interests, provide treatment alternatives through which the interests can be served, and assist the patients in deciding which alternative is best.

Shared decision making is a variation on that theme, in which physicians bring their knowledge and expertise to bear and patients share their own preferences and values in an effort to decide which option is best for them. Brock[19] describes the process:

> ...[t]he idea here is that, on one hand, uninformed patient choices or consent will lead to decisions that fail to best serve patient interests—thus, the need for physician participation. On the other hand, decisions guided by physician's values will fail to reflect patients' self-determination interest in making important decisions about their lives for themselves—thus the need for patient participation.

Hallmarks of shared decision making include provision of the clinician's perspective, the patient's perspective, and some type of decision aid that provides information to the patient about the various treatment choices.[20] Shared decision making has been specifically embraced in situations in which there are multiple reasonable treatment options and legitimate uncertainty about which option would be best for a certain patient. One relevant example is the decision whether to pursue surgical or medical management for lumbar spinal stenosis, a decision that patients at Dartmouth-Hitchcock Medical Center (DHMC) often make with the assistance of the DHMC Center for Shared Decision Making.

There are different perspectives on how shared decision making fits into the medical decision framework. Whitney and colleagues[21] have suggested that informed consent and shared decision making be treated as separate processes, with informed consent applicable to situations in which a "single correct clinical response exists" and shared decision making is reserved for circumstances in which two or more "medically reasonable" choices exist. King and Moulton,[3] on the other hand, have suggested that shared decision making is a more appropriate governing paradigm than informed consent for all medical decision making and should replace informed consent as the legal and ethical standard for sharing medical information.

We believe that shared decision making is best viewed as a natural evolution of the doctrine of valid consent, not as a separate decision-making framework. Not every medical encounter lends itself to or permits the type of extensive information sharing and deliberative processes that take place in dedicated centers for shared decision making. Clinicians should, however, incorporate the spirit of shared decision making into their practices and seek to provide care that represents a meeting of their knowledge and medical perspective with their patients' priorities and values.

## SPECIFIC EXAMPLES OF CONSENT ISSUES IN NEUROLOGY

Difficult ethical issues involving consent arise routinely in the practice of neurology. The authors have chosen three examples: (1) the use of intravenous tissue-type plasminogen activator (tPA) in ischemic stroke patients, (2) the referral of patients for carotid endarterectomy (CEA) for internal carotid artery stenosis, and (3) the implementation of DNR orders.

### Intravenous Tissue-type Plasminogen Activator in Ischemic Stroke

It is well understood that, although intravenous tPA may be autonomy saving for sufferers of ischemic stroke, it is not life saving and carries significant risks of intracranial hemorrhage. The seminal study, done by the National Institute of Neurologic Disorders (NINDS) and the Stroke rt-PA Stroke Study Group found improvement in functional outcome at 6 months in selected patients in whom intravenous tPA had been administered within 3 hours of the first symptom of an ischemic stroke, with an absolute risk reduction in poor outcomes of 13.1%. The rate of symptomatic intracranial hemorrhage was, however, 10 times as high in patients receiving intravenous tPA as it was in patients not receiving the therapy. There was no difference in 3-month mortality rates between the treatment and placebo groups.[22]

The outcomes of additional studies at the community hospital level have raised concerns about the ability of community hospitals to implement intravenous tPA in ways that replicate the benefits seen in the NINDS trial and minimize the risks of intracranial hemorrhage. In a 1-year study of area hospitals in Cleveland, for example, 15.7% of patients treated with tPA had a symptomatic intracranial hemorrhage and the in-hospital mortality rate for those patients treated with tPA (15.7%) was more than double that of the matched patients who did not receive tPA (7.2%).[23] Nevertheless, it has become common practice in certain institutions to administer intravenous tPA within 3 hours of onset of ischemic stroke once hemorrhage has been ruled out and other risk factors have been excluded. The American Heart Association lists intravenous tPA within 3 hours of onset of ischemic stroke symptoms as a class IA recommendation ("definitely recommended").

The neurologic impairments of some ischemic stroke patients and the time constraints on the use of intravenous tPA can make it challenging to assess capacity and secure valid consent before the administration of tPA. In light of these difficulties and of the benefits demonstrated by the NINDS trial, some observers have suggested that the administration of intravenous tPA in ischemic stroke should be covered by the emergency exemption to the informed consent doctrine discussed above.[9,24] Although the American Heart Association lists intravenous tPA as a class IA recommendation in appropriate candidates, other professional associations have questioned whether the use of intravenous tPA in acute ischemic stroke should be considered standard of care. The American Academy of Emergency Medicine (AAEM) has stated:

> It is the position of the American Academy of Emergency Medicine that objective evidence regarding the efficacy, safety, and applicability of tPA for acute ischemic stroke is insufficient to warrant its classification as standard of care. Until additional evidence clarifies such controversies, physicians are advised to use their discretion when considering its use. Given the cited absence of definitive evidence, AAEM believes it is inappropriate to claim that either use or non-use of intravenous thrombolytic therapy constitutes a standard of care issue in the treatment of stroke.[25]

In 1999, the American Academy of Neurology Ethics and Humanities Subcommittee took the position that intravenous tPA for acute ischemic stroke should not be considered the unequivocal standard of care. The subcommittee found the emergency treatment doctrine that permits presumed consent is inapplicable because many patients or surrogates refuse the therapy based on the risk/benefit profile. Accordingly, the subcommittee concluded that patient or surrogate consent is required before the administration of intravenous tPA to ischemic stroke patients.[26] With additional studies of efficacy, safety, and patient and surrogate preferences that have been published over the past decade, it plans to revisit this recommendation.

The essence of the emergency exception is the assumption that the vast majority of patients would consent to the treatment if time and circumstances permitted a proper capacity assessment and disclosure of the risks and benefits. The risk/benefit analysis associated with tPA in ischemic stroke is simply too personal to make that assumption. Notwithstanding the evident difficulties of obtaining consent in the context of acute stroke, this is exactly the type of situation in which a valid consent process is critical. The decision whether to accept an increased risk of death in the short term in exchange for the avoidance or amelioration of severe neurologic disability in the long term is an extremely personal decision that depends on an individual's own values and priorities. Acceptance and rejection of tPA are both completely rational choices and the appropriate decision for any given individual requires that individual to weigh of risk of death against risk of neurologic disability.

White-Bateman and colleagues[9] suggest that there are three major contraindications to direct informed consent in stroke patients: (1) impaired consciousness, (2) significant Wernicke aphasia, and (3) striking deficiency in executive function. In the absence of such circumstances, it is ethically imperative that clinicians assess the capacity of the patient using tools that determine whether the patient understands that he or she is being asked to make a choice about medical treatment. As White-Bateman and colleagues suggest, physicians should use concise structured oral presentations that focus on the fact that tPA is not life saving, but autonomy saving. If the patient lacks capacity, a surrogate should be called on to make a decision on the patient's behalf. If no surrogate is present or willing to make a decision, then intravenous tPA should not be administered.

It would be ideal for physicians to discuss with high-risk patients the issue of intravenous tPA administration before a stroke and to elicit the patient's preferences for the use of intravenous thrombolytic drugs as part of a broader process of health care planning and advance directive discussion. Some commentators have also suggested community education with solicitation of community preferences as a way of establishing a presumption for or against the use of intravenous tPA for stroke patients in that community.[9,24]

### Carotid Endarterectomy for Carotid Artery Stenosis

Like intravenous tPA for ischemic stroke, CEA provides the prospect of long-term benefit for certain patients in return for the assumption of increased short-term risk. Large randomized clinical trials done in the late 1980s and early 1990s (the North American Symptomatic Carotid Endarterectomy Trial [NASCET] and the European Carotid Surgery Trial [ECST]) showed that CEA for symptomatic patients with severe (>70%) stenosis was associated with an absolute reduction of approximately 16% in the risk of ipsilateral stroke at 2 years. It was also, however, associated with significant risks of perioperative stroke and death (5.8% in NASCET and 7% in ECST).[27–29] A recent meta-analysis conducted by Rerkasem and Rothwell[30] suggests that the risk of perioperative stroke and death in symptomatic patients has remained nearly constant since those initial studies and is approximately 5.6%.

The picture is more complicated for symptomatic patients who do not have severe stenosis and for asymptomatic patients. For symptomatic patients with moderate stenosis (50%–69%), a recent meta-analysis by Rothwell and colleagues[31] suggests an absolute risk reduction of 4.6% with a $P$ value of .04. It is unclear whether there are any significant long-term benefits for asymptomatic patients, although the risk of perioperative stroke in asymptomatic patients is lower than that in symptomatic patients (3.35% for asymptomatic and 5.18% for symptomatic stenosis in one meta-analysis by Rothwell and colleagues).

The risks and benefits associated with CEA are known to vary significantly as a function of the surgeon performing the procedure. The American Heart Association and American Stroke Association recommend CEA for symptomatic patients with severe stenosis (70%–99%) only if the predicted combined perioperative morbidity and mortality rate is less than 6%.[32] For asymptomatic patients with stenosis greater than 60%, the perioperative risks of stroke and death should be less than 3%.[32]

Given the complex risk-and-benefit profile associated with CEA, a patient who wants to make a truly informed decision about whether to have the surgery must know with as much specificity as possible the absolute reduction in his or her long-term risk of stroke that will result from the procedure and the specific risks of perioperative stroke and death. To the extent they have the information, clinicians discussing CEA with patients have an ethical obligation to give relevant risk and benefit information specific to the surgeon who would be performing the operation, and to refer patients to surgeons with the best outcomes. Specific numbers needed to treat and numbers needed to harm should be discussed whenever possible. If local outcomes data are not available, clinicians should attempt to provide information for surgeons with roughly the same level of experience as that of the local surgeons, so that the information will be as useful as possible to the patient. Clinicians are also obligated to provide information about viable alternatives, such as medical therapy and, in appropriate circumstances, carotid angiography and carotid artery stenting (CAS). The relative risks and benefits of CAS are the subject of ongoing randomized controlled trials. Currently CAS is thought to be appropriate only for symptomatic patients with severe stenosis who are poor surgical candidates.[33]

A recent study of vascular surgery trainees at one hospital in London showed that many trainee surgeons competent to perform a CEA were not obtaining valid consent. Specifically, only a minority of trainees discussed the personal- or hospital-specific risk of stroke with the patient.[34] Some physicians might be tempted to downplay the risk of perioperative stroke and death in an effort to protect patients from anxiety or to ensure that the patient makes what the physician believes is the best decision under the circumstances. As with intravenous tPA, however, the balancing of the benefits of long-term risk reduction against short-term risk assumption is individualized and clinicians should not assume that patients will favor long-term risk reduction. The decision-making process should be guided by principles of shared decision making in which the physician lays out the facts as clearly as possible as applied to the patient's individual circumstances, and the patient makes a decision based on personal priorities.

### Do-not-resuscitate Orders

In the absence of a DNR order, consent to perform CPR in the event of a cardiac or respiratory arrest is presumed. Only competent patients or their surrogates can authorize physicians to sign DNR orders, which generally prohibit chest compressions, defibrillation, endotracheal intubation, mechanical and mouth-to-mouth ventilation, and the administration of vasopressor and cardiac stimulant drugs.

The presumption in favor of CPR is based on the assumption that, given the choice, most people would want every effort to be made to save their lives and restore them to health. In reality, however, CPR is rarely successful in restoring prior health. Patients who have out-of-hospital cardiac arrests have a 3% to 14% of surviving to hospital discharge and those who suffer in-hospital arrests have a 10% to 20% chance of survival to hospital discharge.[35] Patients with significant comorbidities fare much worse; in two studies, none of the patients with metastatic cancer, acute stroke, sepsis, or pneumonia survived to hospital discharge following CPR administration.[36,37] Evidence suggests that, of those who survive to discharge, most have diminished global functioning.[37]

Possibly more than in any other context, the framing of the discussion about DNR orders profoundly affects the patient's understanding of options related to the decision about whether to sign a DNR order. Often, the choice of whether to enter a DNR order is framed as a decision between life and death. Patients or their surrogates might be asked something like the following: "If your [his or her] heart were to stop beating, would you want us to do everything we could to save you [him or her]?" This type of framing, with no specifics regarding the mechanics of CPR and mechanical ventilation, or any discussions of the likelihood that the interventions ultimately will prove life saving, deprives patients of the opportunity to make truly informed decisions about what they would want done in the case of a life-threatening emergency. Murphy and Finucane[38] found that, almost uniformly, patients who initially requested resuscitation when asked in the above terms, ultimately opposed resuscitation after being told about the mechanics of CPR, the intensive care unit experience, and the probability of rehabilitation.

In discussing resuscitation status, clinicians are ethically obligated to give patients or their surrogates relevant, specific information regarding CPR and mechanical ventilation, including outcome statistics that are as directly relevant to the patient as possible, taking into account the patient's age and comorbidities. Just as patients should be given numbers needed to treat and be told about the risks associated with any given treatment, they should be told directly about the low success rates of CPR, the probability that their functioning will be impaired following CPR, and the physical invasion that CPR and mechanical intubation require so that they can make a truly informed decision about whether to consent to CPR. It is particularly critical to convey this information in the setting of resuscitation discussions in light of the general public misperception, fueled in large part by deceptive imagery in the media, that CPR routinely and instantly restores patients to good health.

With honest and open communication between clinicians, patients, and family members, it is usually possible to reach a decision regarding resuscitation that is acceptable to the medical team, patient, and patient's family or other surrogates. At the extreme, however, cases arise in which patients (or, more typically, their surrogates) insist on full resuscitation when clinicians feel that the resuscitation would be futile and, in some cases, cruel. A physician might ultimately feel that to resuscitate a particular patient would actually do harm to that patient in violation of the physician's ethical duty of nonmaleficence. The question remains: Is it ever ethically acceptable for a clinician to unilaterally enter a DNR order for a patient?

Clinicians have no ethical duty to offer or provide futile therapies for patients. Defining futility is problematic, but it is generally understood that, although certain treatments may confer the intended physiologic benefit and therefore be technically effective (eg, restarting a patient's heart with a defibrillator), they may not confer any significant therapeutic benefit (eg, providing the patient with any significant additional meaningful life). Lawrence Schneiderman and his colleagues,[8] who have written extensively on the subject, suggest that the essence of futility is overwhelming improbability in the face of possibility. Under their analysis, "an act is futile if the desired outcome, while empirically possible, is so unlikely that its exact probability may be incalculable."[8]

Given the low success rates of CPR, particularly for patients with significant comorbidities, some observers have suggested that the current presumption in favor of resuscitation should be abandoned in certain categories of patients and that CPR should not be offered to patients whose chances of successful resuscitation are very low. Murphy and Finucane[38] suggested that patients with metastatic cancer, class C cirrhosis, AIDS with at least two episodes of *Pneumocystis carinii* pneumonia, dementia requiring long-term care, coma lasting longer than 48 hours, multiple organ system failure without improvement after at least 3 days in the intensive care unit, or unsuccessful out-of-hospital cardiopulmonary resuscitation should not be offered resuscitation. They proposed that in such cases where CPR would be a futile form of therapy, physicians should be permitted to unilaterally enter DNR orders without discussing this with the patient or the patient's surrogates.[38]

Although the idea that physicians should have the authority to unilaterally enter DNR orders follows logically from the general principle that clinicians are not required to offer futile treatment, there are several features of CPR that make it unique. First, there is a widely held perception among patients and families, supported by actual hospital policies, the advance directive movement, and pervasive media images, that patients will be resuscitated unless they or their surrogates specify otherwise. Regardless of how society has gotten to this point and whether cultural reeducation to change the default position on CPR might be beneficial, it would be a radical departure from patient and family expectations to sanction the unilateral entry of DNR orders for broad categories of patients in the absence of patient or family consultation.

Second, the difficulty in defining futility is particularly problematic in cases where the alternative to treatment is immediate death. Although in many cases in which CPR would be considered futile by physicians, patients are likely to be actively dying, patients or their surrogates might still consider any additional life to be beneficial. Even if physicians ultimately should have the right to reject this characterization and refuse to resuscitate certain patients, allowing physicians to enter DNR orders without consulting patients or their families seems to be an unnecessarily blunt solution.

If a physician feels that CPR would be futile in a particular case, the physician should explain to the patient or the patient's surrogate specifically why the physician thinks resuscitation would not be beneficial to the patient and make every effort to convince the patient or surrogate to consent to a DNR order. If necessary and available, the physician should engage the resources of ethics committee consultants, chaplains, and palliative care staff. If disagreement persists, the physician should explain that he or she is entering a DNR order for the patient because the physician believes that CPR would not be beneficial to the patient. The physician should advise the patient and family that they can try to find another hospital or facility that would be willing to provide the care they seek. This approach respects the decision-making authority of the patient, while still allowing physicians to refuse treatment in cases in which they believe treatment would be inappropriate.

Because many DNR discussions take place in the context of serious illness or incapacitation, it is common for clinicians to hold discussions regarding resuscitation status with surrogate decision-makers. Surrogates are asked and are ethically obligated to make the decision they believe the patient would have made about CPR if the patient were competent. Yet studies have shown that spouses, who are the most likely surrogates for incapacitated patients, have limited ability to predict whether a patient would want to have CPR. Specifically, in a study of spouses' predictions of patients' choices regarding CPR, one third of the spouses incorrectly identified the patient's preference, most often stating that the patient would want CPR when in fact the patient did not want to be resuscitated.[39]

The most effective way to ensure that a patient's wishes regarding resuscitation are respected is for the patient to execute a legal document appointing an agent to make health care decisions on his or her behalf that is annotated to request or to refuse CPR. This written instruction to the health care agent provides clarity that can avoid unwanted CPR.

## SUMMARY

The doctrine of informed consent has evolved since it was first articulated as a legal doctrine in the early to mid–twentieth century. The modern ethical ideal is that physicians and patients will collaborate in shared medical decision making, with the physician contributing his or her knowledge and expert opinion and the patient providing his or her values and priorities. The goal is a course of medical treatment that reflects what is best for the patient in his or her own medical and personal context. Decisions about resuscitation efforts, intravenous tPA, and CEA present particular challenges to this modern ideal. In all of these situations, physicians are obligated to provide direct, detailed, and relevant information about the proposed intervention, the associated risks, and the likely outcomes.

## REFERENCES

1. Gert B, Culver CM, Clouser KD. Bioethics: a return to fundamentals. New York: Oxford University Press; 1997. p. 176.

2. Miller LJ. Informed consent. Part I. JAMA 1980;244:2100–3.

3. King JS, Moulton BW. Rethinking informed consent: the case for shared medical decision making. Am J Law Med 2006;32:429–501.

4. 105 NE 92, 93 (NY 1914).

5. Beresford R. Neurology and the law: private litigation and public policy. Philadelphia: F.A. Davis; 1998. p. 37.

6. Gert B, Culver CM, Clouser KD. Bioethics: a systematic approach. New York: Oxford University Press; 2006. p. 112–7.

7. Luce JM, White DB. A history of ethics and law in the intensive care unit. Crit Care Clin 2009;25:221–37.

8. Bernat JL. Ethical issues in neurology. 3rd edition. Philadelphia: Lippincott Williams & Wilkins; 2008. p. 24.

9. White-Bateman SR, Schumacher HC, Sacco RL, et al. Consent for intravenous thrombolysis in acute stroke: review and future directions. Arch Neurol 2007; 64(6):785–92.

10. Malenka DJ, Baron JA, Johansen S, et al. The framing effect of relative and absolute risk. J Gen Intern Med 1993;8:543–8.

11. Mazur DJ, Hickam DH, Mazur MD, et al. The role of doctor's opinion in shared decision making: what does shared decision making really mean when considering invasive medical procedures? Health Expect 2005;8(2):97–102.

12. Mazur DJ, Hickam DH. Patients' preferences for risk disclosure and role in decision making for invasive medical procedures. J Gen Intern Med 1997;12(2): 114–7.

13. Gert B, Nelson WA, Culver CM. Moral theory and neurology. Neurol Clin 1989;7: 691.

14. Tversky A, Kahneman D. The framing of decisions and the psychology of choice. Science 1981;211:453–8.

15. Murphy DJ. Do-not-resuscitate orders: time for re-appraisal in long-term care institutions. JAMA 1988;260:2098–101.

16. Manthous CA, DeGirolamo A, Haddad C, et al. Informed consent for medical procedures: local and national practices. Chest 2003;124:1978–84.

17. Fleck LM, Hayes OW. Ethics and consent to treat in acute stroke therapy. Emerg Med Clin North Am 2002;20:705.

18. Emanuel EJ, Emanuel LL. Four models of the physician-patient relationship. JAMA 1992;267:2221–6.

19. Brock DW. The ideal of shared decision making between physicians and patients. Kennedy Inst Ethics J 1991;1(1):31.

20. Weinstein JN, Clay K, Morgan TS. Informed patient choice: patient-centered valuing of surgical risks and benefits. Health Aff 2007;26:726–30.

21. Whitney SN, McGuire AL, McCullough LB. A typology of shared decision making, informed consent and simple consent. Ann Intern Med 2004;140:54–9.

22. The National Institute of Neurological Disorders and Stroke rt-PA Stroke Study Group. Tissue plasminogen activator for acute ischemic stroke. N Engl J Med 1995;333:1581–7.

23. Katzan IL, Furlan AJ, Lloyd LE, et al. Use of tissue-type plasminogen activator for acute ischemic stroke: the Cleveland area experience. JAMA 2000;283:1151–8.

24. Ciccone A. Consent to thrombolysis in acute stroke: from trial to practice. Lancet Neurol 2003;2:375–8.

25. Goyal DG, Li J, Mann J, et al. Position statement of the American Academy of Emergency Medicine on the use of intravenous thrombolytic therapy in the treatment of

stroke. Available at: http://www.aaem.org/positionstatements/thrombolytic therapy. php. Accessed December 8, 2009.

26. American Academy of Neurology. Consent issues in the management of cerebrovascular diseases: a position paper of the American Academy of Neurology, Ethics and Humanities Subcommittee. Neurology 1999;53:9–11.

27. Rothwell PM, Gutnikov SA, Warlow CP. Reanalysis of the final results of the European Carotid Surgery Trial. Stroke 2003;34:514–23.

28. Barnett HJ, Taylor DW, Eliasziw M, et al. North American symptomatic carotid endarterectomy trial collaborators. Benefit of carotid endarterectomy in patients with symptomatic moderate or severe stenosis. N Engl J Med 1998;339:1415–25.

29. Rothwell PM, Eliasziw M, Gutnikov SA, et al. Analysis of pooled data from the randomized controlled trials of endarterectomy for symptomatic carotid stenosis. Lancet 2003;361:107–16.

30. Rerkasem K, Rothwell PM. Temporal trends in the risks of stroke and death due to endarterectomy for symptomatic carotid stenosis: an updated systemic review. Eur J Vasc Endovasc Surg 2009;37:504–11.

31. Rothwell PM, Slattery J, Warlow CP. A systematic comparison of the risks of stroke and death due to carotid endarterectomy for symptomatic and asymptomatic stenosis. Stroke 1996;27:266–9.

32. Biller J, Feinberg WM, Castaldo JE. Guidelines for carotid endarterectomy: a statement for healthcare professionals from a special writing group of the Stroke Council, American Heart Association. Circulation 1998;97:501–9.

33. Lanzino G, Rabinstein AA, Brown RD. Treatment of carotid artery stenosis: medical therapy, surgery or stenting? Mayo Clin Proc 2009;84:366.

34. Black SA, Nestel D, Tierney T, et al. Gaining consent for carotid surgery: a simulation-based study of vascular surgeons. Eur J Vasc Endovasc Surg 2009;37: 134–9.

35. Choudry NK, Choudry S, Singer PA. CPR for patients labeled DNR: the role of the limited aggressive therapy order. Ann Intern Med 2003;138:65–8.

36. Taffet GE, Teasdale TA, Lucho RJ. In-hospital cardiopulmonary resuscitation. JAMA 1988;260:2069–72.

37. Bedell SE, Delbanco TL, Cook EF, et al. Survival alter cardiopulmonary resuscitation in the hospital. N Engl J Med 1983;309:569–76.

38. Murphy DJ, Finucane TE. New do-not resuscitate policies: a first step in cost control. Arch Intern Med 1993;153:1641–8.

39. Uhlmann RF, Pearlman RA, Cain KC. Physicians' and spouses' predictions of elderly patients' resuscitation preferences. J Gerontol 1988;43(5):M115–21.

# Neurology Education: Current and Emerging Concepts in Residency and Fellowship Training

Barney J. Stern, MD[a,*], Ralph F. Józefowicz, MD[b], Brett Kissela, MD[c], Steven L. Lewis, MD[d]

**KEYWORDS**

- Education • Neurology • Residency • Fellowship
- Training program

Neurology training continues to evolve to accommodate changing Accreditation Council for Graduate Medical Education (ACGME) requirements and neurology education imperatives. Key stakeholders for neurology graduate education include prospective neurology residents, neurology residents and fellows (subspecialty residents), residency and fellowship program directors, the Neurology Review Committee (NRC) under the auspices of the ACGME, the American Board of Psychiatry and Neurology (ABPN),[1] the American Academy of Neurology (AAN), the American Neurological Association (ANA), the Child Neurology Society (CNS), the Association of University Professors of Neurology (AUPN), and the Professors of Child Neurology (PCN). Among these constituencies, there are intricate relationships that reflect the continuing efforts to coordinate and advocate for improved graduate education. This article gives updates on current trends in neurology graduate education and highlights challenges that the stakeholders are addressing.

## ATTRACTING STUDENTS TO NEUROLOGY: THE MATCH

Neurologists are in competition with all other specialties in the desire to attract "the best and the brightest" to the field. Efforts to channel medical students into neurology are greatly influenced by the experiences students have in their preclinical years and neurology clerkships. Increasingly, medical schools require a neurology clerkship

[a] Department of Neurology, University of Maryland, 110 South Paca Street, 3-N-139, Baltimore, MD, USA
[b] Department of Neurology, University of Rochester School of Medicine and Dentistry, Rochester, NY 14642, USA
[c] Department of Neurology, University of Cincinnati, Cincinnati, OH 45267, USA
[d] Department of Neurological Sciences, Rush University Medical Center, Chicago, IL 60612, USA
* Corresponding author.
*E-mail address:* bstern@som.umaryland.edu (B.J. Stern).

Neurol Clin 28 (2010) 475–487
doi:10.1016/j.ncl.2009.11.011
0733-8619/10/$ – see front matter © 2010 Elsevier Inc. All rights reserved.
**neurologic.theclinics.com**

because exposure to clinical neurology is thought to be important in helping students consider a career in neurology.[2] Several programs are sponsored by the AAN to enhance student entry into neurology: (1) The Student Interest Group in Neurology program brings together students and faculty at participating medical schools and encourages home grown activities to promote neurology, (2) the Undergraduate Education Subcommittee of the Education Committee advocates for enhanced medical school neurology education and has developed a clerkship core curriculum, (3) medical student scholarships and awards related to the annual meeting are available (https://www.aan.com/go/education/awards; accessed August 22, 2008), and (4) sponsorship of the Consortium of Neurology Clerkship Directors, which brings clerkship directors together to discuss and advocate for common concerns.

## ADULT NEUROLOGY RESIDENCY TRAINING

Application to adult neurology residency programs begins through the services of the Association of American Medical College's Electronic Residency Application Service (ERAS). ERAS is a multifaceted Internet-based tool that facilitates the acquisition and collation of supporting documentation for the applicant; moreover, it allows program directors and staff to securely access the data and communicate with applicants. Following the interview process, both applicants and programs submit a rank list to the National Resident Match Program (NRMP), which ultimately establishes a match between an applicant's and residency program's mutually acceptable highest rated choices. The NRMP has a strictly enforced code of conduct to insure a fair process for all concerned. Participation in the NRMP has been especially valuable for applicants participating in the couples match. Furthermore, applicants for neurology positions can customize their postgraduate year one (internship) selection options depending on where they have matched for their neurology residency.

The NRMP has published statistics applicable to the 2009 match (www.nrmp.org/data/chartingoutcomes2009v3.pdf; accessed August 17, 2009). There was a total pool of 751 applicants for 385 neurology residency positions offered by 87 programs in the NRMP match. Of these positions, 192 (50%) were filled by United States senior medical student candidates; the remaining positions were filled by Independent Applicants. Of the matched United States seniors, 11.4% were members of Alpha Omega Alpha and 11% had PhDs. The mean United States Medical Licensing Examination Step 1 score, which assesses whether the applicant can understand and apply important concepts of the sciences basic to the practice of medicine, was 225 for United States seniors and 224 for matched Independent Applicants

## CHILD NEUROLOGY RESIDENCY TRAINING

The specialty of child neurology was formalized in 1969 when the ABPN awarded the first certificate in Neurology with Special Competency in Child Neurology. As of December 2008, more than 1700 child neurologists had been certified by the ABPN. There are currently 69 child neurology residency training programs, and 290 filled positions. Since child neurology training encompasses 3 years, the average program size is 1.4 residents per year per program.

The duration of child neurology training is 5 years, and consists of the following: 2 years of preliminary training, which may include 2 years of pediatrics; 1 year of pediatrics and 1 year of internal medicine, or 1 year in pediatrics and 1 year in research; and 3 years of neurology training, including 1 year of adult neurology, 1 year of child neurology and 1 chief resident year. Child neurologists who wish to be double-boarded in both pediatrics and child neurology must select the first preliminary tract, which includes 2 years of pediatrics.

Child neurology does not belong to the NRMP and does not use the ERAS, since neither the NRMP nor the ERAS can match students for positions that begin more than 1 year following medical school graduation. Rather, child neurology participates in the San Francisco Match and uses its own application service, the Central Application Service. According to the 2009 San Francisco Match data, 88 of 123 first year child neurology training positions were filled through the match.

In 2002, the CNS surveyed its members and nonmember child neurologists and reported that 904 full-time patient care child neurologists were practicing in the United States that year.[3] No growth in the supply of child neurologists was projected over the next 20 years, and wait times for an appointment averaged 53 and 44 days for a new and return visit, respectively. Thus, workforce issues remain a major challenge for the specialty of child neurology.[4]

There has been much discussion concerning shortening the duration of preliminary training in pediatrics from 2 years to 1 year. An informal poll of chiefs of academic child neurology divisions concerning shortening this training was inconclusive.[3,4] Since many academic child neurologists also take general pediatric call in their departments, board certification in pediatrics is necessary for this subgroup. Because one of the 2 years of preliminary pediatric training may be substituted by a year of internal medicine or research, one could argue that this second year of preliminary training be made optional.

## ADVANCED TRAINING: FELLOWSHIPS

Approximately three-quarters of graduating residents pursue advanced, subspecialty training, and the authors suspect that this proportion will increase over time.[5] This reflects the increasing trend for subspecialty training throughout medicine, and is a concern to some.[6] There are essentially three pathways to advanced training: unaccredited subspecialties, ABPN-accredited programs, and the United Councils for Neurologic Subspecialties (UCNS)-accredited programs. Subspecialty training opportunities continue to evolve to reflect new opportunities (http://www.aan.com/education/fellowships/; accessed August 22, 2008), such as the recent interest in a career path as a neurohospitalist or specialist in pediatric neurocritical care.[7,8]

ABPN-accredited programs function under ACGME and NRC guidelines (http://www.acgme.org/acWebsite/RRC_180/180_prIndex.asp; accessed August 22, 2008); therefore, trainees are referred to as subspecialty residents, rather than as fellows. Specialty certification is available in clinical neurophysiology, neuromuscular medicine, pain medicine, sleep medicine, and vascular neurology (http://www.abpn.com/; accessed August 22, 2008).

The UCNS is sponsored by five constituent organizations: AAN, ANA, AUPN, CNS, and the PCN (http://www.ucns.org/go/about; accessed August 22, 2008). It offers certification in autonomic disorders, behavioral neurology and neuropsychiatry, clinical neuromuscular pathology, geriatric neurology, headache medicine, neurocritical care, neuroimaging, and neuro-oncology.

Overall, there is an accelerating trend toward subspecialty program accreditation and subspecialist certification. Currently, there are several paths available for advanced training. It remains unclear whether a consolidation process will occur or multiple tracks will persist. Furthermore, accreditation and certification for subspecialties that require multidisciplinary training (eg, interventional neuroradiology [endovascular surgical neuroradiology]), will necessitate a continuing dialog among stakeholders.[9]

## PROGRAM DIRECTORS CONSORTIUM

The Consortium of Neurology Program Directors (CNPD) was formed in 1997 in response to the rapidly changing environment of neurology graduate medical education and the perceived need for a group in which program director issues could be discussed and information distributed. Furthermore, it was recognized that this group was the perfect vehicle to facilitate communication between program directors and organizations of importance such as the NRC and the ABPN. The CNPD was formed with the assistance of the AAN, which has provided financial and staff member support for the CNPD since inception. The CNPD is a subcommittee of the AAN's Graduate Education Subcommittee, which in turn is a subcommittee of the Education Committee. Its leadership is voted upon every 2 years by the subcommittee membership. To date, there have been seven chairs of the CNPD. Around the time in which the CNPD was being formed, the AAN also assisted with the development of the Consortium of Neurology Clerkship Directors (CNCD) and, later, the Consortium of Neurology Residents and Fellows (CNRF). The CNPD now meets biannually and presents the Clerkship Directors or Program Directors course, which is codirected by the chairs of the CNPD and the CNCD.

A pivotal development has been the creation of the CNPD listserv, which has facilitated a robust dialog allowing program directors to ask questions of their colleagues across the United States via informal surveys and to solicit advice on a variety of topics. The CNPD has also become a valuable group for those within neurology graduate medical education. It strives to enhance the professional development and career satisfaction of neurology residency program directors. The group is devoted to bidirectional communication between program directors and regulatory groups (NRC, ABPN, etc), sharing of best practices among program directors, and development of collegiality among program directors. Furthermore, the organization strives to be action oriented. In recent years, the CNPD, in collaboration with the CNRF, has been successful in generating consensus against the requirement of the use of a NRC case log system, and in taking on research projects, such as the study of the ABPN-mandated clinical competency examinations.

In the future, the CNPD hopes to incorporate fellowship directors into the organization, given their significant role in neurology graduate medical education after residency. Program administrators (formerly called program coordinators), also essential, can now be certified (Training Administrators of Graduate Medical Education, http://www.tagme.org/neurology.htm). The CNPD has tried to foster their professional development in this manner. Some progress has been made toward organizing a group specifically for program administrators. Finally, some members of the CNPD have been advocating that the group be split off from AAN. While this idea has been entertained several times since the CNPD was formed, no compelling rationale has been found to justify such a move, given the generous financial support and staff assistance the AAN has provided over the years.

## ACGME NEUROLOGY REVIEW COMMITTEE

The ACGME, established in 1981 when a consensus in the academic medical community determined the need for an independent accrediting organization for residency programs, is a private, nonprofit council that evaluates and accredits medical residency programs in the United States. The mission of the ACGME is to improve health care by assessing and advancing the quality of resident physicians' education through accreditation. There are currently over 8000 ACGME-accredited residency programs in 126 specialties and subspecialties. The number of active full-time and part-time residents exceeds 100,000.

The ACGME has 28 review committees (one for each of 26 specialties, one for the 1-year transitional program, and one for institutional review). Each residency committee is comprised of about 6 to 15 volunteers. Members of the residency review committees are appointed by the American Medical Association Council on Medical Education and the appropriate medical specialty boards and organizations.

The NRC consists of 11 members: eight current or former program directors, one resident member, and two ex officio members representing the ABPN and the AAN, respectively. The nominating organizations for the NRC include the AMA, the ABPN, and the AAN. The NRC is responsible for accrediting and regularly reviewing residency programs in two primary specialties (neurology and child neurology), and four subspecialties (clinical neurophysiology, vascular neurology, neuromuscular medicine, and neurodevelopmental disabilities). Four interdisciplinary neurologic subspecialties are accredited by other review committees: endovascular surgical neuroradiology, hospice and palliative medicine, pain medicine, and sleep medicine.

There are currently 126 adult neurology training programs that train over 1,800 residents, and 69 child neurology residency training programs that train almost 300 residents. The number of programs and residents for the neurologic subspecialties are: neurophysiology, 90 programs and 214 residents; neuromuscular medicine, 21 programs and 30 residents; neurodevelopmental disabilities, 8 programs and 15 residents; and vascular neurology, 64 programs and 55 residents.

The NRC creates and periodically reviews program requirements for the primary specialties and subspecialties in neurology. These program requirements are posted on the ACGME Web site (www.acgme.org). Incorporated into these individual specialty and subspecialty-specific program requirements are the common program requirements, which are written by the ACGME and apply to all medical specialties. All residency programs are expected to comply completely with each of the common and specialty-specific program requirements. To insure that this occurs, the NRC periodically reviews each neurology residency program by means of a site visit conducted by an ACGME field staff member. To prepare for such a review, each program must complete and submit a program information form (PIF), a detailed analysis of the scope and quality of the training program. The PIF is loosely organized around the program requirements, thereby insuring that all program requirements are met. During the site visit, the ACGME site visitor verifies the contents of the PIF by meeting with the program director, department chairperson, key faculty, and all of the neurology residents in the program. The NRC then reviews the PIF and the site visit report, and determines if any citations need to be levied against the residency program for failure to comply with the program requirements. Residency programs with substantial compliance receive continued full accreditation for a period of 4 to 5 years. Programs with substantial citations may only be reaccredited for 2 or 3 years with a subsequent review scheduled for the end of that time. Programs with egregious citations may be placed on probation. The accreditation report from the NRC is sent to the designated institutional official (generally, the Graduate Medical Education dean), the residency program director, and the department chairman; and is shared with all of the residents in the program. The final accreditation decision and the review cycle (years until the next review) are also posted on the ACGME Web site. Program citations that frequently result in adverse accreditation decisions include violation of duty hours, lack of resident supervision by faculty, lack of competency-based goals and objectives, and low first-time pass rates for the ABPN certification examination.

The future direction of the ACGME and each residency review committee will be to focus more on outcomes of the residency program, the Milestones initiative, as opposed to process.[10,11] Specifically, instead of evaluating whether each residency program has the potential to train residents in a specialty, the ACGME will determine whether the residency program is actually training the residents adequately. In other words—rather than focusing on the size and breadth of the faculty, the scope of the didactic curriculum, an adequate patient population, a list of conferences, and so forth—the new evaluation system will focus on outcomes such as board pass rates, ability for residency graduates to secure top notch fellowships or practice positions, participation in Maintenance of Certification following completion of the residency program, and, eventually, patient outcomes. This last metric, patient outcomes, is the most problematic to measure, since many other factors besides the role of the physician influence the health of the patient.

## THE CORE COMPETENCIES

The ACGME common program requirements list six core competencies (**Table 1**) required for resident education.[12] These competencies grew out of the ACGME Outcome Project,[13] an initiative begun by the ACGME more than 10 years ago which, in turn, was developed in response to the focus on educational outcomes by the US Department of Education that began in the 1980s.[14] Since 2002, all ACGME-accredited training programs, in all specialties and subspecialties, have been required to demonstrate that they are teaching these six core competencies to their trainees within the curriculum, with ongoing assessment of each resident's or fellow's competencies within each of these domains. **Table 1** provides a brief description and summary of each of these competencies from the ACGME Common Program Requirements (2007). In 2003, the ABPN[14] published a monograph outlining the history and development of the Core Competencies and their usefulness as a concept in residency education and life-long assessment and credentialing of neurologists. In this regard, currently all CME activities of the AAN also include a list of which core competencies are being taught or assessed with each program, with the assumption that this competency-based subdivision of educational activities may be useful or necessary in current or future professional maintenance of certification programs.

As noted by Elkind,[15] many if not all of these competencies were likely taught and evaluated, at least implicitly, within residency programs even before the ACGME definition of the six core competencies. The mandate of the ACGME outcome project is for the program director to explicitly show that these competencies have been taught by the program and achieved by the trainee before entering unsupervised practice. At the time of each program's review by the Residency Review Committee of the ACGME, each program director must provide evidence of where and how these competencies are taught (formally or informally) and evaluated—that is, through personal observation by faculty and 360-evaluations by faculty, other health care providers, and even patients[14], or through more formal testing as appropriate. Currently the NRC and the ACGME do not define when, where, and how these competencies should be taught and assessed; it is the responsibility of the individual program to create its own outline for instruction and assessment of these general competencies. This lack of standardization is akin to each residency director being in the position of recreating the wheel, without the director knowing whether the program's approach to teaching and assessment of the competencies and, perhaps equally

| Table 1 | |
|---|---|
| **The ACGME competencies** | |
| **Competency** | **Brief Summary of Common Program Requirements** |
| Patient care | Residents must be able to provide patient care that is compassionate, appropriate, and effective for the treatment of health problems and the promotion of health. |
| Medical knowledge | Residents must demonstrate knowledge of established and evolving biomedical, clinical, epidemiologic, and social-behavioral sciences; and the application of this knowledge to patient care. |
| Practice-based learning and improvement | Residents must demonstrate the ability to investigate and evaluate their care of patients, appraise and assimilate scientific evidence, and continuously improve patient care based on constant self-evaluation and life-long learning. |
| Interpersonal and communication skills | Residents must demonstrate interpersonal and communication skills that result in the effective exchange of information and collaboration with patients, their families, and health professionals. |
| Professionalism | Residents must demonstrate a commitment to performing professional responsibilities and an adherence to ethical principles. |
| Systems-based practice | Residents must demonstrate an awareness of and responsiveness to the larger context and system of health care, and the ability to call effectively on other resources in the system to provide optimal health care. |

*Data from* The Common Program Requirements: General Competencies, Approved by the ACGME Board February 13, 2007 (ACGME Outcome Project Webpage 2007).

important, documentation of the process, are adequate until after the NRC completes a review of the program.

It must be emphasized that the ACGME views the core competencies as those skills that are required of a minimally competent practitioner ready to enter the unsupervised practice of their specialty or subspecialty. They are not requirements that can be done or met by a resident early in training. For example, a resident viewing an online module on professionalism, followed by successful completion of a multiple-choice question quiz, does not prove that a resident is competent in the domain of professionalism. The six core competencies of the ACGME are an attempt to represent definable outcomes that require ongoing observation and assessment during residency or fellowship training, with the expectation that a minimally competent practitioner must show that he or she has achieved competence in these domains (appropriate to their specialty or subspecialty) before entering the unsupervised practice of their specialty or subspecialty.

In addition to the concern described above regarding the ACGME's lack of a standardized approach to the core competencies within all programs of a specialty, a more serious overriding concern may be fact that the ACGME Outcome Project was not itself assessed for effectiveness before its initiation. It remains unclear and unproven whether physician training and competence have been or will be improved by the incorporation and documentation of teaching and assessment of the ACGME's six defined core competencies in training programs.

The newest competency initiative by the ACGME is the Milestones initiative.[10,11] Currently in development, this initiative is being described as the next step in the outcomes-based accreditation project.[10] Specifically, the Milestones initiative is being described as an attempt to have each specialty develop its own set of desired educational outcomes and the methods of assessment of these outcomes, with more specificity regarding the levels of performance required for clinical competence during specific points in training and at the point of proficiency in a specialty or subspecialty.[10,11,13] This project is expected to involve close interaction between the ACGME (and its residency review committees) and the corresponding specialty boards of the ABMS.[11] On the positive side, it seems that the Milestones initiative involves more standardization of an assessment tool within all programs of a specialty. However, implementation of a (likely) expensive, time-consuming (both for faculty and trainees), national initiative without evidence for effectiveness remains a concern.

## ACGME-MANDATED DUTY HOURS

It has been widely recognized that excessive fatigue can lead to preventable errors in many professions, including medicine.[16,17] For safety reasons, duty hour limitations have been in development for some medical specialties since the 1980s. The ACGME Board of Directors approved the common duty hour standards for programs in all specialties in February 2003. According to the ACGME Web site (www.acgme.org; accessed September 8, 2009), the current duty hour standards are as follows:

An 80-hour weekly limit, averaged over 4 weeks. Review committees for various specialties may set more restrictive standards. Moonlighting done in the sponsoring institution counts toward the weekly limit. In addition, program directors must ensure that external and internal moonlighting does not interfere with the resident's achievement of the program's educational goals and objectives.

Adequate rest between duty periods.

A 24-hour limit on continuous duty time, with an additional period up to 6 hours permitted for continuity of care and educational activities.

One day in 7 free from all patient care and educational obligations, averaged over 4 weeks.

In-house call no more than once every 3 nights, averaged over 4 weeks.

The supervision of the ACGME with regard to these duty hour standards is via:

Confidential Internet resident surveys.

Interviews with program directors, staff, and residents during accreditation site visits, and review of duty hour documentation, such as time sheets and call schedules.

ACGME Monitoring Committee assessment of the performance of all review committees in applying and enforcing the accreditation standards.

Education of residents, program directors, and other audiences about resident duty hours.

Owing to the nature of our specialty (as compared with surgical specialties) and diligence of neurology program directors, duty hour violations are generally uncommon during neurology training. Mechanisms for coping with the duty hour regulations include shifting work done by residents to others (eg, hiring physician extenders or hospitalists) or modifying resident work into shifts (eg, instituting a night float or day float system). In the January 2009 ACGME Newsletter, in which the most common citations for the previous year (2008) were listed, duty hours was not among them. The newsletter also stated that no neurology programs required a site visit during 2008 because of duty hours.

It should be noted that the Resident Survey remains the standard mechanism by which compliance with duty hours is measured. The Resident Survey questions can be found online (http://www.acgme.org/acWebsite/Resident_Survey/sample_report. pdf) along with a sample report demonstrating results that an ACGME site visitor and NRC would ultimately see (http://www.acgme.org/acWebsite/Resident_Survey/ sample_report.pdf). The survey contains 13 questions regarding duty hours (questions 20–32 out of 32 questions). If a program is not 100% compliant according to the survey, then extra attention is devoted to this topic during the site visit process when the site visitor will ask all parties to confirm or deny compliance. Noncompliance is unfavorably reviewed during the NRC review process.

### The Future of Duty Hours: Institute of Medicine Report of 2008

In December of 2008, the Institute of Medicine (IOM) released a report titled "Resident Duty Hours: Enhancing Sleep, Supervision, and Safety." This somewhat controversial report suggested further limitations on resident duty hours as described in the summary (**Fig. 1**) from IOM Web site (http://www.iom.edu/Object.File/Master/60/ 471/one%20pager%20revised%20for%20web%202.pdf). The CNPD leadership sent a letter to the ACGME in which concerns were raised, including (1) stricter duty hour limits preventing continuity of care (with a significant impact on learning), (2) patient care errors from handoffs due to shift work, (3) decreased opportunity for educational conferences due to expected increases in shift work such as night float rotations, and (4) training environments that do not mirror actual practice after graduation with the concern that residents will not be equipped to handle real life stresses. Furthermore, the more restrictive limitations would be a significant hardship for small residency programs, and the CNPD estimates that many might not be able to comply. Other general concerns include the cost of implementing such a system. The CNPD estimates that a 35% increase in neurology physician extenders would be required for nationwide neurology training program compliance, which would be exceedingly difficult regardless of cost. There is an inadequate supply of neurology-specific physician extenders and, currently, neurohospitalists are not widely available. Thus, no pool of talent exists to fill the needs of training programs if the IOM rules are adopted. Furthermore, most neurology programs would not have sufficient budgets to allow such hiring. On a larger scale, the IOM report suggested that the cost to implement these new restrictions would be "in the ballpark of $1.7 billion." A subsequent article has estimated that the costs of implementing such a system for all residency training programs in the United States would range from $1.1 to $2.5 billion. In addition, cost-effectiveness modeling raised questions about the value of these new regulations given that there is no proof that these recommendations will lead to reduced errors.[18] Another concern is that such changes, should they come to pass, would lead to erosion of academic practice. It is feared that pushing work currently done by residents onto academic faculty might lead them to leave academia. While many who are directly involved with residency training are generally not in favor of these changes, there is pressure from the general public and governmental officials to take all measures necessary to prevent medical errors related to physician fatigue. Finally, Blanchard and colleagues[19] opine that "in this era of evidence-based medicine and comparative effectiveness, such a major policy change should be based not only on the recommendations of an expert committee but also on careful studies and evidence that improvements in both patient and educational outcomes will result."

## AMERICAN BOARD OF PSYCHIATRY AND NEUROLOGY

One major change recently instituted by the ABPN is the elimination of the Part II oral examination and consolidation of candidate testing into one comprehensive

# RESIDENT DUTY HOURS: ENHANCING SLEEP, SUPERVISION, AND SAFETY

| COMPARISON OF IOM COMMITTEE ADJUSTMENTS TO CURRENT ACGME DUTY HOUR LIMITS | | |
|---|---|---|
| | 2003 ACGME Duty Hour Limits | IOM Recommendation |
| Maximum hours of work per week | 80 hours, averaged over 4 weeks | No change |
| Maximum shift length | 30 hours (admitting patients up to 24 hours then 6 additional hours for transitional and educational activities) | • 30 hours (admitting patients for up to 16 hours, plus 5-hour protected sleep period between 10 p.m. and 8 a.m. with the remaining hours for transition and educational activities)<br>• 16 hours with no protected sleep period |
| Maximum in-hospital on-call frequency | Every third night, on average | Every third night, no averaging |
| Minimum time off between scheduled shifts | 10 hours after shift length | • 10 hours after day shift<br>• 12 hours after night shift<br>• 14 hours after any extended duty period of 30 hours and not return until 6 a.m. of next day |
| Maximum frequency of in-hospital night shifts | Not addressed | 4 night maximum; 48 hours off after 3 or 4 nights of consecutive duty |
| Mandatory time off duty | • 4 days off per month<br>• 1 day (24 hours) off per week, averaged over 4 weeks | • 5 days off per month<br>• 1 day (24 hours) off per week, no averaging<br>• One 48-hour period off per month |
| Moonlighting | Internal moonlighting is counted against 80-hour weekly limit | • Internal and external moonlighting is counted against 80-hour weekly limit<br>• All other duty hour limits apply to moonlighting in combination with scheduled work |
| Limit on hours for exceptions | 88 hours for select programs with a sound educational rationale | No change |
| Emergency room limits | 12-hour shift limit, at least an equivalent period of time off between shifts; 60-hour workweek with additional 12 hours for education | No change |

Fig. 1. IOM Proposal for revised duty hours. (*From* Institute of Medicine of the National Academies. Resident Duty Hours: Enhancing Sleep, Supervision, and Safety. Washington DC: National Academies Press, 2008; with permission.)

examination.[20] As part of this process, the neurology residency programs now have to assess clinical skills competency during residency using the Neurology Clinical Evaluation Exercise (NEX) and provide the ABPN with documentation that a resident has demonstrated competency in medical interviewing, the neurologic examination, humanistic qualities, professionalism, and patient counseling skills. Residents are required to demonstrate competency by being observed by at least three faculty members in their own department while they evaluate five patients during their 36-month residency. The five patients must represent problems in critical care, neuromuscular, ambulatory with an episodic disorder, neurodegenerative, and child neurology (http://www.abpn.com/downloads/forms/NEX%20Clinical%20Skills%20Evaluation%20Instructions.pdf).

Questions have been raised about the validity of the process, especially given that the examiners and examinees are in the same department. The hope is that early supervision and, potentially, repeated testing will result in greater resident competency because shortcomings can be addressed during residency training.[20]

## FUTURE ISSUES FACING NEUROLOGY RESIDENCY EDUCATION

As we look forward to 2010 and beyond, many changes, in addition to those previously described in duty hour limitations, are anticipated to occur in neurology residency training. Regardless of whether the IOM suggestions are adopted by the ACGME under pressure from the public, it is clear that a zero-tolerance approach to duty hour violations will become the standard.

The role of the CNPD will likely be expanded as time goes on. The CNPD has already begun to collaborate on education research,[21] and it is expected that this effort will increase over time. Furthermore, it is apparent that sharing of resources between program directors in the CNPD will continue, for the benefit of program directors and trainees alike. The CNPD community has begun to embrace educational tools created by a variety of groups, such as the American Headache Society's headache training simulation program and the AAN Evidence Based Medicine curriculum. The AAN has used results from a recurring survey of program directors to define areas of need across many programs that might be filled in the future by development of adaptable curricula, such as the Evidence Based Medicine Toolkit, which can be shared. The ACGME has also begun to post "Notable Practices," demonstrating excellent examples that program directors can consider and perhaps adapt for their own use.

The ACGME will continue to strive for outcomes-based evaluations, with a focus on the end result of competent trainees and with greater flexibility regarding the process of education. One of the stated goals of the ACGME is to reduce the burden of work required for program accreditation. In the future, it is anticipated that the PIF will become much shorter and easier to complete (the PIF is currently being edited by the NRC), and perhaps supplemented by more interval data, such as more frequent resident surveys. To facilitate an overhaul of the PIF, the NRC has completed a major edit of the Neurology-specific Program Requirements (NPR). The edited NPR are currently waiting for approval from the ACGME. The NRC has been very open to input from program directors and has been increasingly transparent about the process and results of NRC accreditation decisions. The improved communication between the NRC and neurology program directors was facilitated by the development of the CNPD, and has been of great benefit to both parties.

One important change that has been written into the revised NPR is mandatory salary support for program directors at the level reflecting an effort of 20% plus 1% per resident in the program as a line item proportion of total salary. The intention of this change was to ensure that all program directors receive the adequate support that is necessary to carry out the duties required to stay in compliance with the many ACGME and NRC regulations and to serve the educational needs of trainees. This has been a topic of debate among program directors, who realize that this intention is at odds with the realities of local funding availability within their home departments. At the time of this writing, it is not clear whether the ACGME will approve this new requirement and how strictly the NRC will enforce it in the future.

The ABPN has mandated the use of NEX during training to determine competency to sit for the ABPN board examination. This change was made for many reasons, not the least of which was the unpopular system of a one-time, high stakes examination that did not necessarily correlate well with true competency. Another benefit of the NEX is to guarantee that all programs observe clinical encounters during training, as this has not occurred consistently in past. While this program has been adopted by all training programs, uncertainty exists in the reliability and validity of the NEX examinations.[21] In the future, change may be necessary in the number and format of the examinations or in requirements for training and certification of local examiners.

## SUMMARY

As the complexity of requirements and demands pertinent to the education of neurologic trainees has increased, those involved in the day-to-day supervision of graduate education have become more organized and an active interaction has developed between the providers and regulatory organizations. There are increasing indications that increased transparency and collaboration has enhanced the education process. Many challenges remain and many more will appear, but a foundation and strategy has evolved over the past few years to leverage the energies of all stakeholders for the benefit of neurologic trainees and their patients.

## REFERENCES

1. Pascuzzi RM. Opinion/Education: the ABPN is the neurology resident's best friend. Neurology 2008;70:e16–9.
2. Corboy JR, Boudreau E, Morgenlander JC, et al. Neurology residency training at the millennium. Neurology 2002;58:1454–60.
3. Polsky D, Weiner J, Bale JF, et al. Specialty care by child neurologists, a workforce analysis. Neurology 2005;64:942–8.
4. Werner R, Polsky D. Comparing the supply of pediatric subspecialists and child neurologists. J Pediatr 2005;146:20–5.
5. FitzGerald DB, Mitchell AL. Career choices: the fellowship search. Neurology 2008;70:e5–8.
6. Aminoff MJ. Training in neurology. Neurology 2008;70:1912–5.
7. Freeman WD, Gronseth G, Eidelman BH. Invited article: is it time for neurohospitalists? Neurology 2008;70:1282–8.
8. LaRovere KL, Riviello JJ. Emerging subspecialties in neurology: building a career and a field: pediatric neurocritical care. Neurology 2008;70:e89–91.
9. Chen M, Nguyen T. Emerging subspecialties in neurology: endovascular surgical neuroradiology. Neurology 2008;70:e21–4.
10. Nasca TJ. The CEO's first column—the next step in the outcomes-based accreditation project. ACGME Bulletin May 2008;2–4.
11. Nasca TJ. Where will the "Milestones" take us? The next accreditation system. ACGME Bulletin September 2008;3–5.
12. ACGME Outcome Project Webpage. Common program requirements: general competencies. Approved by the ACGME board 2007. Available at: http://www.acgme.org/outcome/comp/GeneralCompetenciesStandards21307.pdf. Accessed May, 2009.
13. Philibert I. The competencies: the ACGME and the community in 2008 and beyond. ACGME Bulletin September 2008;1–2.
14. Scheiber SC, Kramer TAM, Adamowski SE. Core competencies for neurologists. What clinicians need to know. Philadelphia: Butterworth Heinemann; 2003.

15. Elkind MSV. Strangelove, or how I learned to stop worrying and love the core competencies. Neurology 2005;64:e3–6.
16. Lockley SW, Cronin JW, Evans EE, et al. Effect of reducing interns' weekly work hours on sleep and attentional failures. N Engl J Med 2004;351:1829–37.
17. Rothschild JM, Landrigan CP, Cronin JW, et al. The Critical Care Safety Study: The incidence and nature of adverse events and serious medical errors in intensive care. Crit Care Med 2005;33:1694–700.
18. Nuckols TK, Bhattacharya J, Wolman DM, et al. Cost implications of reduced work hours and workloads for resident physicians. N Engl J Med 2009;360:2202–15.
19. Blanchard MS, Meltzer D, Polonsky KS. To nap or not to nap? Residents' work hours revisited. N Engl J Med 2009;360(21):2242–4.
20. Pascuzzi RM. A dinosaur roars. Assessing clinical skills in residency. Neurology 2009;73:826–7.
21. Schuh LA, London Z, Neel R, et al. Education research: bias and poor interrater reliability in evaluating the neurology clinical skills examination. Neurology 2009;73:904–8.

# Using Evidence-Based Medicine in Neurology

Janis M. Miyasaki, MD, MEd, FRCPC, FAAN

**KEYWORDS**

- Neurology • Evidence-based medicine
- Critical appraisal • Guideline

## HISTORICAL CONTEXT

A recent Kaiser Health Tracking Poll for presidential candidates policies reported that after the war in Iraq, Americans were most interested in health care.[1] Within the category of health care, those polled wanted candidates' plans to expand health insurance coverage and reduce health care costs. It can be inferred that Americans do not want more health care; rather, they want better health care. According to the Agency for Healthcare Quality and Research, quality and effectiveness of health care means "providing the right care to the right patient at the right time and getting it right the first time."[2] The agency further articulates that its mission is to conduct and support health services research that "reduces the risk of harm from health care services by using evidence-based research and technology to promote the delivery of the best possible care; transforms research into practice to achieve wider access to effective health care services and reduce unnecessary health care costs; and improves health care outcomes by encouraging providers, consumers and patients to use evidence-based information to make informed treatment choices/decisions."

Evidence-based medicine (EBM) is an old concept whose time has come. Efficiency in health care is a long-cherished goal dating to the nineteenth century. In modern times, Archibald Cochrane influenced medical research profoundly with his book published in 1971, *Effectiveness and Efficiency: Random Reflections on Health Services*.[3] Cochrane's premise was that resources are always scarce and, therefore, the most reliable evidence should be used to guide health care delivery. In particular, he advocated for the use of randomized controlled trials (RCTs) as least likely to be biased in their conclusions.

A common misconception is that EBM views RCTs as the only valid source of evidence. This is perhaps perpetuated by the Cochrane Collaboration's exclusive use of RCTs in their reports. Guyatt and colleagues,[4] however, first used the term, *evidence-based medicine*, and defined it as "conscientious, explicit and judicious

The Morton and Gloria Shulman Movement Disorders Centre, Toronto Western Hospital, University of Toronto, 399 Bathurst Street, 7 McL, Toronto, ON M5T 2S8, Canada
*E-mail address:* miyasaki@uhnresearch.ca

Neurol Clin 28 (2010) 489–503
doi:10.1016/j.ncl.2009.11.010
0733-8619/10/$ – see front matter © 2010 Elsevier Inc. All rights reserved.

**neurologic.theclinics.com**

use of the best available evidence in making decisions about the care of individual patients." Therefore, other forms of evidence also guide practice.

To begin with what EBM is not, it is not cookbook medicine; it does not seek to limit physician autonomy; it is not a sword in the courtroom (however, it is also not a shield); it is not limited to RCTs; and it does not obviate clinical experience.

Critics deride EBM as cookbook medicine—an effort to make every treatment uniform and to remove the "art" of medicine. This aversion dates back to early American history when experienced physicians individualized care whereas traveling salesmen provided one-cure-fits-all potions. The latter were a snake oil salesmen whereas the former became the first gentlemen physicians. Contemporary culture also values individuality and, in particular, the maverick. EBM challenges these heroes by making knowledge explicit, systematic, and democratic. Rather than knowledge being hold by an olite few (expert opinion), following EBM principles enables even novices to obtain the best evidence. The evidence typically applies to those in clinical trials—ideal patients from a narrow spectrum of illness that may have only passing resemblance to individual patients in an office. Even guidelines that synthesize large volumes of information do not provide simple algorithms for each situation. Most guidelines state that the information does not replace clinical judgment and decision making by individual clinicians and their specific patients. Therefore clinical judgment remains an essential part of decision making for patient care.

Guidelines, a common EBM tool, can be taken as a standard of practice. Courts recognize, however, that it is only one standard of practice—multiple guidelines on a single topic and, therefore, multiple standards of practice may exist. The practice pattern of peers is another standard. Further complicating the issue is the knowledge that most guidelines are out of date within 2 years of publication. Therefore, the most recent information may not be incorporated in a guideline. Ignoring the existence of a guideline is not wise, but slavishly following a guideline does not serve patients well either. Awareness and familiarity with up-to-date information and the incorporation of patient preferences are the best defenses in practice.

What is EBM, then? It is the practice of taking information needs and formulating an answerable question, searching the literature for the best evidence, critically appraising the evidence for validity, applying the evidence, and evaluating the results. This requires multiple competencies: abilities to formulate good questions (harder than it initially seems), search the literature, critically appraise literature, extract useful information, and then reflect on the results when put into practice. Therefore, common clinical questions lend themselves best to this method due to the time and effort required.

## A WORKING EXAMPLE

In this article, a hypothetical case demonstrates the steps in EBM. Dr Jones sees Ms Smith, a 55-year-old woman, for Parkinson disease. She notes a left hand tremor at rest for 1 year. Examination reveals cogwheel rigidity in the left arm and bradykinesia. Ms Smith does not swing her arm on the left side but otherwise her examination is normal. Dr Jones confirms a diagnosis of parkinsonism, most likely Parkinson disease. Ms Smith asks how certain he is of the diagnosis.

Dr Jones turns to scientific literature with the question, "For patients diagnosed with Parkinson disease (patient population), how often is the diagnosis confirmed (diagnostic accuracy) on autopsy (gold standard)?" Dr Jones wants to refine his question by adding limits to the search. Which study design criteria should he impose?

Dr Jones checks the American Academy of Neurology (AAN) Web site for the Clinical Practice Guideline Process Manual and notes the criteria (listed in **Box 1**).[5]

The question of diagnostic accuracy is complicated because a diagnostic test does not exist for Parkinson disease and the diagnostic gold standard continues to be autopsy confirmation. Dr Jones uses the criteria for Parkinson disease diagnosis that two of the three features—tremor, bradykinesia, and rigidity—should be present to make the diagnosis. He finds a retrospective study (class III) where autopsy confirmation was the gold standard and clinical criteria are the same as his criteria.[6] The investigators report 99% sensitivity but only 8% specificity. The positive predictive value is 77% and the negative predictive value is 67%.

$$\text{Sensitivity} = \frac{\text{True Positives}}{\text{True Positives} + \text{False Negatives}}$$

Sensitivity answers the question, "Given the presence of the disease, what is the likelihood of having a positive test?" Specificity is the ability to detect the disease-free state or answers the question, "Given the absence of the condition, what is the likelihood the test is negative?" Usually, diagnostic criteria should have high specificity. In the instance of diagnosing Parkinson disease, the alternative disorders are mostly parkinsonian and patients with these diagnoses should also have a trial of levodopa. Therefore, diagnostic criteria can be more sensitive because applying treatment still is appropriate in the absence of Parkinson disease at autopsy.

Dr Jones then looks at the positive predictive value and knows that this tells him, if the test is positive, what the likelihood is that the condition is present. The negative predictive value tells him, if the test is negative, what the likelihood is that the condition is absent. In numeric terms,

$$\text{Positive Predictive Value} = \frac{\text{True Positives}}{\text{True Positives} + \text{False Positives}}$$

---

**Box 1**
**American Academy of Neurology criteria for diagnostic article quality**

Class I: Evidence provided by a prospective study in a broad spectrum of persons with the suspected condition, using a reference (gold) standard for case definition, where test is applied in a blinded evaluation enabling the assessment of appropriate tests of diagnostic accuracy. All patients undergoing the diagnostic test have the presence or absence of the disease determined.

Class II: Evidence provided by a prospective study of a narrow spectrum of persons with the suspected condition or a well-designed retrospective study of a broad spectrum of persons with an established condition (by gold standard) compared with a broad spectrum of controls where test is applied in a blinded evaluation enabling the assessment of appropriate tests of diagnostic accuracy.

Class III: Evidence provided by a retrospective study where persons with the established condition or controls are of a narrow spectrum and where the reference standard, if not objective, is applied by someone other than the person who performed the test.

Class IV: Any design where test is not applied in an independent evaluation or evidence provided by expert opinion alone or in descriptive case series (without controls).

*From* Edlund W, Gronseth G, So Y, Franklin G. AAN Clinical Practice Guideline Process Manual. St. Paul: American Academy of Neurology. 2005; with permission.

$$\text{Negative Predictive Value} = \frac{\text{True Negative}}{\text{True Negative} + \text{False Negative}}$$

If Dr Jones had the original data, he would like to know the diagnostic accuracy (efficiency) of the test or the proportion of correct results, true positives and true negatives.

$$\text{Diagnostic Accuracy (Efficiency)} = \frac{\text{True Positives} + \text{True Negatives}}{\text{No. of All Test Results}}$$

The same investigators applied the criteria for Parkinson disease diagnosis (ie, that all three features [tremor, bradykinesia, and rigidity] must be present) and found 65% sensitivity and 71% specificity, with a positive predictive value of 88% and a negative predictive value of 40%.

Dr Jones prefers criteria that have relatively good sensitivity and good specificity. The article further applies the criteria of asymmetric findings and the absence of atypical features. The sensitivity increases to 75% and specificity is 75% whereas the positive predictive value is 93% and the negative predictive value is 49%. Therefore, Dr Jones reports that he is 93% certain that she has Parkinson disease. The most common misdiagnoses are multiple systems atrophy, progressive supranuclear palsy, dementia with Lewy bodies, and other parkinsonian disorders.

At a later visit, Ms Smith is concerned about what the future holds for her. She asks, "What is my risk for dementia with Parkinson disease? How quickly will I progress?"

Dr Jones searches the literature to answer the question, "For a patient with initial tremor and Parkinson disease, what is the risk of dementia?" This demonstrates how to formulate a question for literature searches. A good memory aid to develop the question is the acronym PICO: specific Patient population, Intervention (in this case, prognostic factor), Control, and Outcome desired. Dr Jones recalls that the least biased information for therapies is provided by RCTs with objective outcomes or double-masked assessment. He wonders about comparable criteria for a high-quality prognostic article. Trying to minimize the risk of bias, Dr Jones determines that a prognostic article should have a broad spectrum of patients observed over a predetermined length of time for the outcome. The outcome should be objective or at least measured by an investigator who is blinded to the presence or absence of the predictor.

To provide Ms Smith with prognostic information, Dr Jones searches for studies that follow all subtypes of patients with Parkinson disease with clear assignment to tremor dominant or akinetic rigid without tremor, using the Unified Parkinson's Disease Rating Scale. Motor progression should be assessed by a rater blinded to the assignment of tremor dominant or akinetic rigid groups. Alternatively, he would accept a prospective study of tremor dominant patients whose progression over time was assessed by a blinded rater. At the last hospital meeting with administrators, he learned that they grade evidence on the four A's: accessible, accurate, applicable, and actionable.[7] Although easy to remember, it does not help him grade the quality of the evidence to allow him to make recommendations to his patient.

Dr Jones checks the criteria for prognostic studies from the AAN Web site (**Box 2**).[5] He finds that the articles retrieved are of low quality. The criteria for inclusion, duration of follow-up, masking to important prognostic variables, and transparent figures to allow calculation are all missing.

The important question for Dr Jones is, "Given a specific presentation, what is the risk of progressing to impaired walking due to imbalance" He would calculate the

---

**Box 2**
**American Academy of Neurology classification of prognostic evidence**

Class I: Evidence provided by a prospective study of a broad spectrum of persons who may be at risk for developing the outcome. The study measures the predictive ability using an independent gold standard for case definition. The predictor is measured in an evaluation that is masked to clinical presentation and the outcome is measured in an evaluation that is masked to the presence of the predictor. All patients have the predictor and outcome variables measured.

Class II: Evidence provided by a prospective study of a narrow spectrum of persons at risk for having the condition or by a retrospective study of a broad spectrum of persons with the condition compared with a broad spectrum of controls. The study measures the prognostic accuracy of the risk factor using an acceptable independent gold standard for case definition. The risk factor is measured in an evaluation that is masked to the outcome.

Class III: Evidence provided by a retrospective study where the persons with the condition or the controls are of a narrow spectrum. The study measures the predictive ability using an acceptable independent gold standard for case definition. The outcome, if not objective, is determined by someone other than the person who measured the predictor.

*From* Edlund W, Gronseth G, So Y, Franklin G. AAN Clinical Practice Guideline Process Manual. St. Paul: American Academy of Neurology. 2005; with permission.

---

following: the absolute risk reduction (or increase) for reaching (for example) Hoehn and Yahr stage 3 (bilateral signs with postural instability) disability in 5 years with a tremor presentation compared with patients with an akinetic rigid–no tremor presentation. Similarly, he would want to provide Ms Smith with the figure of absolute risk reduction (or increase) for a tremor dominant patient to develop dementia over the course of illness compared with progression for a patient with an akinetic rigid–no tremor presentation.

$$\text{Absolute Risk Reduction } (\%) = \text{Event rate for Control group} \\ - \text{Event rate for the treatment group}$$

$$\text{Relative Risk Reduction } = \frac{\text{Control Event rate} - \text{Treatment Event Rate}}{\text{Control Event Rate}}$$

Because the relative risk reduction is relative to the control group, the relative risk reduction may seem impressive for little gain. For example, a treatment for syncope is significantly better than placebo in a trial of 500 patients. The placebo group has a 4% rate of syncope and the treatment group has a 3% rate of syncope, the absolute reduction in syncope for the treatment group is 1% but the relative risk reduction is 25%—a much more impressive, but misleading, number.

For the syncope example,

$$\text{Number Needed to Treat } = 1/\text{Absolute Risk Reduction } = 1/0.04 - 0.03 = 100$$

The large number needed to treat result tells Dr Jones that the effect of the syncope treatment is minimal.

Dr Jones recalls that the $P$ value, or significance, may also be misleading. He knows that a $P$ value of 0.05 means that there is a 1 in 20 chance that the results are due to chance alone rather than a real difference between no treatment and the experimental drug. A smaller $P$ value does not mean that the results are more meaningful—the $P$ value reflects the risk that the results or difference between control and experimental group are due to chance alone and not a real effect of the experimental treatment. A smaller *P* value means the result is less likely to be a random occurrence and more likely a true treatment effect.

Dr Jones wonders what has a more accurate reflection of the precision of the study results. He reviews the definition of a confidence interval (CI). He learns that a CI puts an upper and lower limit on where the true treatment effect lies with 95% confidence. Put another way, the CI quantifies the effect of interest and also the uncertainty of this effect.[8] He also learns that a biased study with a large sample size can have a narrow CI. Dr Jones must first assess the quality of the study before calculating the CI.

When calculating the CI, the data used and the equation depends on the data analyzed. The reader may use online statistics calculators to estimated CIs.

Dr Jones sees that the CI is mostly affected by the sample size. For instance, if 25% of patients with a tremor presentation progress to instability in 5 years, and the number of tremor dominant patients followed is 200, the 95% CI is 19, 31. That is, there is a 95% certainty that the true percentage of tremor dominant patients progressive to instability in 5 years lies between 19 and 31%. Therefore, the effect of tremor is clinically important and there is little uncertainty that this result is true.

If the sample size were much smaller—say 20—the 95% CI is 8–42% meaning the result is less precise.

The smaller sample size means that the 95% CI now ranges from 15 to 35 making the result less precise.

Dr Jones returns to the available evidence for tremor and progression of illness. He learns from a recent review that there is strong evidence for higher age at onset (>57 years), predicting more disability, and that patients with predominantly axial symptoms, as indicated by the postural instability gait disorder composite score, have more disability compared with those with tremor as a significant problem. He is not able to give further information to Ms Smith because the required data are missing.[9] Dr Jones tells Ms Smith that tremor dominant patients and younger-onset patients have a better prognosis than those without tremor or with onset after 57 years.

After 2 years, Ms Smith returns reporting more disability. Previously, she used exercise to manage symptoms but now requests medication to improve motor function. Ms Smith finds writing on the chalkboard slow and laborious. Marking students' work is slow and she must arrive at work 1 hour earlier to prepare for work.

Dr Jones recalls studies comparing levodopa and dopamine agonists for the treatment of motor symptoms in Parkinson disease. He poses the following question, "For Parkinson disease patients not yet on medication requiring motor benefit, is a dopamine agonist or levodopa better for relief of motor disability?" Searching the literature, he identifies several articles and a guideline on initiating treatment in Parkinson disease. Reviewing the guideline, he notes that almost all the articles for levodopa compared with dopamine agonists are included. Checking the publication date of the guideline, he is concerned about its validity because it was published in 2002.[10] Dr Jones checks the AAN Web site and notes that on October 15, 2005, the guideline was reaffirmed.[11]

Dr Jones reviews the methodology for this particular guideline recognizing that guidelines have different degrees of rigor in development. Even more frustrating, he finds that there are multiple criteria for a good guideline. He reviews the criteria for a good guideline from the National Guideline Clearinghouse. All guidelines on this Web site must fulfill all four criteria: (1) have systematically developed statements that include recommendations, strategies, or information; (2) be produced by a medical specialty association; relevant professional society; public or private organization; government agency at the federal, state, or local level; or health care organization or plan; (3) be able to produce documentation and verify that a systematic literature search and review of existing scientific evidence published in peer-reviewed journals was performed; and (4) have a full-text guideline available on request in print or electronic format in the English language that was developed, reviewed, or revised within the past 5 years.

Dr Jones feels these criteria are not rigorous enough for him to recommend treatment. He checks the AGREE (Appraisal of Guidelines for Research and Evaluation) Instrument by the AGREE Collaboration.[12] The AGREE Instrument consists of 23 items in six domains: scope and purpose, stakeholder involvement, rigor of development, clarity and presentation, applicability, and editorial independence. Each item is graded on a four-point scale (**Box 3**). He decides it is too labor intensive for him to use more than once. Dr Jones reads an article on grading existing systems of guidelines.[13] He finds questions (listed in **Box 4**) to grade guideline process.

Dr Jones determines that the AAN guideline fulfills most of these criteria, indicating that the process is sound and conclusions are therefore valid.

Reading the conclusions, he sees that there is good quality evidence that levodopa or dopamine agonists can be used as initial therapy to address motor disability. The choice depends on individual patients because levodopa has superior motor benefit but has an increased risk of dyskinesias whereas dopamine agonists have a markedly reduced risk of dyskinesias.

---

**Box 3**
**AGREE Instrument**

*Scope and Purpose*

1. The overall objectives, clinical questions and patients to whome the guideline is meant to apply are specifically described.

*Stakeholder Involvement*

2. The guideline development group includes representatives from all relevant professional groups and defines clearly the target users, pilots the guidelines with the target users and takes into account patients' views and preferences.

*Rigor of Development*

3. Systematic methods using clear, explicit criteria for selection and the manner by which recommendations are formulated are clearly described. There is a clear link between the evidence used and the conclusions and recommendations. When making recommendations, the health benefits, side effects and risks are considered. There is an explicit link between the recommendations and the supporting evidence.

4. A clear process exists for updating the guideline.

*Clarity and Presentation*

5. The recommendations are specific and unambiguous and discuss different treatment options. Tools for endusers are supplied.

*Applicability*

6. The potential barriers to application including cost implications are considered.

7. The guideline proposes quality improvement measures based on conclusions.

*Editorial Independence*

8. The guideline is editorially independent from the funding body and all potential conflicts of interest are available for review.

*Adapted from* The Agree Collaboration. Appraisal of guidelines for research and evaluation: AGREE instrument. Available at www.agreecollaboration.org.

---

**Box 4**
**GRADE Working Group Critique of Existing Systems**

1. Is the process applicable to different types of clinical questions? Effectiveness, harm, diagnosis and prognosis.

2. Is the end product useful for patients, professionals and policy makers?

3. Is the process clear and logical?

4. How subjective are the steps in analysis or formulation?

5. Are there explicit levels of evidence or strengths of recommendation?

6. Are there important dimensions omitted?

7. Is the system successful in discriminating between high and low levels of evidence or strong and weak recommendations?

8. Are assessments reproducible?

*Data from* Atkins D, Eccles M, Flottorp S, et al. Systems for grading the quality of evidence and the strength of recommendations I: critical appraisal of existing approaches The GRADE Working Group. BMC Health Services Research 2004;4:38–45.

---

Dr Jones wants more specific information. He wants to understand the magnitude of benefit or risk reduction with the different drugs. Dr Jones retrieves one of the original articles.[14] The study reports that those starting levodopa (the control drug) have a 31% rate of dyskinesias after 5 years. In comparison, the subjects starting pramipexole first develop dyskinesias 10% of the time. He recalls that the number needed to treat tells him the number of patients he would have to treat with a dopamine agonist to avoid one case of dyskinesias. This is calculated as

$$\text{Number Needed to Treat} = 1/\text{Absolute Risk Reduction}$$
$$= 1/\% \text{ Dyskinetic Levodopa Subjects}$$
$$- \% \text{ Dyskinetic Pramipexole Subjects}$$
$$= 1/31\% - 10\% = 5$$

Therefore, Dr Jones tells Ms Smith that using pramipexole will result in an absolute risk reduction of 21%. That is, the likelihood of her developing dyskinesias if she uses pramipexole first is 10% compared with 31% for those starting levodopa treatment. The effect is such that Dr Jones would need to start five patients on pramipexole to avoid one patient developing dyskinesia in 5 years.

After learning this information, she asks about neuroprotective treatment in Parkinson disease. Searching PubMed, Dr Jones learns that there are several studies on neuroprotection in Parkinson disease and one guideline, again published by the AAN.[15] He already assessed the AAN guidelines as fulfilling the majority of criteria for good quality in the process. He uses the guideline as background information and formulates these questions: "For patients with Parkinson disease, does selegiline or rasagiline result in slower disease progression?" "For patients with Parkinson disease, are there other treatments that result in slower disease progression?"

Reviewing the guideline, Dr Jones concludes that levodopa is possibly neuroprotective over 9 months and that rasagiline may have neuroprotective benefit but that longer-term studies are required. An earlier analysis concluded that selegiline had symptomatic benefit and has not demonstrated neuroprotective benefit.[10] He discusses this with Ms Smith. Given the probability of motor benefit and fewer side effects, Ms Smith chooses levodopa to address her disability. Dr Jones reminds her that although motor benefit is superior with levodopa, the risk of motor complications is approximately 31% compared with 10% for pramipexole-treated patients at 5 years or a 21% risk reduction for dyskinesias with pramipexole as initial therapy.

Four years later, Ms Smith reports disabling dyskinesias through the majority of the waking day despite multiple dose manipulations. His question to guide the literature search is, "For patients with Parkinson disease and dyskinesias, do amantadine, clozapine, or dopamine agonists reduce dyskinesias but maintain motor function?" Dr Jones reviews case series reporting dyskinesia benefit with amantadine, clozapine, and dopamine agonists. Realizing that case series have a higher risk of bias (usually a single center, single physician practice with a narrow spectrum of patients), he seeks out clinical trials for dyskinesia reduction. Dr Jones finds a double-blind placebo-controlled study of amantadine to reduce dyskinesias and one study of clozapine to treat dyskinesias.[16,17] He will grade the studies for quality before basing treatment decisions on their results.

Dr Jones realizes there are multiple systems for grading evidence. He reads the Grading of Recommendations Assessment, Development and Evaluation Working Group (GRADE) assessment and notes that the criteria allow for consideration of study quality, but he cannot locate a single source to explain what constitutes a "serious limitation" (**Box 5**).[18] He turns to the AAN process and notes that for treatments, the criteria listed in **Box 6** apply.[5]

Using the two systems, he grades the first study for amantadine to treat dyskinesias. The study was randomized and placebo controlled, with a 92% completion rate (class I by AAN treatment criteria), but all subjects were from a single center (narrow spectrum of patients resulting in a downgrade to class II). Therefore, using the AAN criteria, Dr Jones concludes that amantadine is possibly effective to reduce dyskinesias in Parkinson disease and, therefore, may be considered to treat dyskinesias in Parkinson disease. Using the GRADE system, the limitations of a moderate likelihood of reporting bias from the single center and the short duration of the study mean the quality of evidence moves from high to low. This translates to "further research is likely to have an important impact on our confidence in the estimate of effect and is likely to change the estimate."[19] The recommendations that correspond to this level of evidence depend on the risk versus benefit of amantadine for dyskinesias. The study reports neither group had adverse events; however, the study was only 3 weeks in duration. Therefore, the risk versus benefit is unclear. Based on GRADE criteria, amantadine received a 2C recommendation (**Box 7**)[20]; that is, amantadine can be weakly recommended for the treatment of dyskinesias based on low-quality evidence and with uncertainty in the estimates of benefits versus risks. The recommendations using the AAN and GRADE criteria are similar.

Trying to compare the two studies, Dr Jones summarizes the following: amantadine resulted in a 24% reduction in dyskinesia severity as measured by the Goetz scale, decreased time "on" with dyskinesia, and improved motor "off" scores. The clozapine study measured time with dyskinesia and reported a 1.7-h reduction in dyskinesia time without changes in motor on or off scores. Three of 25 subjects receiving clozapine developed eosinophilia (a precursor to agranulocytosis) that quickly resolved. More subjects dropped out of the placebo arm than the clozapine arm. The relative risk of blood count abnormalities using clozapine is calculated as

$$\text{Risk of Eosinophilia} = \frac{\text{No. of Patients with Eosinophilia}}{\text{No. of Patients Exposed to Clozapine}} = 3/25 = 12\%$$

Both studies used small subject numbers over short periods of time (3 weeks for amantadine in a crossover design and 10 weeks for clozapine). Dr Jones takes this information to Ms Smith and gives his opinion that because clozapine has potential

---

**Box 5**
**Assessing Evidence from the GRADE pilot study**

1. Quality of evidence across studies for each outcome

    Evidence quality is High from a RCT

    Evidence quality is Moderate from a Quasi-RCT (not further specified)

    Evidence quality is Low from an observational study

    Evidence quality is Very Low from any other sources

    −1 grade: serious flaws; important inconsistency; or some uncertainty about the applicability to your question

    −2 grades: Very serious flaws; major uncertainty regarding applicability to your question

    +1 grade if: association is strong and there are no plausible confounders, the association is consistent and direct

    +2 grades if: Extremely strong association with no plausible confounders, the association is consistent and direct

2. Relative importance of outcomes

    For each outcome studied, the relative importance of this outcome for making a decision about the clinical question should be assessed. For instance, benefit of a treatment may be strong, but the risk of death is indeterminate. The risk might overshadow any treatment benefit. This does not change the judgment of the overall quality of evidence.

3. Overall quality of evidence across the important outcomes

    The overall quality of the evidence across the important outcomes, should be based on the lowest quality of evidence for the outcomes that are *critical* to making a decision.

4. Balance of the benefits and harms

    Presumed benefit should be weighed against the probable harms or possible harms where the outcome is serious (such as mortality).

5. Recommendation

    This should be based on the quality of evidence, the ability to incorporate the recommendation into practice and risk versus likely benefit

    Estimates for recommendations are:

        If 90–100% of people likely to do it = do it

        60–90% of people likely to do it = probably do it

        40–60% of people likely to do it = maybe do it

        30–40% of people likely to do it = probably don't do it

        0–30% of people likely to do it = don't do it

*Data from* Atkins D, Briss PA, Eccles M, et al. Systems for grading the quality of evidence and the strength of recommendations II: Pilot study of a new system. BMC Health Services Research 2005;5:25–37.

---

serious side effects (agranulocytosis, therefore requiring weekly blood monitoring) whereas the amantadine study had meaningful data (reduction in dyskinesia severity and reduction in motor off scores), he suggests amantadine. Ms Smith agrees with this treatment plan.

She experiences good dyskinesia control for 6 months but then reports she has disabling dyskinesias for the majority of the waking day. Dr Jones decides to research

---

**Box 6**
**American Academy of Neurology criteria for treatment**

Class I: Prospective RCT with masked outcome assessment, in a representative population. The following are required:

a. Primary outcomes clearly defined

b. Exclusion/inclusion criteria clearly defined

c. Adequate accounting for dropouts and crossovers with numbers sufficiently low to have minimal potential for bias

d. Relevant baseline characteristics are presented and substantially equivalent among treatment groups or there is appropriate statistical adjustment for differences

Class II: Prospective matched group cohort study in a representative population with masked outcome assessment that meets criteria listed in a–d or a RCT in a representative population that lacks one criteria listed in a–d.

Class III: All other controlled trials (including well-defined natural history controls or patients serving as own controls) in a representative population, where outcome is independently assessed or independently derived by objective outcome measurement.

Class IV: Evidence from uncontrolled studies, case series, case reports, or expert opinion.

*From* Edlund W, Gronseth G, So Y, Franklin G. AAN Clinical Practice Guideline Process Manual. St. Paul: American Academy of Neurology. 2005; with permission.

---

surgical options for Ms Smith, who is now 59 years old. He is aware that surgical treatments have evolved considerably since his training when pallidotomy was the treatment of choice. He limits his PubMed search to 2003 onwards, English language, RCT, guideline, or meta-analysis. His question is "for patients with disabling dyskinesias, does subthalamic nucleus stimulation result in dyskinesia reduction?" Thirty-three abstracts fulfill these criteria (July 22, 2008). Dr Jones retrieves one article to review in full.[21] The investigators report 178 subjects randomized to surgery or best medical treatment. Motor improvement was significantly greater for those undergoing subthalamic nucleus stimulation compared with best medical treatment, and a quality-of-life scale showed a similar improvement. Dr Jones notes that whereas the subjects were randomized to surgery or best medical therapy, the raters of the outcome were not blinded to treatment assignment. Therefore, the risk of bias is significant. A meta-analysis of the subject reveals the same deficiency—studies included used outcomes measured by unblinded assessors, thus leaving the results at risk for bias.[22]

Dr Jones calculates the number needed to harm because surgery is an invasive treatment. From Deuschl and colleagues[21] article, he notes that 12.8% of the surgery group had serious adverse events compared with 3.8% of the best medical therapy group.

Number Needed to Harm = 1/Absolute Risk Increase
= 1/(%Subthalamic Nucleus Deep Brain Stimulation-Subjects with Serious Adverse Events - % Controls with Serious Adverse Events)
= 1/(12.8% − 3.8%) = 1/9% = 11

Therefore, for every 11 patients receiving subthalamic nucleus deep brain stimulation, one additional patient has a serious adverse event.

---

**Box 7**
**GRADE system for evidence and recommendations**

Grade 1A: Strong recommendation (applying to most patients in most circumstances without reservation) with high-quality evidence

> Benefits clearly outweigh risk and burdens

> High-quality evidence from RCTs without important limitations or overwhelming evidence from observational studies

Grade 1B: Strong recommendation (can apply to most patients in most circumstances without reservation) with moderate-quality evidence

> Benefits clearly outweigh risk and burdens

> Moderate-quality evidence from RCTs with important limitations (inconsistent results, methodologic flaws, indirect or imprecise) or exceptionally strong evidence from observational studies

Grade 1C: Strong recommendation (but may change when higher-quality evidence becomes available) from low- or very low–quality evidence

> Benefits clearly outweigh risk and burdens

> Low-quality or very low–quality evidence from observational studies or case series

Grade 2A: Weak recommendation (best action may differ depending on circumstances or patients' or societal values) with high-quality evidence

> Benefits closely balanced with risks and burden

> RCTs without important limitations or overwhelming evidence from observational studies

Grade 2B: Weak recommendation (best action may differ depending on circumstances or patients' or societal values) with moderate-quality evidence

> Benefits closely balanced with risks and burden

> Evidence from RCTs with important limitations (inconsistent results, methodological flaws, indirect or imprecise) or exceptionally strong evidence from observational studies

Grade 2C: Very weak recommendation (other alternatives may be equally reasonable) from low-quality or very low–quality evidence

> Uncertainty in the estimates of benefits, risks and burden or benefits, risks and burden may be closely balanced

> Low- or very low–quality evidence from observational studies or case series

*Created from* Guyatt G, Gutterman D, Baumann MH, et al. Grading strength of recommendations and quality of evidence in clinical guidelines: report from an American College of Chest Physicians Task Force. Chest 2006;129:174–81; with permission.

---

The investigators report paired results (each surgical patient was matched to a best medical therapy patient) and found that for 55 of the 78 pairs, the surgical subject had better improvement. From the data, he could not tell what the likelihood of being dyskinesia-free is for Ms Smith should she undergo surgery (absolute risk reduction). To derive this figure, Dr Jones would need to know what qualifies as a good response for Ms Smith (completely free of dyskinesias or no disabling dyskinesias or less severe on time) and then be able to find the number of surgical patients fulfilling this criterion as compared with the number of best medical therapy patients fulfilling this criterion.

Ms Smith considers the information and decides to adjust her physical demands. She retires from teaching and elects to continue medical management. Nearly 10

> **Box 8**
>
> http://www.cche.net/usersguides/main.asp
>
> http://www.poems.msu.edu/InfoMastery/ (course on EBM with estimated times to complete modules)
>
> http://www.jr2.ox.ac.uk/bandolier/index.html (Bandolier for definitions and discussion of EBM)
>
> http://www.cmaj.ca/cgi/collection/evidence_based_medicine_series?page=2 (EBM web resources)

years after her diagnosis, Ms Smith returns to Dr Jones accompanied by her husband. He reports episodes of confusion and poor memory. Mr and Mrs Smith wonder if she has dementia and if there is treatment to improve cognition.

To answer these questions, Dr Jones needs to first diagnose Mrs Smith. He looks for information on screening tests for dementia in Parkinson disease. He is able to find one study using an exhaustive test instrument (Cambridge Cognitive Examination [Cam-Cog] compared with a screening test, the Mini–Mental Status Examination.[23] The study had Parkinson patients with dementia by *Diagnostic and Statistical Manual of Mental Disorders* (Fourth Edition) criteria (clinical gold standard) and those without dementia. Therefore, the tests were used in a broad population of patients that Dr Jones is also interested in. The tests perform similarly for detecting dementia. He concentrates on the numbers for the Mini–Mental Status Examination, because he feels this can be adopted in his practice (fulfilling the criteria applicability). The investigators report a sensitivity of 98% and specificity of 77% for a cutoff score of 23 of 30 points.

Dr Jones recalls that sensitivity is the proportion of true positives for a test. Specificity is the proportion of true negatives or, in mathematical terms,

$$\text{Sensitivity} = \frac{\text{True Positives}}{\text{True + False Positives}}$$

$$\text{Specificity} = \frac{\text{True Negatives}}{\text{True + False Negatives}}$$

Hence, the sensitivity should be high for a screening test to identify all possibly affected individuals and then apply the more specific test to identify all truly affected individuals. Specificity should be high for a diagnostic test, because this is the test used to definitely diagnose affected individuals for treatment. In the instance of dementia in Parkinson disease, the lengthy Cambridge Cognitive Examination performs well as a screening test and diagnostic test (95% sensitivity and 94% specificity).

Armed with this information, Dr Jones applies the Mini–Mental Status Examination and finds that Mrs Smith scores 21 of 30. He concludes, therefore, with reasonable certainty that Mrs Smith is cognitively impaired and counsels Mr and Mrs Smith further.

## SUMMARY

Mrs Smith's history demonstrates multiple opportunities to put EBM into practice. EBM is not using RCTs, algorithms, or practice by committee. EBM comprises a group of skills that are transparently applied to aid treatment decisions. Using available scientific evidence to provide clinically relevant and reliable information for clinicians and patients is an important arm of EBM practice. To further develop EBM skills, refer to the Web sites listed in **Box 8.**

Health care providers are challenged more than ever to provide evidence for their decisions. As the Agency for Healthcare Research and Quality explicitly states, EBM plays and will continue to play a crucial role in improving health care quality. Every neurologist should master EBM skills to provide patients with the best possible care.

## REFERENCES

1. Available at: http://www.kff.org/kaiserpolls/upload/7625.pdf. Accessed July 30, 2008.
2. Available at: http://www.ahrq.gov/about/highlt07.htm. Accessed July 30, 2008.
3. Cochrane AL. Effectiveness and efficiency: random reflections on health services. 2nd edition. London: Nuffield Provincial Hospitals Trust; 1971.
4. Guyatt G, Cairns J, Churchill D, et al. Evidence-based medicine working group evidence-based medicine. A new approach to teaching the practice of medicine. JAMA 1992;268:2420–5.
5. American Academy of Neurology. Clinical practice guideline process manual. 2004 edition. Available at: http://www.aan.com/globals/axon/assets/3749.pdf. Accessed July 30, 2008.
6. Hughes AJ, Daniel SE, Kilford L, et al. Accuracy of clinical diagnosis of idiopathic Parkinson's disease: a clinico-pathological study of 100 cases. J Neurol Neurosurg Psychiatr 1992;55:181–4.
7. Rundall TG, Martelli PF, Arroyo L, et al. The informed decisions toolbox: tools for knowledge transfer and performance improvement. J Healthc Manag 2007;52: 325–42.
8. Sackett DL, Richardson WS, Rosenberg W, et al. Evidence based medicine. London: Churchill Livingstone; 1998.
9. Post B, Maruschka P, Merkus P, et al. Prognostic factors for the progression of Parkinson's disease: a systematic review. Mov Disord 2007;22:1839–51.
10. Miyasaki JM, Martin W, Suchowersky O, et al. Practice parameter: initiation of treatment for Parkinson's disease: an evidence-based review. Neurology 2002; 58:11–7.
11. Available at: http://www.aan.com/index.cfm?axon=redirect&;&path=/go/practice/guidelines. Accessed July 30, 2008.
12. Available at: www.agreecollaboration.org. Accessed July 30, 2008.
13. Atkins D, Eccles M, Flottorp S, et al. Systems for grading the quality of evidence and the strength of recommendations I: critical appraisal of existing approaches The GRADE Working Group. BMC Health Serv Res 2004;4:38–45.
14. Parkinson Study Group. Pramipexole versus levodopa as initial treatment for Parkinson disease. JAMA 2000;284:1931–8.
15. Suchowersky O, Gronseth G, Perlmutter J, et al. Practice parameter: neuroprotective strategies and alternative therapies for Parkinson disease and evidence-based review. Neurology 2006;66:976–82.
16. Snow BJ, Macdonald L, McAuley D, et al. The effect of amantadine on levodopa-induced dyskinesias in Parkinson's disease: a double-blind, placebo-controlled study. Clin Neuropharmacol 2000;23:82–5.
17. Durif F, Debilly B, Galitzky M, et al. Clozapine improves dyskinesias in Parkinson disease: a double-blind, placebo-controlled study. Neurology 2004;62:381–8.

18. Atkins D, Briss PA, Eccles M, et al. Systems for grading the quality of evidence and the strength of recommendations II: pilot study of a new system. BMC Health Serv Res 2005;5:25–37.

19. Guyatt GH, Oxman AD, Vist GE, et al. GRADE: an emerging consensus on rating quality of evidence and strength of recommendations. BMJ 2008;336:924–6.

20. Guyatt G, Gutterman D, Baumann MH, et al. Grading strength of recommendations and quality of evidence in clinical guidelines: report from an American College of Chest Physicians Task Force. Chest 2006;129:174–81.

21. Deuschl G, Schade-Brittinger C, Krack P, et al. A randomized trial of deep-brain stimulation for Parkinson's disease. N Engl J Med 2006;355:896–908.

22. Kleiner-Fisman G, Herzog J, Fisman DN, et al. Subthalamic nucleus deep brain stimulation: summary and meta-analysis of outcomes. Mov Disord 2006;21: 290–304.

23. Hobson P, Meara J. The detection of dementia and cognitive impairment in a community population of elderly people with Parkinson's disease by use of the CAMCOG neuropsychological test. Age Ageing 1999;28:39–42.

# Pay for Performance and the Physicians Quality Reporting Initiative in Neurologic Practice

James C. Stevens, MD, FAAN[a,b,c,]*

---

**KEYWORDS**

- Pay for performance
- Physicians Quality Reporting Initiative
- Quality improvement • Health reform

---

Our nation's dedicated health care providers—physicians, nurses, hospitals, and others—work tirelessly to provide care to millions of Americans. Quality and efficiency of care, however, vary significantly across the country.[1] It has become increasingly evident to those paying for and receiving medical care that our system does not always encourage the right care at the right time for each and every patient.[2] Today's fee-for-service payment system perversely rewards providers for the quantity of care delivered, including the number of tests and procedures performed, irrespective of the quality and value of the treatment and evaluation decisions being made. While most people agree that America's health care system needs significant change, opinions on exactly how to reform it have divided policymakers and the public for decades. The Institute of Medicine (IOM) defines quality health care as care that is safe, timely, effective, and patient-centered, and that is delivered in an equitable, efficient manner.[3] A meaningfully reformed health care delivery system will reorient payment incentives toward services and activities that improve patient care in those areas outlined by the IOM, while at the same time slowing the pace of growth in national health care spending.

Pay for performance (P4P) is one strategy for moving from payment based solely on the quantity of services rendered to payment for quality or efficiency of care. Such

---

[a] Department of Neurology, Indiana University School of Medicine, 1701 North Senate Boulevard, Indianapolis, IN 46206, USA
[b] Practice Committee for the American Academy of Neurology, 1080 Montreal Avenue, St Paul, MN 55116, USA
[c] Department of Neurology, Fort Wayne Neurologic Center, 7956 West Jefferson Boulevard, Fort Wayne, IN 46804, USA
* Department of Neurology, Fort Wayne Neurologic Center, 7956 West Jefferson Boulevard, Fort Wayne, IN 46804.
*E-mail address:* JCS@FWNC.com

Neurol Clin 28 (2010) 505–516
doi:10.1016/j.ncl.2009.11.013
0733-8619/10/$ – see front matter
**neurologic.theclinics.com**

payment systems are now being used in private health plans as well as in government-run insurance plans. The most recent government-run, physician-centric plan is a pay-for-reporting effort, entitled the Physicians Quality Reporting Initiative (PQRI). This article reviews information concerning the what, why, how, pitfalls, and promise of these programs with the goal of gaining understanding of the role of such programs in health care reform in the United States.

## WHAT IS A PAY-FOR-PERFORMANCE PROGRAM AND WHY SHOULD IT BE CONSIDERED FOR HEALTH REFORM?

P4P programs are based on the practice of giving incentives (primarily financial) to providers to improve the quality of care they give their patients. These programs are intended to reward high clinical quality, well-coordinated, patient-centered, and efficient care. Quality care is defined above by the IOM,[3] as well as by the US Agency for Healthcare Research and Quality as "doing the right thing, at the right time, in the right way, for the right person—and having the best possible results."[4] Efficient care is defined as delivering the highest quality care for the least cost.[3]

The level of quality health care provided is determined by the use of standardized "performance measures," also called "quality indicators" or "quality measures." These measures are a defined set of criteria used to determine whether a service provided to a patient is consistent with the best available evidence on how to approach the specific issue or condition.[5] The measures typically are evidence-based (from medical literature, including practice guidelines), with numerator and denominator definitions, exclusions, and transparency of process. Good performance measures should truly reflect quality of care and fairly differentiate clinicians and institutions. They should have scientific validity without undue administrative or financial burden. Successful P4P programs require valid statistical methods transparent to all involved.[6] They should have the capability to determine whether these quality improvement efforts lead to change in the desired direction, whether efforts contribute to unintended consequences in other parts of the system or in patient results, and whether additional efforts are necessary to bring a process back to "acceptable" ranges.[7] Using the sample of success as the numerator and total opportunities as the denominator, events can be tracked over time by the monitoring organization.

These measures may be categorized as structural measures, process measures, and outcome measures (to be defined later in the text). They can be recorded from the medical chart, from claims data, or from electronic health record submissions to be used by the payer implementing the program. P4P programs can take on many forms. Various models may have different effects on provider motivation, collaboration, and team building. Some programs target primary care while others engage specialists or focus on hospitals rather than physicians. The form of payment may be an enhanced fee schedule, a straight bonus, or a block grant. Payment may also be indirect, through reduced administrative costs, reduced patient copays, or increased numbers of patients due to enhanced reputation.[6] Programs may give rewards for absolute levels of performance, or may reward by grading providers on a "curve" relative to peers. Fixed targets and absolute thresholds have the advantage of providing a predictable opportunity for reward. The amount of financial "skin" in these programs and the timeliness of reimbursement will especially affect participation.

Why should P4P programs be considered as part of a health reform initiative in the first place? As stated in the introduction, the current health care system is exceedingly expensive with no proof to date that the added costs lead to improved patient outcomes. Employers and consumers who pay these ever-increasing costs have rightly demanded evidence of value in the health care they are purchasing. In 2008, the United States spent more than 17% of its gross domestic product (GDP) on health care, which is more than any industrialized country in terms of per-capita spending.[1] By 2017, health expenditures are projected to consume almost 20% of the GDP, or $4.3 trillion annually.[1] Many United States businesses are having a difficult time competing globally when faced with paying billions of dollars to provide health insurance for employees and their families.[8] Rising costs are threatening the budgets in both the public and private sectors and, consequently, the affordability of health insurance.[9] Meanwhile, despite these enormous costs, several reports suggest that our health care system ranks low in several measures of quality. Both public and private payers are demanding increased accountability.

In 2001, the IOM report estimated that medical errors cause between 44,000 and 98,000 deaths annually.[3] The gap between what physicians know should be done and what is actually done accounts for more than $9 billion per year in lost productivity and $2 billion per year in hospital costs.[10] While the nation spends lavishly on many services that lack evidence for effectiveness (overuse), it fails to deliver effective services (underuse) that improve health. Typical patients may receive only 55% of recommended services, while disadvantaged patients and minorities often fare far worse.[11] Health outcomes in the United States, such as infant mortality rates and life expectancy, are below average when compared with those of other developed countries.[12] Examination of regional differences within the United States suggests that there is often an inverse correlation between outcomes and expenditures.[13] More than half of Americans are dissatisfied with their health care, an approval rating lower than that of citizens from the United Kingdom, Canada, and New Zealand.[14] Overuse is encouraged by such practice conditions as advertising campaigns that promote marginally effective drugs, lucrative reimbursement for procedures, and the threat of medico-legal liability for those providers who withhold therapies. These circumstances fuel spending and consume resources that would provide greater health gains if directed instead to quality and efficacious care.

Many perceive that we get exceedingly poor value for the dollars we spend on health care. Performance measurement should direct our attention and resources to where they will do the most good. As long as health care money is spent without apparently discriminating between low-priority, ineffective care and high-priority, effective care, the United States health care system will continue to worsen.[15] The ultimate public policy goal is to increase value for America's health care consumers. A step toward that goal would be to ensure that the highest quality care is being delivered in the most efficient manner possible. That means paying for quality of care rather than quantity of care. This can be done only through much-needed payment reforms. There is a need to shift from the complete autonomy of our current health care system to one of accountability. Accountability on the basis of clinical evidence is a "watchword" for health care reform in the United States.[16] Since the IOM report in 2001, which called for an alignment of payment incentives with quality improvement, P4P has been pushed to the forefront of health reform discussions. P4P is seen as one piece of the health care solution, although perhaps only an interim one. While P4P is by no means a panacea for escalating costs, the federal government and private insurers see P4P as an important catalyst for change and are therefore generating momentum behind efforts to establish P4P programs.

## HOW ARE QUALITY IMPROVEMENT, PAY FOR PERFORMANCE, AND THE PHYSICIANS QUALITY REPORTING INITIATIVE IMPLEMENTED?

Quality has long been measured to provide information to health care organizations. The public distribution of information on the quality of health care dates back at least to the 1860s when Florence Nightingale publicized the mortality rates of patients in London hospitals.[17] In 1914, Ernest A. Codman,[18] a surgeon at the Massachusetts General Hospital, established the first morbidity and mortality conferences. He wanted to compare hospitals, but the administration at Massachusetts General Hospital refused to give Codman permission to make such comparisons and subsequently revoked his staff privileges. He responded by starting his own hospital, named the End Result Hospital, and published outcomes and error data on a series of 337 patients.[19] Later, he became a founder of the Hospital Standardization Program, which eventually developed into the Joint Commission on Accreditation of Healthcare Organizations (JCAHO), now known as the Joint Commission.

Quality was initially studied as an industrial process in the United States by Walter A. Shewhart[20] in 1931. His concepts included identifying customer needs, reducing variation in processes, and minimizing inspections. Influenced by Shewhart's work, W. Edwards Deming recognized quality as a primary driver for industrial success and later introduced these methods to post–World War II Japanese engineers and executives.[21] Applied strategically, these approaches resulted in considerable growth in the Japanese automobile industry and its subsequent worldwide recognition for quality.

Formal quality improvement (QI) principles in the United States health care complex were not adopted until decades after they were first proposed. Not until the 1980s, when the JCAHO mandated quality improvement and performance measures for hospital accreditation, did QI in health care become a national mandate. By the 1990s, QI had entered the outpatient arena as some managed care organizations began basing payments to primary care practitioners on such performance measures as immunization rates, mammography screening, and other Health Plan Employer Data and Information Set (HEDIS) measures.[22] These measures were initially designed to be implemented by purchasers of health care and managed care organizations, and now are widely applied in employer-based managed care organizations.

Payers employ a wide range of performance measures when composing their scorecards. Most include some widely accepted clinical quality metrics (eg, the previously mentioned HEDIS measures), as well as other types of metrics, including patient satisfaction. In 1998, the federal government's growing interest in QI led to the development of a National Forum for Health Care Quality Measurement and Reporting, which later became the National Quality Forum (NQF). This group was designated to be "the principal body that endorses national healthcare performance measures, quality indicator or quality or care standards" by acting as a liaison between the Centers for Medicare and Medicaid Services (CMS) and the medical industry (including consumer groups and provider organizations) to set standards for health care quality.[23] The NQF is currently working to promulgate standardized performance measures that will be accepted across the industry, particularly in light of the fact that many health plans are already relying to a greater degree on medical specialty societies and their own physician networks to provide and select their P4P measures.

Valid, implementable, evidence-based measures of health care quality are required to improve the performance of our health care system. Only through such robust measures will it be possible to demonstrate that changes in practice or payment policies improve quality.[24] A comprehensive QI program should include measures that address structure, process, and outcomes.[25] Structural measures deal with the availability and quality of resources, management systems, and policy guidelines. An example of a health care structural component is the presence of an electronic prescribing system. Process measures evaluate the activities of physicians or other health care providers to determine if established evidence-based recommendations are being followed. An example of a process measure is the percentage of patients admitted to the hospital with a noncardioembolic ischemic stroke who are subsequently discharged on an antiplatelet agent. Outcome measures evaluate the end result of health care, and are typically based on group results rather than individual cases. An example of an outcome measure is the 90-day stroke and mortality rate following carotid endarterectomy.

Although many performance measures have been developed for the primary care physician with respect to chronic diseases, such as diabetes, heart failure, and chronic obstructive pulmonary disease, relatively few measures specifically address neurologic care. The only measure sets currently in use in a public program are those developed for stroke care.[22] In 2008, it was estimated that over 160 P4P programs were being used by private payers, covering over 85 million Americans, to measure and reimburse their participating providers. These are seen predominantly in health maintenance organizations with primary care providers, not-for-profit ownership, and payment by capitation systems.[26] Many of the payers were tying more than 5% of their overall reimbursement to the individual physician for their performance in the P4P program. The vast majority (over 95%) of hospitals participate in the government-run hospital quality reporting initiative, and accept P4P as an inevitability.[23] As more evidence regarding the results of the government-directed P4P demonstration programs become available, commercial plans will likely follow suit in an attempt to adopt "best practices."

A study of community health centers (where many indigent and minority patients receive care) by the Health Disparities Collaboratives of the Health Resources and Services Administration demonstrated an improvement in selected processes of care, such as foot examinations in diabetic patients, use of anti-inflammatory medications in patients with asthma, and routine checks of hemoglobin A1C levels, for those centers that had fully implemented quality measures versus centers that had not.[27] There was, however, no demonstrable improvement in the patients' clinical outcomes (ie, need for urgent care for asthma attacks, lowered hemoglobin A1C levels, better control of blood pressure in hypertensive patients).

In a hospital-based demonstration study by the Hospital Quality Alliance, 207 hospitals that participated in a P4P incentive program were compared with 406 hospitals that only reported performance (ie, they were not paid) on 10 individual performance measures and 4 composite measures of quality.[28] When comparing composite measures dealing with heart failure, acute myocardial infarction, and pneumonia, the hospitals that were paid (P4P) improved to a greater degree than those facilities that only reported. The improvements ranged from 2.6% to 4.1% over a 2-year period. Baseline performance was inversely associated with improvement.

The US Congress, as part of the Medicare Prescription Drug, Improvement, and Modernization Act of 2003, directed the IOM to identify and prioritize options for aligning performance with payment in the Medicare program. As a result of this mandate, the IOM developed three reports that formed a series called *Pathways to Quality*

*Health Care*, which offered strategies for implementing care deemed safe, effective, patient-centered, timely, efficient, and equitable.[29] Ten recommendations from the final report in the series resulted are included in the current PQRI. Those recommendations are:

1. P4P should be implemented in Medicare, using a phased approach, as a stimulus to foster comprehensive and system-wide improvements in the quality of health care.
2. Congress should derive the initial funding (over 3–5 years) for a P4P program in Medicare largely from existing funds.
3. Congress should give the Secretary of the Department of Health and Human Services (DHHS) the authority to aggregate the pools of money for different care settings into one consolidated pool from which all providers would be rewarded when new performance measures allow (shared accountability and care coordination).
4. The P4P program should reward health care that is of high quality, patient-centered, and efficient.
5. The program should reward both providers who improve performance significantly and those who achieve high performance.
6. Incentives should be offered to providers for the submission of performance data, which should be transparent and be made public in ways that are meaningful to consumers.
7. P4P for physicians should initially begin as a voluntary program, relying on financial incentives sufficient to ensure broad participation. Three years after the release of this August 2006 report, the Secretary of DHHS should determine if stronger actions—such as mandating provider participation—are required.
8. The P4P program should reward improved coordination of care across providers and through entire episodes of illness.
9. The Secretary of DHSS should explore a variety of approaches for assisting providers in the implementation of electronic data collection and reporting systems.
10. The Secretary of the DHHS should implement a monitoring and evaluation system for the Medicare P4P program.

As a result of the aforementioned IOM report, the 2006 Tax Relief and Health Care Act (Public Law No. 109–432) required the establishment of a physician quality reporting system that would include an incentive payment, which would be based on a percentage of the allowed Medicare charges for all such covered professional services, to eligible professionals who satisfactorily report data on quality measures.[1] CMS named the program the PQRI. The Medicare Improvements for Patients and Providers Act of 2008 (Public Law No. 110–275) (MIPPA) made this program permanent and extended the bonuses through 2010: The incentive was increased from 1.5% in 2007 to 2.0% for the 2008 through 2010 programs. No additional bonus payments were specified for the years following 2010. The professionals eligible to participate in the PQRI include Medicare physicians, physician assistants, nurse practitioners, nurse-midwives, nurse anesthetists, clinical social workers, registered dieticians, nutritional professionals, clinical psychologists, and therapists.

As directed by the legislation within the MIPPA, CMS is currently developing a plan for transitioning PQRI to a value-based purchasing program that will financially reward physicians based on their performance, rather than simply for reporting quality data. CMS is required to report to Congress by May 2010.

The initial PQRI program of 2007 (in which providers participated from July 1 through December 31, 2007) contains 74 performance measures.[30] They each consist of a numerator and a denominator that permit the calculation of the percentage of a defined patient population that receives a particular process of care or achieves a particular outcome. The denominator population is defined by certain *International Classification of Diseases, 9th Revision (ICD-9)* and *Current Procedural Terminology (CPT)* Category I codes specified in the measure and submitted as part of a claim for Medicare Physician Fee Schedule services by eligible professionals. When the patient is part of the denominator population, then the applicable *CPT* Category II code that defines the numerator is submitted.

When a patient falls in the denominator population, but specifications define circumstances in which a patient may be excluded from the numerator population, *CPT* Category II code modifiers 1-P, 2-P, or 3-P are available to describe a medical, patient, or system reason, respectively, for such exclusion.

To successfully report a measure under the PQRI program, it is necessary to report a numerator code (*CPT* Category II) with or without an applicable modifier. The performance measures that could be used by neurologists in the original PQRI program included screening for future fall risk, use of antidepressant medication during the acute phase for patients suffering a new episode of depression, medication reconciliation, advanced care plan, eight measures related to treatment of acute stroke, and two neuroimaging measures.

For 2008 and 2009, the PQRI program was modified with the addition of some measures and the elimination of others. For example, registry data can now be used for quality measure reporting and reports now can be include "groups" of measures that have been developed. To qualify for a "bonus" for reporting, the provider must submit at least three measures (fewer are allowed if the provider does not see Medicare patients who would qualify for reporting three or more measures) on at least 80% of the cases in which a measure is reportable. If successful, the provider receives a bonus (1.5% of all the Medicare fee-for-service submissions during the reporting period for the 2007 program, increased to 2% for the 2008 and 2009 programs). The provider could submit the information electronically or manually (via the CMS 1500 paper claim form). The program requires accurate and consistent use of the National Provider Identifier on claims, with the bonus being paid to the holder of record of the Taxpayer Identification Number. CMS made the determination that PQRI data were not to be reported publicly. A survey conducted by the American Academy of Neurology in 2009 of its membership determined that only 6.5% of neurologists participated in the 2007 PQRI program, dropping to 4.4% in 2008.[31]

CMS has decided in the 2010 PQRI program to accept only performance measures endorsed by the NQF, with allowance for grandfathering of prior performance measures from the American Quality Alliance. The measures submitted for approval to the NQF can come from a variety of sources, although in reality the majority comes from the Physicians Consortium for Performance Improvement (PCPI), which is the American Medical Association's committee for performance measure development, or from the National Committee for Quality Assurance. The process for selecting and approving the performance measures includes consideration of gaps in care, gaps in measures, care coordination, misuse, overuse, expenditures, and feasibility testing (whether they can be realistically measured and reported).[32] The process the PCPI uses for measure development is as follows:

1. Identify the topic.
2. Identify guidelines and the evidence base.

3. Define the evidence-based measures.
4. Send out for public comment.
5. Develop a portfolio of tools for implementation.
6. Pilot test the measures.
7. Forward to NQF-CMS for approval.

The PCPI Stroke and Stroke Rehabilitation Workgroup, which was led by a neurologist, produced eight measures meeting criteria for approval for PQRI implementation.[32] The performance measures now in the process of being developed or approved deal with epilepsy, Parkinson disease, multiple sclerosis, and headache.

## PITFALLS OF PAY-FOR-PERFORMANCE PROGRAMS

Although there has been much activity in the private and public sectors concerning the development and implementation of P4P programs over the last decade, these programs have faced numerous justifiable criticisms concerning their value. While the government spends a significant resources for biomedical research ($28 billion to the National Institutes of Health in 2006), relatively few dollars are spent on quality improvement development, implementation, and assessment (in 2006, $319 million were allocated to the Agency for Healthcare Research and Quality).[12] This results in a ratio of one dollar spent on the development of treatments and diagnostic tests compared with one penny spent to ensure that patients actually receive the appropriate care. Mandating certain treatment or diagnostic approaches to patient care, without anchoring a physician's judgment with regard to the particulars of the specific situation (eg, patient comorbidities, patient preferences, compliance concerns due to financial or cultural considerations), invites the risk that such mandates will be perceived as obstacles to good patient care, and may result in poor physician involvement in these programs.[9,15,33,34] It has been noted that many P4P programs are woefully incomplete (not comprehensive), providing performance measures for very few of the many key aspects of health care.[16,17] There is currently a lack of standardization of performance measurement among various private health plans, thereby creating a nightmare of confusion for those providers asked to participate in multiple P4P programs.[17,23]

There has been significant concern that the performance measures currently placed in P4P programs are not meaningful to good patient outcomes. The connection between structural or process measures and patient outcomes is often simply presumptive.[17,24,26] Defining problems and solutions concerning patient safety and performance measures can also be quite problematic.[24] It is acknowledged that many solutions in health care do not require an evidence-based performance measure to know the answer of what is the "right thing" to do for a patient (eg, the necessity of conducting a randomized trial to determine whether jumping from an airplane with a parachute is better than jumping without one).[35] The shortcomings of the previously mentioned HEDIS measures have been acknowledged: The measures are seen as inefficient and at times even counterproductive to improving clinical outcomes.[15] Much of the care recommended is of modest or unproven value, making mandatory adherence ineffective in improving the quality of care delivered. It has been noted that many P4P programs choose to measure what is easy to follow rather than what is most important to improving patient outcomes.[23] The use of "consensus-based" measures also is potentially fraught with problems, as our currently held "beliefs" may, in fact, have little to do with the reality of improving patient care.[17] We have an important need, therefore, to evaluate the effectiveness of implementing any performance measure. A systematic approach of study, similar to the way we conduct biomedical research, should be employed to avoid unintended consequences when incorporating these measures into our day-to-day management of patients.[7,9,16,24] Yet, in most circumstances, this is still not being done.

Allowing for appropriate risk adjustment is also a concern when participating in a P4P program. The results of these programs (if made available to the public) could mislead consumers and give health providers an incentive to avoid caring for those who are extremely ill or who are unlikely to follow through with recommendations (so-called "gaming" the system).[6,16,17]

Implementation of these programs is not without challenges and costs. These may be represented, for example, by the financial burden of acquiring software and increased personal or personnel time for the documentation required to ensure that the data submitted and received accurately reflect the work done.[9,17,24,26] The validity of claims data and even electronic health record data has come into question.[26,36] In a recent study, the use of electronic health record data missed many exclusion criteria for medications documented in providers' notes. As a result, there was an underestimation of performance on a medication-based performance measure (use of warfarin in patients with atrial fibrillation and heart failure).[36]

There is also the question of whether the financial incentives offered by the P4P programs are significant enough to generate widespread involvement of health care providers.[9,26] With the offer of a 2% bonus on the Medicare fee for service charges during the reporting period, the CMS voluntary reporting program (PQRI) has attracted relatively little interest from providers of neurologic care.[31] Apart from using mandates, a significant amount of "skin" will need to be placed in these programs as a motivation for adequate participation (akin to the 30% of total annual reimbursement seen in the United Kingdom's P4P offering).[22] Unless these issues are adequately addressed, mandated performance measures may never work as intended and could lead to ineffectual health care delivery.

## THE PROMISE OF PAY-FOR-PERFORMANCE PROGRAMS

Despite the concerns outlined above, there is the potential for considerable improvement in health care delivery by using P4P as one of many tools for reforming health care. Several studies demonstrate that, as the focus is placed on quality improvement, physicians and patients benefit.[37] Quality improvement does not necessarily lead to higher costs and in fact quite often leads to lower costs of care.[38] A large percentage of physician time is wasted by poor coordination, redundancy of effort, and poor sharing of information, resulting in great variability in how care is delivered. With P4P, there exists the potential, with appropriate incentives, to increase value for patients through improvements in the entire sequence of activities involved in their care.[23] Using performance measures based solidly on evidence and validated for their utility in improving patient outcomes, physicians and other health care providers can be properly motivated, via a P4P system, to reorganize their services around the integrated care of medical conditions.[26,39] The US Congress approved in 2009 an allocation of $1 billion dollars for comparative effectiveness research.[34] This will involve over 100 projects that promise to add significantly to our database to develop meaningful, evidence-based performance measures. Both public and private payers could use approved performance measures from a central body, such as the NQF, to develop a standardized system of measurement. By better identifying areas of overuse and underuse and thus enabling more precise targeting of health care dollars to where they do the most good, P4P could play a key role in repairing our fundamentally flawed payment system.[15]

## SUMMARY

Transforming our current health care system requires long-term behavioral change. P4P is only one of many reforms needed to establish a sustainable health system in the United States. The ultimate public policy goals are to increase value for America's health care consumers, to ensure that the highest quality of care is being delivered in the most efficient manner possible, and to pay for quality of care and not just for quantity of care. It is unknown whether P4P and PQRI will affect behavior enough to improve patient outcomes. Measurement and feedback, as well as public transparency, can create incentives that go beyond those related to finances. Physicians are motivated in varying degrees by professionalism, altruism, duty to patients, regret from bad outcomes, risk aversion, desire for enhanced reputation, and other intangible rewards and punishments. It is not certain whether monetary rewards will add enough additional incentive to improve performance. Physicians will need to remain vigilant, and payers should be encouraged to closely monitor and examine the consequences of these programs. For any P4P program to succeed, the performance measures must be valid, and the providers must be engaged and reasonably rewarded. The data collection and reporting should not be complicated, and ongoing analysis of P4P outcomes must be included to ensure that unintended consequences do not arise and that appropriate outcome goals are achieved.

P4P is certainly not a panacea for our escalating medical costs, which are driven variously by structural issues, including the number of the uninsured, the rapid increase in our aging population, and the costs of advances in medical technology and therapeutics. Nevertheless, the federal government and private payers are building momentum for P4P as a catalyst for change and health care reform.

## REFERENCES

1. Senate Finance Committee Report. Transforming the health care delivery system: proposals to improve patient care and reduce health care costs. Washington, DC: National Academy Press; 2009. p. 2–10.
2. Varkey P, Reller K, Resar R. Basics of quality improvement in health care. Mayo Clin Proc 2007;82(6):735–9.
3. Institute of Medicine. Crossing the quality chasm: a new health system for the 21st century. Washington, DC: National Academy Press; 2001.
4. Agency for Healthcare Research and Quality, US Department of Health and Human Services. Your guide to choosing quality healthcare: a quick look at quality. Available at: www.ahrq.gov/consumer/qnt/qntqlook.htm. Accessed August 25, 2009.
5. Rosenthal MB, Landon BE, Normand SLT, et al. Pay for performance in commercial HMO's. N Engl J Med 2006;355(18):1895–902.
6. Brush J, Krumholtz H. Pay for performance: hype or key to quality? Cardiosource 2007;7:201–6.
7. Shine KI. Health care quality and how to achieve it. Acad Med 2002;77:91–9.
8. Cortese D, Smoldt R. Healing America's ailing heath care system. Mayo Clin Proc 2006;81(4):492–6.
9. Health Reform Dialogue. A dialogue on US health reform. March, 2009.
10. National Committee for Quality Assurance. The state of healthcare quality: 2004. Available at: www.ncqa.org/communications/SOMC/SOHC2004.pdf. Accessed August 25, 2009.
11. McGlynn EA, Asch SM, Adams J, et al. The quality of health care delivered to adults in the United States. N Engl J Med 2003;348(2):2635–45.

12. Woolf SH. Potential health and economic consequences of misplaced priorities. JAMA 2007;297(5):523–6.
13. Wennberg JE, Cooper MM, edltors. The Dartmouth atlas of health care in the United States. (IL): American Hospital Association Press; 1999. p. 143–7.
14. Schoen C, Osborn R, Huynh PT, et al. Primary care and health system performance: adults experience in 5 countries. Health Aff 2004;4:487–503.
15. Hayward R. Performance measurement in search of a path. N Engl J Med 2007; 356(9):951–3.
16. Fisher E. Paying for performance—risks and recommendations. N Engl J Med 2006;355(18):1845–7.
17. Epstein A. Performance reports on quality—prototypes, problems, and prospects. N Engl J Med 1995;337(1):57–61.
18. Codman EA. The product of a hospital. Surg Gynecol Obstet 1914;18:491–6.
19. Codman EA. A study in hospital efficiency: as demonstrated by the case report of the first five years of a private hospital 1916. Private printing. (IL): Reprinted by JCAHO; 1996.
20. Shewhart WA. Economic control of quality of manufactured product. New York: D. Van Nostrand Co; 1931.
21. Deming EW. Out of crisis. Cambridge (MA): MIT Center for Advanced Engineering Study Publishing; 1982.
22. Bever CT, Holloway RG, Iverson DJ, et al. Neurology and quality improvement: an introduction. Neurology 2008;70:1636–40.
23. Keeping score: a comparison of pay for performance programs among commercial insurers. Baltimore (MD): PriceWaterhouse Coopers' Health Insurance Institute; 2008. p. 1–22.
24. Auerbach AD, Landefed CS, Shojania KG. The tension between needing to improve care and knowing how to do it. N Engl J Med 2007;357(6):608–13.
25. Donabedian A. The quality of car. How can it be assessed? Arch Pathol Lab Med 1997;121:1145–50.
26. Endsley S, Baker G, Kershner B, et al. What physicians need to know about pay for performance. Fam Pract Manag 2006;3:69–73.
27. Landon BE, Hicks LS, O'Malley AJ, et al. Improving the management of chronic disease at community health centers. N Engl J Med 2007;356(9):921–34.
28. Lindenauer PK, Remus D, Roman S, et al. Public reporting and pay for performance in hospital quality improvement. N Engl J Med 2007;356(5):486–96.
29. Institute of Medicine. Rewarding provider performance: aligning incentives in Medicare. Washington, DC: National Academy Press; 2006.
30. Centers for Medicare and Medicaid Services. 2007 physicians quality reporting initiative. Available at: www.cms.hhs.gov/PQRI/01Overview.asp#TopOfPage. Accessed August 27, 2009.
31. American Academy of Neurology. 2009 membership survey. Available at: www.aan.com. Accessed August 27, 2009.
32. Centers for Medicare and Medicaid Services. Overview of physicians quality reporting initiative. Available at: www.cms.hhs.gov/PQRI/02Overview.asp#TopOfPage. Accessed August 27, 2009.
33. Greene RA, Beckman HB, Mahoney T. Beyond the efficiency index: finding a better way to reduce overuse and increase efficiency in physician care. Health Aff 2008;27(4):250–9.
34. Hatzband P, Groopman J. Keeping the patient in the equation—Humanism and health care reform. N Engl J Med 2009;361(6):554–5.

35. Health A. Athenahealth helps physicians maximize revenue under new national Medicare pay for performance program. Available at: www.athenahealth.com. Accessed August 27, 2009.

36. Baker D, Persell S, Thompson BA, et al. Automated review of electronic health records to assess quality of care for outpatients with heart failure. Ann Intern Med 2007;146(4):270–8.

37. Porter ME, Teisberg EO. Redefining health care. (MA): Harvard Business School Press; 2006. p. 149–228.

38. Premiere, Inc. Centers for Medicare and Medicaid Services. Premiere hospital quality incentive demonstration (HQID) project: findings from year two. Charlotte (NC): Premiere, Inc; 2006.

39. Batalden P, Splaine M. What will it take to lead the continual improvement and innovation of health care in the twenty-first century? Qual Manag Health Care 2002;11:45–54.

# Patient Education in Neurology

Andrea N. Leep Hunderfund, MD, J.D. Bartleson, MD*

**KEYWORDS**

- Education • Patient education • Communication
- Health literacy • Neurology

Patient education is a critical component of the medical encounter—so much so that it has been deemed a fundamental patient right.[1] Patients increasingly want to participate in their own health care. In order to make the best health decisions for themselves or their family members, patients need to clearly understand the diagnosis, prognosis, treatment options (with their attendant risks), and principles of disease prevention. It is the responsibility of health care providers to ensure that this information is given and that effective patient education occurs. The ever-expanding number of diseases, diagnostic modalities, and treatments in neurology make this responsibility more important and more challenging than in the past.

Although physicians have always provided such information to patients, the type and amount of information varies greatly, frequently consisting of what a physician considers important rather than information that a patient needs or wants. Patient surveys consistently find that patients are dissatisfied with the information health care providers give them[2–4] and that they desire better communication.[5] Communication breakdowns between physicians and patients are frequent. For example, studies have shown that half of psychosocial and psychiatric problems are missed,[6] that physicians interrupt patients an average of 18 seconds into patient description of the presenting problem,[7] that 54% of patient problems and 45% of patient concerns are neither elicited by physicians nor disclosed by patients,[8] that patients and physicians do not agree on the main presenting problem in 50% of visits,[9] that patients and doctors often disagree on the key messages that should be taken away from a consultation,[10] and that physicians often underestimate patients' desire for information.[11] Such communication breakdowns are frequently the basis for complaints to licensing bodies and for malpractice suits.[12]

Patients often do not understand or recall what a physician has told them.[13–16] Recall is further decreased when the information given to patients is upsetting.[3] Disorders affecting sight, hearing, language, or cognition—all commonly seen in neurology—create additional obstacles. For example, in one study, approximately one quarter of patients

Department of Neurology, Mayo Clinic College of Medicine, 200 First Street SW, Rochester, MN 55905, USA
* Corresponding author.
*E-mail address:* bartleson.john@mayo.edu (J.D. Bartleson).

Neurol Clin 28 (2010) 517–536
doi:10.1016/j.ncl.2009.11.002
0733-8619/10/$ – see front matter
**neurologic.theclinics.com**

discharged from the hospital after suffering a stroke could not differentiate between stroke and heart attack.[17] Another study showed that approximately one quarter of stroke patients lacked the basic understanding that stroke was caused by damage to the brain.[18] Despite these observations, obstacles to learning frequently go unrecognized by health care providers and only rarely is any assessment made of whether or not patients actually understand or recall the information given. The consequence of poor understanding or recall is that patients often feel they lack information. This in turn leads to feelings of uncertainty, anxiety, depression, and frustration.[3]

Physicians generally assume that patients will follow directions but often fail to identify potential barriers to their implementation, despite the fact that there are many reasons for nonadherence. These include problems with the prescribed or recommended regimen (such as adverse effects), poor instructions, poor provider-patient relationship, poor memory, patients' disagreement with the need for treatment, patients' inability to afford care, and many others.[19-21] Lack of adherence is then blamed on patient noncompliance rather than prompting a critical appraisal of the initial patient education provided or a search for obstacles that may be interfering with adherence to treatment recommendations.

Although it is generally accepted that patient education is important,[22-24] health care providers often receive little or no formal training in this discipline. The implicit assumptions are that knowledge of medical facts automatically translates into the ability to explain them to patients and that patients will in turn understand the information that is provided. Simple knowledge of medical facts, however, does not automatically translate into the ability to effectively explain them to patients. This is demonstrated by the fact that health care providers remain deficient in communication skills[25,26] and rate their knowledge and expertise in this area as lacking.[27] Fortunately, medical communication skills—a fundamental component of effective patient education—can be successfully taught and learned.[28-31]

The purpose of this review is to provide a definition of patient education, to examine the potential benefits and effectiveness of patient education, to build a general framework for approaching patient education, and to summarize representative studies of patient education in selected neurologic conditions.

## WHAT IS PATIENT EDUCATION?

In practical terms, patient education can be viewed as any advice or information (verbal, written, audiovisual, or otherwise) given by health care professionals to improve patients' understanding of their health condition and potential treatment options.[32] Van den Borne defines patient education more precisely as a "systematic experience in which a combination of methods is generally used, such as the provision of information and advice and behavior modification techniques, which influence the way the patient experiences his illness and/or his knowledge and health behaviors, aimed at improving or maintaining or learning to cope with a condition, usually a chronic one."[33] The American Academy of Family Physicians defines patient education as "a process that changes or enhances a patient's knowledge, attitudes, or skills to maintain or improve health."[34] These definitions underscore the need to impart not only facts but also sufficient understanding of a condition and its treatment such that patients will demonstrate behavioral changes that in turn lead to positive health outcomes.

## BENEFITS OF PATIENT EDUCATION

Patient education can justifiably be regarded as valuable in its own right. As with many other complex interventions in health care, the effectiveness of patient education is difficult to study. This is due in part to the widely variable nature of patient education interventions, which can be characterized according to six dimensions (**Box 1**).[35] One patient education intervention can vary from the next based on any combination of these six dimensions. They can even vary within a given dimension (eg, the effectiveness of verbal education is influenced by the social skills, communication skills, and clinical experience of the educator; the effectiveness of written materials is dependent on how the material has been developed and presented and how much time patients spend reading the material). For these reasons, it is difficult to draw broad conclusions from or perform pooled analyses of available patient education research.

Keeping these limitations in mind, studies have shown that patient education can have a positive impact on patient satisfaction,[36] health-related quality of life and mood,[37–40] adherence to treatment plans,[41,42] disease self-management skills,[43,44] and improved medical outcomes.[45–48] High-quality provider-patient communication—a fundamental component of effective patient education—also has many benefits, including improved patient satisfaction,[49–53] better adherence to treatment plans,[54] decreased risk of malpractice suits,[55] improved medical outcomes,[4,56] and decreased burnout and work-related stress among health care providers.[57]

Providing information through patient education efforts can also prevent unnecessary use of health care resources and enhance patient self-care through the use of active coping strategies.[43,44] Active coping strategies help patients learn to deal with a problem using resources available to them or to function in spite of the problem. Passive coping strategies, in contrast, permit patients to relinquish control of a problem and allow it to adversely affect other areas of life.[58,59] This leads to maladaptive outcomes, such as feelings of helplessness, excessive reliance on others, increased pain, and depression.[60] Active coping strategies may be particularly beneficial in conditions, such as low back or neck pain, which often are associated with substantial health care use and missed time from work despite having a favorable natural history.[61–63]

## GENERAL FRAMEWORK FOR APPROACHING PATIENT EDUCATION

Given the many potential benefits of patient education, it is important for physicians to nurture and develop their skills in this area. The following discussion provides a general framework for approaching patient education—specifically, the use of educational interventions to produce changes in patient knowledge, attitudes, behaviors, or skills needed to maintain or improve their health.

---

**Box 1**
**Six dimensions of patient education interventions, with examples**

1. Relationship of instructor to learner: independent, one-on-one, group

2. Medium: oral, written, audiovisual, Internet

3. Technique: lecture, discussion, demonstration, practice

4. Pedagogic characteristics: degree of structure, duration, frequency, intensity

5. Type of follow-up: use of reminders, feedback, reinforcement

6. Type of behavior change principles considered: motivation, self-efficacy, readiness to change

*Adapted from* Haines T, Gross A, Burnie SJ, et al. Patient education for neck pain with or without radiculopathy. Cochrane Database Syst Rev 2009;1:CD005106; with permission.

A fundamental goal of the typical patient encounter is to evaluate the chief complaint and make an assessment of the patient's health condition. For patients with new problems, this includes determination of the diagnosis, prognosis, and treatment options based on a careful history, physical examination, and diagnostic testing. For patients with established chronic conditions, the focus is on an assessment of the state of the disease process, its impact on patients, and the effectiveness of its management to date. This should be done in a patient-centered way rather than an illness-centered way.[64]

As a patient's chief complaint and health condition are being evaluated, it is important to also assess the patient's baseline knowledge, attitudes, behaviors, and skills as they pertain to this condition. This helps the health care provider identify and prioritize the patient's education needs. Questions to consider during this process include the following:

1. Is the patient lacking knowledge about current diagnosis, prognosis, or treatment options or disease prevention? General questions patients should be able to answer at the end of every office visit are outlined in **Box 2**.[65]
2. Does the patient have an attitude or behavior that needs to be changed or developed to maintain or improve his or her health? Common examples encountered in clinical practice include lifestyle changes, such as smoking cessation, moderation of alcohol intake, weight loss, dietary modifications, exercise or stretching programs, sleep hygiene, and driving restrictions. Adherence to treatment recommendations (eg, prescribed medications; follow-up appointments; use of devices, such as continuous positive airway pressure machines or gait aids; and so forth) is also highly dependent on patient attitudes and behaviors.[66]
3. Is the patient lacking a skill important to the prevention or management of disease? Certain diseases require mastery of a skill for optimal management. Examples

---

**Box 2**
**Questions patients should be able to answer at the end of an office visit**

What health problems do I have, and what should I do about them?

Where do I go for tests, treatment, and follow-up?

How should I take my medications?

    When do I take them?

    What will they do?

    How do I know if they are working?

    What are the possible side effects?

Are there any other instructions?

    What to do?

    How to do them?

    When to do them?

What are the next steps?

    When do I need to be seen again?

    Do I have another appointment? If so, what are the date and time?

Whom do I call if I have questions? What are the phone numbers to call?

*Adapted from* Weiss BD. Health literacy: a manual for clinicians. Chicago: American Medical Association Foundation and American Medical Association; 2003. p. 40; with permission.

include checking blood sugar, administering an injection (eg, immunotherapy for multiple sclerosis [MS]), responding to an acute event (eg, first aid for seizures), using devices (eg, blood pressure cuff, orthotic, gait aid, pill container, communication device, feeding tube, deep brain stimulator, or vagal nerve stimulator), or learning adaptive or therapeutic techniques (such as those taught by physical, occupational, speech, and cognitive behavioral therapists). Less readily apparent examples include the ability to understand written materials, navigate the medical system, access needed information, or develop active coping skills.

It is important to take into account patients' readiness to learn, their values and priorities, and any potential barriers or obstacles that could interfere with the achievement of a given educational goal. Such barriers may be related to age, level of education, ethnicity, low cognitive abilities, low income, and other patient-specific factors.[67–70] The concept of low health literacy has gained attention in recent years as a significant obstacle to effective patient education and a predictor of poorer health outcomes, including mortality.[71–73]

Health literacy is defined as "the degree to which individuals have the capacity to obtain, process, and understand basic health information and services required to make appropriate health decisions."[74] Low health literacy limits patients' ability to comprehend, retain, recall, and act on health care information provided. Research suggests that health literacy is a stronger predictor of health status than socioeconomic status, age, or ethnic background.[75–77] More than a third of English-speaking patients and more than half of primarily Spanish-speaking patients seen at United States public hospitals have low health literacy.[72]

All domains of literacy—listening, speaking, reading, writing, and numeracy—influence health literacy, as does a patient's cultural and conceptual knowledge of health.[70] Other factors that contribute to low health literacy include older age, decreased general cognitive skills, limited education, limited English language proficiency, lack of experience in the current health care system, the complexity of information being presented, and how the information is communicated.[78–80] Although most adults read at an eighth-grade level and 20% of the population reads at or below a fifth-grade level, the majority of health care materials are written at or above a 10th-grade level.[81,82] Thus, even well-educated patients can be relatively illiterate when it comes to medical conditions. For example, only 67% to 91% of patients can correctly understand medication label instructions, and even patients with the highest literacy levels err between 5% and 27% of the time.[83]

Three questions can be used to rapidly determine if a patient has poor health literacy. These include (1) How often do you have someone help you read hospital materials? (2) How confident are you filling out medical forms by yourself? and (3) How often do you have problems learning about your medical condition because of difficulty understanding written information?[84] Certain behaviors and responses can also suggest poor health literacy. These include filling out forms incompletely or inaccurately, frequently missing appointments, being unable to name medications or explain their purpose, allowing a family member to intervene in the conversation, and claiming to have forgotten glasses to avoid reading in front of a health care provider.[78,79]

Comorbid conditions can also pose significant obstacles to effective patient education. These include depression, anxiety, other psychiatric disease, physical limitations, hearing or vision impairments, learning disabilities, language dysfunction, and dementia or other brain injury.[69] Neurologists may be especially likely to encounter these in routine clinical practice.

Once a patient's education needs are identified, appropriate educational goals and objectives can be set. These goals and objectives are then used to direct and focus education efforts. These should focus on enabling patients to improve knowledge, change an attitude or behavior, or acquire a skill. Education interventions can take many forms according to the six dimensions outlined in **Box 1**. The ideal educational effort is one that is tailored to patients' educational needs, is guided by their values and priorities, and takes into account any obstacles or barriers they may face.

When the goal is to improve patient knowledge, it is important to use effective communication techniques. These include limiting the amount of information provided (and repeating it), speaking slowly, using plain nonmedical terminology (**Table 1**), employing multiple methods of conveying the key messages (drawing or using pictures, providing written material, and so forth),[85] and creating a positive, shame-free environment to encourage questions.[86,87] Using the simple phrase, "What else?" for example, allows patients to express all of their concerns openly.[88]

Effective patient education also requires finding out what patients already know and believe—then building on that understanding and correcting it when necessary. This has been promoted as the "ask, tell, ask" or "teach-back" strategy: (1) ask patients to explain the issue, problem, or treatment in their own words; (2) provide patients with relevant information; and (3) ask patients to rephrase in their own words the information that was just provided or to voice additional questions and concerns.[89] This strategy was found to provide a more accurate clinical assessment of patients' problems and to shorten office visits.[31]

Such strategies can also help reveal any preconceived ideas patients may have about their condition. Studies have shown that the most common sources of medical information for patients are family and friends followed by mass media and the Internet.[90,91] This is important to recognize, because portrayals of neurologic disease in the media are often misleading and inaccurate.[92,93] Finally, it is helpful to find out what patients have heard from other health care providers, as patients can become confused and distressed when they hear conflicting advice from different doctors.

Throughout this process, it is important to keep in mind that patients may differ in how much information they desire about their health condition.[94] Some patients, for example, may prefer a nonparticipatory role.[95] Although younger, white, middle-class, educated patients tend to ask more questions,[96] older, less-educated patients do not view themselves as less involved.[97] When asked, patients of different socioeconomic classes do not differ in how much information they say they want.[96]

When the goal is to change patient attitude or behavior, the first step is to assess a patient's readiness to change. This can be done using the transtheoretic or Stages of Change model of health behavior change.[98] According to this model, there are five stages of change: (1) precontemplation (not yet acknowledging that there is a problem or behavior that needs to be changed), (2) contemplation (acknowledging that there is a problem but not yet ready or sure of wanting to make a change), (3) preparation (getting ready to change), (4) action (actively changing), and (5) maintenance (maintaining the behavior change over time). The potential for relapse (abandoning new changes and returning to old behaviors) is recognized throughout.

The next step is to employ effective strategies for encouraging patient behavior change. In general, this should be done using a collaborative, patient-centered approach rather than a direct, confrontational approach. One example of such an approach is motivational interviewing.[99] This technique advocates the use of reflective listening to elicit and selectively reinforce a patient's own self-motivational statements.

The FRAMES model serves as a useful mnemonic that summarizes key principles underlying most approaches to behavior change.[100] These include (1) *Feedback* (giving feedback on the risks and negative consequences of a given behavior), (2) *Responsibility* (emphasizing that patients are responsible for their own behaviors and decisions), (3) *Advice* (giving straightforward advice about behavior change), (4) *Menu* of options (providing various available strategies, treatments, or programs to assist with behavior change), (5) *Empathy* (being empathetic, respectful, and nonjudgmental), and (6) *Self-efficacy* (expressing confidence in patients' ability to change if they choose).

The Five A's mnemonic provides an easy way to remember steps in encouraging patient behavioral change.[101] These include (1) *Assessing* patient behaviors, beliefs, and motivations; (2) *Advising* patients based on their personal health risks; (3) *Agreeing* with patients on a realistic set of goals; (4) *Assisting* to anticipate barriers and develop a specific action plan to address identified barriers; and (5) *Arranging* follow-up support. This approach also emphasizes a patient-centered rather than a confrontational style.

When the goal is to acquire a skill, key patient education principles include the use of demonstration, simulation, and practice. Skills should be broken down into simple individual steps. Patients also need to be told how to obtain any needed resources and supplies. Often this is not done directly by physicians but by nurses, physician assistants, pharmacists, social workers, and physical, occupational, speech, or cognitive behavioral therapists. Pharmaceutical companies and medical device manufacturers can also serve as potential resources for patient education and support services.[102–105]

Important to any educational effort is the ability to identify and appropriately use effective patient education strategies and resources. Key attributes of effective health communication strategies include accuracy, availability, consistency, cultural competency, reliability, timeliness, and understandability. In addition, content must be balanced (recognizing different but valid perspectives on an issue), evidence based, and designed to reach the largest number of people possible. Finally, the strategy should be repeated over time to reinforce its message.[106]

Patient education resources come in many forms. These include verbal communication, printed materials, audiovisual materials, computer-based modules, the Internet, ancillary staff, patient support groups, and consultation tools (such as screening tools or decision aids). Each of these has its advantages and disadvantages. Verbal information is easy and readily provided but can disempower patients because they are unable to refer to the information later and often do not remember what they were told.[107] Printed materials are typically familiar to health care providers, accessible, inexpensive, and convenient but have the disadvantage of being a passive strategy for disseminating information and may not be effective if used alone.[108] They must be written in an easy-to-read way that is appropriate for those with low levels of literacy. Ivnik and Jett provide an excellent review on how to create effective written patient education materials.[109] Although it is easy to find health information on the Internet, patients are often poorly equipped to assess the credibility and validity of what they read. Pictures or audiovisual formats are helpful adjuncts to other forms of patient education. This is especially true for patients with low health literacy.[110] Research suggests that humans in general have a cognitive preference for picture- rather than text-based information.[111] Overall, the more understandable, accessible, personalized, and relevant the information is, the more likely it is that an educational intervention will be successful.[112] Some of the available neurology patient education resources are listed in **Table 2**.

Although often neglected, it is important to gauge the success of any educational effort. This means taking the time to ensure that patients understand their health conditions, proper administration of their medications, and general medical instructions.[113] When the goal is to improve patient knowledge, the teach-back technique

**Table 1**
**Examples of plain, nonmedical words that can be substituted for medical terminology**

| Instead of These Medical Terms | Use These Plain, Nonmedical Words |
|---|---|
| Analgesic | Pain killer |
| Atherosclerosis | Cholesterol build-up in a blood vessel |
| Anticoagulant | Blood thinner |
| Antiepileptic | Seizure medicine |
| Anti-inflammatory | Reduces swelling and irritation |
| Atrial fibrillation | Top of the heart is quivering |
| Atrophy | Muscle shrinkage |
| Bacteria | Germ |
| Benign | Not cancer |
| Carotid artery | Blood vessel (or pipe) that carries blood to the front of the brain |
| Cervical | Neck |
| Cognition | Ability to think and remember |
| Compressing | Pushing on |
| Dementia | Loss of the ability to think and remember |
| Demyelination | Loss of insulation around nerves |
| Disease | Condition |
| Dissection | Tear in the wall of a blood vessel (or pipe) |
| Distal | Lower or farther away |
| Echocardiogram | Pictures of your heart |
| Edema | Swelling |
| Embolus | Blood clot |
| Enlarge | Get bigger |
| Exacerbation | Attack or flare-up |
| Glucose | Blood sugar |
| Hematoma | Collection of blood |
| Hemorrhage | Bleed |
| Hydrocephalus | Extra fluid on the brain |
| Hyperlipidemia | High cholesterol |
| Hypertension | High blood pressure |
| Infarct | Brain cells die |
| Intracerebral | In the brain |
| Lateral | Outer side |
| Lesion | Abnormal spot, often of uncertain cause |
| Lumbar | Low back |
| Lumbar puncture | Put a needle into your back to collect fluid |
| Medial | Inner side |
| Monitor | Keep track of/keep an eye on |
| Metastatic | Cancer has spread |
| Myelopathy | Spinal cord problem |
| Neuropathy | Nerve disease |
| Noninvasive | Without surgery or cutting the skin |
| Occluded | Blocked or plugged up |

(continued on next page)

**Table 1**
*(continued)*

| Instead of These Medical Terms | Use These Plain, Nonmedical Words |
| --- | --- |
| Oral | By mouth |
| Papilledema | Swelling at the back of the eye |
| Proximal | Closer or nearer |
| Radiculopathy | Nerve is damaged where it comes out of spine |
| Radiology | X-ray department |
| Referral | Send you to another doctor |
| Screening | Test to look for a possible abnormality |
| Status epilepticus | Seizures in the brain that do not stop |
| Stenosis | Narrowing or blockage |
| Subarachnoid | Space around the brain |
| Syncope | Faint or pass out |
| Terminal | Going to die |
| Thoracic | Middle of the back |
| Thrombus | Blood clot |
| Tissue plasminogen activator (TPA) | Clot buster |
| Toxic | Poisonous |
| Transesophageal | Down or through the swallowing tube |
| Transient ischemic attack (TIA) | Temporary blockage of blood flow to part of the brain |
| Tumor | Growth |
| Vertebral artery | Blood vessel (or pipe) that carries blood to the back of the brain |

can be used. This involves asking patients to repeat their understanding of the information to ensure accurate comprehension and retention. When the goal is to change an attitude or behavior, patients can be asked to summarize their reasons and motivations for behavior change and to set specific, concrete goals. When the goal is to acquire a skill, patients can be asked to demonstrate adequate performance of the skill. This assessment should be done immediately after the educational intervention and during subsequent interactions with patients. This helps to ensure ongoing retention and application of knowledge, lasting behavior change, and mastery of needed skills. The expectation is that effective patient education will result in improved health outcomes.

Although the efforts of individual health care providers to be effective patient educators are critical, patients can also be equipped to take a more active role in obtaining the education they need. The Ask Me 3 campaign is an example of this. Promoted by the Partnership for Clear Health Communication at the National Patient Safety Foundation, it encourages patients to seek answers to three basic questions every time they talk to a health care provider: (1) What is my main problem? (2) What do I need to do? and (3) Why is it important for me to do this?[114] Individual health care providers can also help assist patients by creating an environment that welcomes questions, encourages patients to make a list of questions they want to discuss before the appointment, provides calendars to chart periodic disorders (eg, headaches, seizures, and so forth), uses questionnaires before appointments to facilitate patient-provider

**Table 2**
**Selected resources for neurology patient education**

| | |
|---|---|
| *Neurology* Patient Page | An online feature of the journal *Neurology* written especially for patients and their families to provide a critical review of groundbreaking discoveries in neurologic research, up-to-date information about many neurologic diseases, and links to other information resources for neurologic patients. Available at: http://www.neurology.org. |
| *JAMA* Patient Page | *JAMA* also publishes succinct descriptions of neurologic and non-neurologic medical conditions aimed at patients and their families. Available at: http://www.jama.com. |
| American Academy of Neurology (AAN) patient brochures, books, and posters | Disease topics researched and written by AAN public education staff and edited by an AAN Practice subcommittee with the goal of introducing patients to their diagnosis, the possible causes of their disorder, and possible treatments. Available at: http://www.aan.com. |
| AAN Patient Web Site http://patients.aan.com/ | Web site created to support patient education that contains disease-specific information, patient stories, and links to other useful sites in an engaging and user-friendly format. |
| AAN *Neurology Now* magazine | Free patient- and family-focused magazine with feature stories and regular sections providing helpful information and support to individuals living with neurologic disease. |
| AAN guideline summaries | Summaries that condense essential information from AAN clinical practice guidelines in a way that is understandable to patients and their families. Available at: http://www.aan.com/go/practice/guidelines. |

discussions,[115] carefully explains the use and purpose of each medication prescribed,[116] and provides guidance on how to assess the credibility and validity of health information on the Internet (**Box 3**).

## PATIENT EDUCATION IN SELECTED NEUROLOGIC DISEASES

As with many other complex interventions in health care, evidence of the effectiveness (or lack thereof) of patient education interventions is needed, even if patient education is regarded as desirable in its own right.[117] Many studies have attempted to show that patient education improves outcomes among patients with diseases, such as diabetes, congestive heart failure, and cancer. Patient education has also been studied, although less extensively, in many common neurologic disorders, including ischemic stroke, migraine, epilepsy, low back pain, neck pain, MS, and others. A review of selected representative studies is presented.

### Ischemic Stroke

Patients are often dissatisfied with the information given them by health care providers, and this is also true for patients with neurologic disease. For example, survivors of

---

**Box 3**
**Questions to assess the credibility or validity of health information on the Internet**

Where does the information come from? Web addresses can be helpful in determining some of this information:

.gov—sponsored by the United States Federal Government

.edu—educational institutions

.org—used by some noncommercial organizations

.com—used by commercial organizations

What is the purpose of the Web site?

Is the information reviewed before it is posted to the Web site?

Does the Web site reflect more than one opinion?

How often is the Web site updated or reviewed?

*Courtesy of* 2009 Mayo Foundation for Medical Education and Research; with permission.

---

stroke or transient ischemic attack and their caregivers often feel that they have not been given enough information about stroke and hence feel unprepared for life after discharge from hospital.[118] This has a negative impact on adherence to secondary prevention recommendations and long-term psychosocial outcomes after stroke.[119]

A systematic review of 17 randomized controlled trials evaluating the effectiveness of providing information to patients affected by stroke or transient ischemic attack or their caregivers found that patient education increased knowledge about stroke, improved patient satisfaction, and reduced patient depression. There was not, however, much evidence that patient education significantly affected other aspects of stroke recovery, such as functional independence or social activities.[38] Better patient education may improve secondary prevention efforts,[120] and enhanced knowledge of stroke care by caregivers has been shown to improve stroke patient satisfaction with their home care after being discharged from the hospital.[121]

### Migraine

Patient education has also been shown to increase patient knowledge and improve health outcomes in patients with migraine headache. For example, Rothrock and colleagues[45] studied the effects of an intensive patient education program on migraine pathogenesis and management. At 6 months, many positive outcomes were noted in the intervention group, including a significantly greater reduction in mean migraine disability assessment scores (MIDAS),[122] reduction in mean headache days per month, reduction in the number of functionally incapacitating headache days per month, decreased analgesic overuse and need for abortive therapy, increased compliance with prophylactic therapy, fewer headache-related calls to health care providers, and fewer unscheduled clinic visits compared with patients receiving routine medical management.[45]

### Epilepsy

Similar intensive patient education efforts can also increase patient knowledge and improve treatment adherence in epilepsy, although effects on seizure frequency have been variable.[123] Helgeson and colleagues[41] evaluated the potential benefits of a 2-day educational treatment program in adult patients with epilepsy. At 4 months, patients who participated in the program had significantly improved epilepsy knowledge, coping skills, and medication adherence. There was, however, no significant difference in seizure frequency compared with those who did not participate. This program remains available to patients and is described in more detail on the Seizures and Epilepsy Education program Web site.[124]

May and Pfäfflin evaluated an intensive 2-day educational program for patients with epilepsy. Participants in this program showed significant improvements at 6 months in epilepsy knowledge, coping with epilepsy, and seizure frequency compared with the control group.[46] A systematic review of self-management strategies for adults with epilepsy, however, concluded that available evidence was still inadequate to strongly advocate for such interventions in the care of adults with epilepsy.[123]

Medication adherence is especially important in the management of epilepsy due to its implications for seizure control. As in other medical conditions, many patients with epilepsy do not take their antiepileptic medications as prescribed and may overestimate their degree of medication adherence.[125] To address this problem, Peterson and colleagues[126] used a combination of strategies to improve medication compliance in patients with epilepsy: patient counseling on the goals of therapy and the importance of compliance, a special medication container, a medication and seizure diary, and prescription refill and appointment-keeping reminder cards sent by mail. After 6 months, this combination of interventions resulted in significantly increased medication compliance and reduced seizure frequency in the intervention group compared with the control group.

### Low Back and Neck Pain

A systematic review of individual patient education for low back pain summarized the results of 24 trials testing the effects of different types of patient education on pain, function, and return-to-work rates.[32] This review concluded that patients with low back pain who receive an individual educational session lasting at least 2 hours in addition to their usual care have better outcomes than patients who only receive usual care.[32,47,48] The effects on short-term and long-term return-to-work rates were large and clinically relevant. For example, in a study by Indahl and colleagues,[47] half as many patients remained on sick leave at 200 and 400 days in the intervention group compared with the control group. This review also concluded that individual education is as effective as noneducational interventions on long-term pain and global improvement for patients with recent-onset low back pain.[32]

Simply providing written information by itself without an in-person education session[127,128] or shorter educational sessions (eg, 20 minutes of patient education provided by a physician[129]) has not been shown to be effective. Similarly, advice to stay active is not effective as a single intervention, even though this recommendation is emphasized in the majority of national and international guidelines on acute low back pain.[130] Patients with chronic low back pain (lasting >12 weeks) are less likely to benefit from patient education than people with acute or subacute pain.[32] Finally, there is no strong evidence that advice to stay active, stress management techniques, or "neck school" (an educational program which typically includes psychological counseling, ergonomics, exercise, self-care, and relaxation) improves symptoms in patients with neck pain.[35]

### Multiple Sclerosis

MS is a disease characterized by many uncertainties, including a course and prognosis that are variable and difficult to predict. Patients with MS are faced with challenging treatment decisions, as several different medically reasonable options exist, each having benefits and harms that people may value differently. For these reasons, MS is a neurologic disease well suited for the study of decision aids as a patient education tool.

Decision aids are patient tools designed to facilitate shared decision making and to enable patients to make informed decisions.[131] Specifically, they help patients understand available options, appreciate scientific uncertainties, and consider the personal importance of possible benefits and harms.[132,133]

Decision aids have been developed to help patients with MS make treatment decisions about immunotherapy[134] and about the management of acute relapses (eg, with no treatment, with oral corticosteroids, or with intravenous corticosteroids).[43] In one study, use of the immunotherapy decision aid did not affect the immunotherapy choices made compared with the control group.[134] Conversely, the same investigators found that training in acute relapse management decision making decreased the number of relapses treated with intravenous steroids and resulted in fewer phone calls to physicians.[43]

A systematic review of randomized controlled trials found that decision aids improve patients' knowledge of the options, create accurate perceptions of their potential benefits and harms, reduce difficulty with decision making, and increase participation in the decision-making process.[133] Use of decision aids did not seem to have a beneficial effect on patient satisfaction with decision making or patient anxiety.

## SUMMARY

Patient education is an important component of quality patient care and offers many potential benefits, including increased patient satisfaction, better patient adherence to treatment plans, and improved medical outcomes. Health care providers are responsible for giving patients the education they need to optimize their health and make health decisions. This requires addressing not only patient knowledge but also their behaviors, attitudes, and skills.

Effective patient education takes into account patients' values and priorities. It also identifies potential barriers to learning or applying information that patients may face. Chief among these barriers is that of low health literacy. Other patient education skills include being an effective communicator, identifying available patient education resources, understanding principles of behavior change, confirming that successful education has occurred, and equipping patients to take an active role in getting the education they need and desire.

Even though patient education is regarded as valuable in its own right, evidence of its effectiveness is needed. Although much study of patient education has already been done, additional research is needed to help health care providers more effectively implement and focus their patient education efforts.

## REFERENCES

1. South Australian Health Commission. Your rights and responsibilities: a charter for consumers of the South Australian public health system. Adelaide (Australia): Government of South Australia; 2008. p. 7–8.
2. Coulter A, Entwistle V, Gilbert D. Informing patients: an assessment of the quality of patient information materials. London: Kings Fund; 1998.
3. Ong LM, de Haes JC, Hoos AM, et al. Doctor-patient communication: a review of the literature. Soc Sci Med 1995;40(7):903–18.
4. Stewart MA. Effective physician-patient communication and health outcomes: a review. CMAJ 1995;152(9):1423–33.
5. Lansky D. Measuring what matters to the public. Health Aff 1998;17(4):40–1.
6. Davenport S, Goldberg D, Millar T. How psychiatric disorders are missed during medical consultations. Lancet 1987;2(8556):439–41.

7. Beckman HB, Frankel RM. The effect of physician behavior on the collection of data. Ann Intern Med 1984;101(5):692–6.

8. Stewart MA, McWhinney IR, Buck CW. The doctor/patient relationship and its effect upon outcome. J R Coll Gen Pract 1979;29(199):77–81.

9. Starfield B, Wray C, Hess K, et al. The influence of patient-practitioner agreement on outcome of care. Am J Public Health 1981;71(2):127–31.

10. Parkin T, Skinner TC. Discrepancies between patient and professionals recall and perception of an outpatient consultation. Diabet Med 2003;20(11): 909–14.

11. Waitzkin H. Doctor-patient communication. Clinical implications of social scientific research. JAMA 1984;252(17):2441–6.

12. Munn I. Poor communication main source of patient complaints in Maritimes, registrars report. CMAJ 1990;143(6):552–4

13. Ley P. Communicating with patients. Improving communication, satisfaction and compliance. London: Chapman and Hall; 1988.

14. Falvo D, Tippy P. Communicating information to patients. Patient satisfaction and adherence as associated with resident skill. J Fam Pract 1988;26(6):643–7.

15. Ziegler DK, Mosier MC, Buenaver M, et al. How much information about adverse effects of medication do patients want from physicians? Arch Intern Med 2001; 161(5):706–13.

16. Schillinger D, Piette J, Grumbach K, et al. Closing the loop: physician communication with diabetic patients who have low health literacy. Arch Intern Med 2003;163(1):83–90.

17. Wellwood I, Dennis MS, Warlow CP. Perceptions and knowledge of stroke amongst surviving patients with stroke and their carers. Age Ageing 1994; 23(4):293–8.

18. Drummond A, Lincoln N, Juby L. Effects of a stroke unit on knowledge of stroke and experiences in hospital. Health Trends 1996;28(1):26–30.

19. Haynes RB, Ackloo E, Sahota N, et al. Interventions for enhancing medication adherence. Cochrane Database Syst Rev 2008;(2):CD000011.

20. Burke LE, Dunbar-Jacob JM, Hill MN. Compliance with cardiovascular disease prevention strategies: a review of the research. Ann Behav Med 1997;19(3): 239–63.

21. Miller NH, Hill M, Kottke T, et al. The multilevel compliance challenge: recommendations for a call to action. A statement for healthcare professionals. Circulation 1997;95(4):1085–90.

22. The Medical School Objectives Writing Group. Learning objectives for medical student education—guidelines for medical schools: report I of the Medical School Objectives Project. Acad Med 1999;74(1):13–8.

23. Simpson M, Buckman R, Stewart M, et al. Doctor-patient communication: the Toronto consensus statement. BMJ 1991;303(6814):1385–7.

24. Makoul G. Essential elements of communication in medical encounters: the Kalamazoo consensus statement. Acad Med 2001;76(4):390–3.

25. Roter DL, Stewart M, Putnam SM, et al. Communication patterns of primary care physicians. JAMA 1997;277(4):350–6.

26. Bensing JM, Roter DL, Hulsman RL. Communication patterns of primary care physicians in the United States and the Netherlands. J Gen Intern Med 2003; 18(5):335–42.

27. Mueller PS, Barrier PA, Call TG, et al. Views of new internal medicine faculty of their preparedness and competence in physician-patient communication. BMC Med Educ 2006;6:30.

28. Roter DL, Hall JA, Kern DE, et al. Improving physicians' interviewing skills and reducing patients' emotional distress: a randomized clinical trial. Arch Intern Med 1995;155(17):1877–84.

29. Roter DL, Hall JA. Improving talk through interventions. In: Doctors talking with patients/patients talking with doctors: improving communication in medical visits. 2nd edition. Westport (CT): Praeger; 2006. p. 165–81.

30. Fellowes D, Wilkinson S, Moore P. Communication skills training for healthcare professionals working with cancer patients, their families and/or carers. Cochrane Database Syst Rev 2003;(2):CD003751.

31. Hahn SR, Lipton RB, Sheftell FD, et al. Healthcare provider-patient communication and migraine assessment: results of the American Migraine Communication Study, phase II. Curr Med Res Opin 2008;24(6):1711–8.

32. Engers A, Jellema P, Wensing M, et al. Individual patient education for low back pain. Cochrane Database Syst Rev 2008;(1):CD004057.

33. Van den Borne HW. The patient from receiver of information to informed decision-maker. Patient Educ Couns 1998;34(2):89–102.

34. Patient education. American Academy of Family Physicians. Available at: http://www.aafp.org/online/en/home/policy/policies/e/educationpatient.html. Accessed September 7, 2009.

35. Haines T, Gross A, Burnie SJ, et al. Patient education for neck pain with or without radiculopathy. Cochrane Database Syst Rev 2009;(1):CD005106.

36. Roter DL. Which facets of communication have strong effects on outcome – a meta-analysis. In: Stewart MA, Roter DL, editors. Communicating with medical patients. Newbury Park (CA): Sage Publications; 1989. p. 183–96.

37. Guo L, Jiang Y, Yatsuva H, et al. Group education with personal rehabilitation for idiopathic Parkinson's disease. Can J Neurol Sci 2009;36(1):51–9.

38. Smith J, Forster A, House A, et al. Information provision for stroke patients and their caregivers. Cochrane Database Syst Rev 2008;(2):CD001919.

39. Macht M, Gerlich C, Ellgring H, et al. Patient education in Parkinson's disease: formative evaluation of a standardized programme in seven European countries. Patient Educ Couns 2007;65(2):245–52.

40. Shimbo T, Goto M, Morimoto T, et al. Association between patient education and health-related quality of life in patients with Parkinson's disease. Qual Life Res 2004;13(1):81–9.

41. Helgeson DC, Mittan R, Tan SR, et al. Sepulveda epilepsy education: the efficacy of a psychoeducational treatment program in treating medical and psychosocial aspects of epilepsy. Epilepsia 1990;31(1):75–82.

42. Grosset KA, Grosset DG. Effect of educational intervention on medication timing in Parkinson's disease: a randomized controlled trial. BMC Neurol 2007;7:20.

43. Köpke S, Kasper J, Mühlhauser I, et al. Patient education program to enhance decision autonomy in multiple sclerosis relapse management: a randomized-controlled trial. Mult Scler 2009;15(1):96–104.

44. Sohng KY, Moon JS, Lee KS, et al. [The development and effects of a self-management program for patients with Parkinson's disease]. Taehan Kanho Hakhoe Chi 2007;37(6):891–901 [in Korean].

45. Rothrock JF, Parada VA, Sims C, et al. The impact of intensive patient education on clinical outcome in a clinic-based migraine population. Headache 2006; 46(5):726–31.

46. May TW, Pfäfflin M. The efficacy of an educational treatment program for patients with epilepsy (MOSES): results of a controlled randomized study. Modular service package epilepsy. Epilepsia 2002;43(5):539–49.

47. Indahl A, Velund L, Reikeraas O. Good prognosis for low back pain when left untampered: a randomized clinical trial. Spine 1995;20(4):473–7.
48. Molde Hagen E, Grasdal A, Eriksen HR. Does early intervention with a light mobilization program reduce long-term sick leave for low back pain? A 3-year follow-up study. Spine 2003;28(20):2309–16.
49. Hulsman RL, Ros WJ, Winnubst JA, et al. Teaching clinically experienced physicians communication skills: a review of education studies. Med Educ 1999; 33(9):655–68.
50. Hall JA, Irish JT, Roter DL, et al. Satisfaction, gender, and communication in medical visits. Med Care 1994;32(12):1216–31.
51. Frederikson LG. Exploring information-exchange in consultation: the patient's view of performance and outcomes. Patient Educ Couns 1995;25(3):237–46.
52. Hall JA, Rotor DL, Katz NR. Meta-analysis of correlates of provider behavior in medical encounters. Med Care 1988;26(7):657–75.
53. Ishikawa H, Takayama T, Yamazaki Y, et al. Physician-patient communication and patient satisfaction in Japanese cancer consultations. Soc Sci Med 2002; 55(2):301–11.
54. Stevenson F, Cox K, Britten N, et al. A systematic review of the research on communication between patients and healthcare professionals about medicines: the consequences for concordance. Health Expect 2004;7(3):235–45.
55. Cole SA. Reducing malpractice risk through more effective communication. Am J Manag Care 1997;3(4):649–53.
56. Stewart M, Meredith L, Brown JB, et al. The influence of older patient-physician communication on health and health-related outcomes. Clin Geriatr Med 2000; 16(1):25–36.
57. Graham J, Potts HW, Ramirez AJ. Stress and burnout in doctors. Lancet 2002; 360(9349):1975–6.
58. Brown GK, Nicassio PM. Development of a questionnaire for the assessment of active and passive coping strategies in chronic pain patients. Pain 1987;31(1): 53–64.
59. Nicholas MK, Wilson PH, Goyen J. Comparison of cognitive-behavioral group treatment and an alternative non-psychological treatment for chronic low back pain. Pain 1992;48(3):339–47.
60. Snow-Turek AL, Norris MP, Tan G. Active and passive coping strategies in chronic pain patients. Pain 1996;64(3):455–62.
61. Burton AK, Waddell G, Burtt R, et al. Patient education material in the management of low back pain in primary care. Bull Hosp Jt Dis 1996;55(3):138–41.
62. Nordin M. Back pain: lessons from patient education. Patient Educ Couns 1995; 26(1–3):67–70.
63. Waddell G. A new clinical model for the treatment of low-back pain. Spine 1987; 12(7):632–44.
64. Mead N, Bower P. Patient-centredness: a conceptual framework and review of the empirical literature. Soc Sci Med 2000;51(7):1087–110.
65. Weiss BD. Health literacy: a manual for clinicians. Chicago: American Medical Association Foundation and American Medical Association; 2003. p. 40.
66. Horne R, Weinman J. Patients' beliefs about prescribed medicines and their role in adherence to treatment in chronic physical illness. J Psychosom Res 1999; 47(6):555–67.
67. Health literacy: report of the Council on Scientific Affairs. Ad Hoc Committee on Health Literacy for the Council on Scientific Affairs, American Medical Association. JAMA 1999;281(6):552–7.

68. Wolf MS, Gazmararian JA, Baker DW. Health literacy and functional health status among older adults. Arch Intern Med 2005;165(17):1946–52.
69. Baker DW, Wolf MS, Feinglass J, et al. Health literacy, cognitive abilities, and mortality among elderly persons. J Gen Intern Med 2008;23(6):723–6.
70. Paasche-Orlow MK, Parker RM, Gazmararian JA, et al. The prevalence of limited health literacy. J Gen Intern Med 2005;20(2):175–84.
71. Dewalt DA, Berkman ND, Sheridan S, et al. Literacy and health outcomes: a systematic review of the literature. J Gen Intern Med 2004;19(12): 1228–39.
72. Marcus EN. The silent epidemic—the health effects of illiteracy. N Engl J Med 2006;355(4):339–41.
73. Baker DW, Wolf MS, Feinglass J, et al. Health literacy and mortality among elderly persons. Arch Intern Med 2007;167(14):1503–9.
74. Ratzan SC, Parker RM. Introduction. In: Selden CR, Zorn M, Ratzan SC, et al, editors. Health literacy, January 1990 through October 1999. Bethesda (MD): National Library of Medicine; 2000. p. 6.
75. Lindau ST, Tomori C, Lyons T, et al. The association of health literacy with cervical cancer prevention knowledge and health behaviors in a multiethnic cohort of women. Am J Obstet Gynecol 2002;186(5):938–43.
76. Schillinger D, Grumbach K, Piette J, et al. Association of health literacy with diabetes outcomes. JAMA 2002;288(4):475–82.
77. Parker RM, Ratzen SC, Lurie N. Health literacy: a policy challenge for advancing high-quality health care. Health Aff (Millwood) 2003;22(4):147–53.
78. Williams MV. Recognizing and overcoming inadequate health literacy, a barrier to care. Cleve Clin J Med 2002;69(5):415–8.
79. Roberts NJ, Ghiassi R, Partridge MR. Health literacy in COPD. Int J Chron Obstruct Pulmon Dis 2008;3(4):499–507.
80. Teutsch C. Patient-doctor communication. Med Clin North Am 2003;87(5): 1115–45.
81. Davis TC, Mayeaux EJ, Fredrickson D, et al. Reading ability of parents compared with reading level of pediatric patient education materials. Pediatrics 1994;93(3):460–8.
82. Davis TC, Crouch MA, Wills G, et al. The gap between patient reading comprehension and the readability of patient education materials. J Fam Pract 1990; 31(5):533–8.
83. Davis TC, Wolf MS, Bass PF 3rd, et al. Literacy and misunderstanding prescription drug labels. Ann Intern Med 2006;145(12):887–94.
84. Chew LD, Bradley KA, Boyko EJ. Brief questions to identify patients with inadequate health literacy. Fam Med 2004;36(8):588–94.
85. Johnson A, Sandford J, Tyndall J. Written and verbal information versus verbal information only for patients being discharged from acute hospital settings to home. Cochrane Database Syst Rev 2003;(4):CD003716.
86. Safeer RS, Kennan J. Health literacy: the gap between physicians and patients. Am Fam Physician 2005;72(3):463–8.
87. Osborne H. Overcoming communication barriers in patient education. Gaithersburg (MD): Aspen Publishers; 2001.
88. Barrier PA, Li JT, Jensen NM. Two words to improve physician-patient communication: what else? Mayo Clin Proc 2003;78(2):211–4.
89. Hahn SR. Communication in the care of the headache patient. In: Silberstein SD, Lipton RB, Dodick DW, editors. Wolff's headache and other head pain. 8th edition. New York: Oxford University Press; 2008. p. 805–24.

90. Stevenson FA, Gerrett D, Rivers P, et al. GPs' recognition of, and response to, influences on patients' medicine taking: the implications for communication. Fam Pract 2000;17(2):119–23.

91. Budtz S, Witt K. Consulting the Internet before visit to general practice. Patients' use of the Internet and other sources of health information. Scand J Prim Health Care 2002;20(3):174–6.

92. Wijdicks EF, Wijdicks CA. The portrayal of coma in contemporary motion pictures. Neurology 2006;66(9):1300–3.

93. Baxendale S. Epilepsy at the movies: possession to presidential assassination. Lancet Neurol 2003;2(12):764–70.

94. Duggan C, Bates I. Medicine information needs of patients: the relationships between information needs, diagnosis and disease. Qual Saf Health Care 2008;17(2):85–9

95. Leydon GM, Boulton M, Moynihan C, et al. Cancer patients' information needs and information seeking behaviour: in depth interview study. BMJ 2000; 320(7239):909–13.

96. Tennstedt SL. Empowering older patients to communicate more effectively in the medical encounter. Clin Geriatr Med 2000;16(1):61–70.

97. Levinson W, Kao A, Kuby A, et al. Not all patients want to participate in decision making. A national study of public preferences. J Gen Intern Med 2005;20: 531–5.

98. DiClemente CC, Velasquez MM. Motivational interviewing and the stages of change. In: Miller WR, Rollnick S, editors. Motivational interviewing: preparing people for change. New York: The Guilford Press; 2002. p. 201–16.

99. Miller WR, Rollnick S. What is motivational interviewing? In: Miller WR, Rollnick S, editors. Motivational interviewing: preparing people for change. New York: The Guilford Press; 2002. p. 33–42.

100. Hester RK, Miller WR. Handbook of alcoholism treatment approaches. 2nd edition. Boston: Allyn & Bacon; 1995.

101. Glasgow RE, Emont S, Miller DC. Assessing delivery of the five 'As' for patient-centered counseling. Health Promot Int 2006;21(3):245–55.

102. AVONEX Services. Avonex (interferon beta-1a). Available at: http://www.avonex. com. Accessed September 7, 2009.

103. MS Lifelines. Rebif (interferon beta-1a). Available at: http://www.mslifelines.com. Accessed September 7, 2009.

104. BETAPLUS. Betaseron (interferon beta-1b). Available at: http://www.betaseron. com/index.jsp. Accessed September 7, 2009.

105. Shared Solutions. Copaxone (glatiramer acetate injection). Available at: http:// www.copaxone.com/supportServices/. Accessed September 7, 2009.

106. U.S. Department of Health and Human Services. Objectives for improving health. In: Healthy people 2010, vol. 1. 2nd edition. Washington, DC: U.S. Government Printing Office; 2000. p. 1–25.

107. Chan Y, Irish JC, Wood SJ, et al. Patient education and informed and consent in head and neck surgery. Arch Otolaryngol Head Neck Surg 2002;128:1269–74.

108. Farmer AP, Légaré F, Turcot L, et al. Printed educational materials: effects on professional practice and healthcare outcomes. Cochrane Database Syst Rev 2008;(3):CD004398.

109. Ivnik M, Jett MY. Creating written patient education materials. Chest 2008; 133(4):1038–40.

110. Giorgianni SJ. Responding to the challenge of health literacy. In: The Pfizer Journal. New York: Impact Communications; 1998. p. 1–37.

111. Katz MG, Kripalani S, Weiss BD. Use of pictorial aids in medication instructions: a review of the literature. Am J Health Syst Pharm 2006;63(23):2391–7.

112. Udermann BE, Spratt KF, Donelson RG, et al. Can a patient educational book change behavior and reduce pain in chronic low back pain patients? Spine J 2004;4(4):425–35.

113. Weiss BD, Coyne C. Communicating with patients who cannot read. N Engl J Med 1997;337(4):272–4.

114. Partnership for Clear Health Communication. National patient safety foundation. Available at: http://www.npsf.org/askme3. Accessed September 7, 2009.

115. Buse DC, Rupnow MFT, Lipton RB. Assessing and managing all aspects of migraine: migraine attacks, migraine-related functional impairment, common comorbidities, and quality of life. Mayo Clin Proc 2009;84(5):422–35.

116. Schillinger D. Misunderstanding prescription labels: the genie is out of the bottle. Ann Intern Med 2006;145(12):926–9.

117. Campbell M, Fitzpatrick R, Haines A, et al. Framework for design and evaluation of complex interventions to improve health. BMJ 2000;321(7262):694–6.

118. Sabari JS, Meisler J, Silver E. Reflections upon rehabilitation by members of a community based stroke club. Disabil Rehabil 2000;22(7):330–6.

119. O'Mahoney PG, Rodgers H, Thomson RG, et al. Satisfaction with information and advice received by stroke patients. Clin Rehabil 1997;11(1):68–72.

120. Battersby M, Hoffmann S, Cadilhac D, et al. 'Getting your life back on track after stroke': a Phase II multi-centered, single-blind, randomized, controlled trial of the Stroke Self-Management Program vs. the Stanford Chronic Condition Self-Management Program or standard care in stroke survivors. Int J Stroke 2009; 4(2):137–44.

121. Evans RL, Bishop DS, Haselkorn JK. Factors predicting satisfactory home care after stroke. Arch Phys Med Rehabil 1991;72(2):144–7.

122. Stewart WF, Lipton RB, Kolodner K, et al. Reliability of the migraine disability assessment score in a population-based sample of headache sufferers. Cephalalgia 1999;19(2):107–14.

123. Bradley PM, Lindsay B. Care delivery and self-management strategies for adults with epilepsy. Cochrane Database Syst Rev 2008;(1):CD006244.

124. Seizures and Epilepsy Education. The S.E.E. program. Available at: http://www. theseeprogram.com. Accessed September 7, 2009.

125. Buelow JM, Smith MC. Medication management by the person with epilepsy: perception versus reality. Epilepsy Behav 2004;5(3):401–6.

126. Peterson GM, McLean S, Millingen KS. A randomised trial of strategies to improve patient compliance with anticonvulsant therapy. Epilepsia 1984;25(4): 412–7.

127. Cherkin DC, Deyo RA, Street JH, et al. Pitfalls of patient education. Limited success of a program for back pain in primary care. Spine 1996;21(3):345–55.

128. Hazard RG, Reid S, Haugh LD, et al. A controlled trial of an educational pamphlet to prevent disability after occupational low back injury. Spine 2000; 25(11):1419–23.

129. Jellema P, van der Windt DA, van der Horst HE, et al. Should treatment of (sub)acute low back pain be aimed at psychosocial prognostic factors? Cluster randomised clinical trial in general practice. BMJ 2005;331(7508):84.

130. Hagen KB, Hilde G, Jamtvedt G, et al. Advice to stay active as a single treatment for low back pain and sciatica. Spine 2002;27(16):1736–41.

131. Charles C, Whelan T, Gafni A. What do we mean by partnership in making decisions about treatment? BMJ 1999;319(7212):780–2.

132. Elwyn G, O'Connor A, Stacey D, et al. Developing a quality criteria framework for patient decision aids: online international Delphi consensus process. BMJ 2006; 333(7565):417–9.

133. O'Connor AM, Stacey D, Entwistle V, et al. Decision aids for people facing health treatment or screening decisions. Cochrane Database Syst Rev 2009;(3): CD001431.

134. Kasper J, Köpke S, Mühlhauser I, et al. Informed shared decision making about immunotherapy for patients with multiple sclerosis (ISDIMS): a randomized controlled trial. Eur J Neurol 2008;15(2):1345–52.

# The Future of Neurology

W. David Freeman, MD[a],*, Kenneth A. Vatz, MD[b]

**KEYWORDS**

- Future • Neurology workforce • Practice • Neurohospitalist
- Neurointensivists • Education

## A BRIEF HISTORY OF NEUROLOGY: "FROM CHARCOT TO CT SCANNER" IN 200 YEARS

The history of neurology and its current state must first be considered to extrapolate future predictions. Neurology's rich history began as early as the 18th century when Jean Martin Charcot, a French neurologist, also known as the "founder of modern neurology," helped distinguish organic diseases from those of hysteria or other psychiatric origin.[1] Charcot's students, including Drs Sigmund Freud, Joseph Babinski, Charles-Joseph Bouchard, and Georges Gilles de la Tourette, continued to separate neurology and psychiatry into distinct fields of study. The 19th century further refined the neurologist's art of "localization" through correlating patient history and clinical examination with postmortem nervous system pathology. Neurologists Hughlings Jackson and Silas Weir Mitchell, and neurosurgeons such as Harvey Cushing, made major contributions to the understanding of neurologic diseases and pathophysiology during this era.[2]

History, examination, and the art of localization remained the mainstay of neurologic diagnosis over the past 100 years. However, technologies emerged during the first half of the 20th Century to supplement the neurologist's clinical acumen, including skull radiographs, lumbar puncture, radionuclide scans, pneumoencephalography,[3] myelography, rudimentary cerebral angiography (Egaz Moniz, 1920s),[4] electroencephalography (4–8 channel, monopolar leads), basic nerve conduction studies, and electromyography. Neuropathology was not obtained until postmortem examination; however, the advent of neurosurgical brain biopsy allowed brain tumors to be examined before death.

Discovery of antibiotics penicillin and streptomycin allowed definitive treatment of neurosyphilis and central nervous system tuberculosis, respectively. Epilepsy was publicly stigmatized but became treatable with phenobarbital in 1904[5] and

The authors have disclosed that they have no financial interests, arrangements, or affiliations with the manufacturers of any products discussed in the article or their competitors.

[a] Mayo Clinic College of Medicine, 4500 San Pablo Road South, Jacksonville, FL 32224, USA
[b] Private practice, Winnetka, IL, USA
* Corresponding author.
*E-mail address:* freeman.william1@mayo.edu (W.D. Freeman).

diphenylhydantoin in 1938,[6,7] bromides or, in the case of petit mal, a ketogenic diet. Cholinergic agents were used for myasthenia gravis, anticholinergics for Parkinson's, and physical therapy for multiple sclerosis. Alzheimer's disease, before modern neuropathology, could be clinically characterized but was otherwise difficult to classify during life as a disease separate from other end-stage dementias, and was largely untreatable. Most patients who had dementia were labeled with the nonspecific term *senility*.

Arthur Nobile's discovery of prednisone in the 1950s was a landmark breakthrough that helped various afflictions, namely rheumatoid arthritis, but also symptomatically improved some inflammatory myopathies and suppressed myasthenia gravis.[8] Before the use of acetylsalicylic acid (circa 1950s to 1970s) and the emergence of anticoagulants such as warfarin in the 1950s, supportive and specific nursing care was the only option for stroke patients because of the lack of medical interventions.

In approximately 1975, modern imaging studies, beginning with CT, first of the brain and later of the spine, revolutionized diagnostic neurology. Concurrently, major advances in treatment began to emerge, including immunologic modulation for multiple sclerosis and myasthenia gravis, L-dopa for Parkinson's disease, and improved antiepileptic drugs. By the mid-1980s, MRI of the brain and spine, along with advancements in electrodiagnostic neurophysiologic techniques, greatly facilitated lesion localization and identification.

Neurosurgery, now aided by neuroimaging and electrophysiologic techniques, would develop interventions for conditions, such as intractable seizures and certain movement disorders, that previously could only be treated medically. By the mid-1990s, recombinant tissue plasminogen activator (rtPA) emerged as a new medical treatment for ischemic stroke. Neuroimaging, notably CT, MRI, and magnetic resonance angiography, and rtPA represent significant advances in neurologic diagnosis and treatment, respectively. Within the past 2 decades, these modalities have transformed the clinical practice of neurology worldwide.

## TRENDS IN THE NEUROLOGY WORKFORCE OVER 3 DECADES

Over the past 30 years the national needs and trends in neurology have been changing more rapidly than the ability to track or predict them. In 1977, Goldstein[9] compared neurologic manpower needs, using three disparate and conflicting reports from 1970 to 1975. He concluded that by 1985, approximately 7000 neurologists would be practicing nationally, resulting in either a modest national shortage of neurologists, or a number that would "approach meeting basic needs."

In 1981, based on the number of residents in neurology training programs and the expected attrition from retirement, Menken[10] projected that by 1990, approximately 10,000 neurologists would be practicing in the United States, for a population ratio of 4.1/100,000, "...with still greater growth into the 1990s." He believed this number represented an "oversupply of neurologists," especially in metropolitan areas. He suggested that the reduced income from this oversupply would lead to neurologists performing primary care along with excessive and expensive procedures, such as electromyography. Furthermore, he suggested that an oversupply of neurologists would also decrease the number of neurologic referrals to academic and training centers. Menken concluded that "it would be wise to reduce the number of training positions and programs [in neurology]." Menken's analysis exemplifies the inherent uncertainty in forecasting future events, especially complex ones.

In contrast, in 1986 Kurtzke and colleagues[11] had a different conclusion. They added to academic needs the number of neurology annual man-hours required to care for 55 identified neurologic conditions, and calculated that by 1990 the United States would require a total of 10,300 neurologists, or 5/100,000 population. The same authors estimated that 6708 neurologists would be practicing in 1986 and, based on estimated incidence of neurologists at the time, projected approximately 11,600 neurologists by 2003, with small yearly increases through 2016.[12]

In 1994, well into the modern era of neuroimaging and managed care, Engstrom and Hauser[13] argued that future neurologists should have primary care training in medicine or pediatrics, and thereby "function comfortably as both consultants and principal physicians." They further stated that "[they] must be trained to apply cost-effective approaches to the use of diagnostic technology and therapy." The authors cited the widely varying estimates of the number of neurologists needed and the wide geographic variation in the United States of neurologists per capita.[11,12] Furthermore, they judged that reliable projections were difficult because of several factors, including variability in how neurologists were currently used, uncertainty about the number of future neurologists to be trained, and the unclear definition of the future role of the neurologist. They concluded by saying, "It would be unfortunate if the role of neurologist in a new health care system were to be confined to consultative services only [since] the unique skills of neurologists place them in a useful position to provide emergency or continuing care of patients with neurologic diseases," noting additionally that the demand of "senior citizens for neurologic services in the future will be considerable."

In 2000, Menken and colleagues,[14] examined the World Health Organization's Global Burden of Disease Study[15,16] and the Initiative on Neurology and Public Policy.[17] Cerebrovascular disease was the second leading cause of disease burden, whereas dementia and other degenerative and hereditary central nervous system disorders were ranked eighth. In terms of death rates, but particularly disability, these investigators calculated that "The proportionate share of the total global burden of disease due to neuropsychiatric disorders…is projected to rise from 10.5% in 1990 to 14.7% in 2020." They also noted that "Of the 10 disorders in the highest disability classes, 8 [including migraine] are neurologic problems," and lamented how little attention had been "given to this study among national and regional organizations of neurologists."

According to a 2004 demographic report and survey of neurologists in the United States,[18] of 15,831 physicians in the American Medical Association Physician Masterfile, 12,498 neurologist members (7010 in practice) of the American Academy of Neurology (AAN) had a primary self-designation of neurology, child neurology, or clinical neurophysiology. Therefore, with a 2008 United States population of approximately 305 million, and assuming approximately the same number of neurologists as in 2003, the population ratio would be at least 5.2/100,000.

The 2004 AAN survey also indicated an uneven geographic distribution of neurologists, ranging from 11.02/100,000 in Washington, DC, to 1.78/100,000 in Wyoming. As shown in **Table 1**,[18] half of the responding clinical neurologists in the United States (approximately 58% of those surveyed) were in private practice, almost evenly divided between solo and group settings. The other half were working in multi-specialty or university-based groups or in HMO- and government-based practices. **Fig. 1**[18] shows that most neurologists are male (5269 vs 1513 female), but also indicates that the distribution of neurologists participating in the survey was skewed toward middle-age. This could be a true representation of that sampled population, but may also suggest either earlier retirement resulting in a high attrition rate in neurology, or under-representation of older neurologists who were either non-AAN members or did not participate in the survey.

**Table 1**
Clinical status of neurologists in the United States

| Clinical Practice Status | All Members | | International Members | | United States' Members[a] | | United States' Neurologists | |
|---|---|---|---|---|---|---|---|---|
| | Count | % of Total | Count | % of Total | Count | % of Total | Count | % of Total |
| Clinical practice | 8527 | 86.5 | 1517 | 93.5 | 7010 | 85.1 | 6346 | 95.1 |
| Solo practice | 1979 | 20.1 | 283 | 17.4 | 1696 | 20.6 | 1571 | 23.5 |
| Neurology group | 2158 | 21.9 | 200 | 12.3 | 1958 | 23.8 | 1874 | 28.1 |
| Multispecialty group | 776 | 7.9 | 45 | 2.8 | 731 | 8.9 | 682 | 10.2 |
| University-based group | 2253 | 22.9 | 497 | 30.6 | 1756 | 21.3 | 1480 | 22.2 |
| Government hospital or clinic | 632 | 6.4 | 278 | 17.1 | 354 | 4.3 | 313 | 4.7 |
| Staff-model HMO | 102 | 1.0 | 4 | 0.2 | 98 | 1.2 | 90 | 1.3 |
| Other public or private hospital or clinic | 627 | 6.4 | 210 | 12.9 | 417 | 5.1 | 336 | 5.0 |
| No clinical practice | 1332 | 13.5 | 105 | 6.5 | 1227 | 14.9 | 330 | 4.9 |
| Total | 9859 | 100.0 | 1622 | 100.0 | 8237 | 100 | 6676 | 100.0 |

[a] Excludes members not residing in the United States.
*Data from* Henry KL, Lawyer BL, Rizzo M, et al. Neurologists 2004: AAN member demographic and practice characteristics. St. Paul (MN): American Academy of Neurology; 2005.

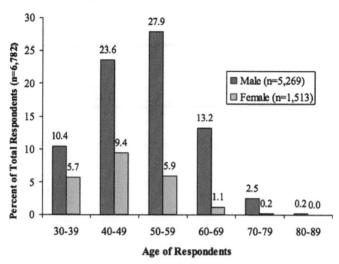

**Fig. 1.** Neurologists in the United States: age and gender. (*Adapted from* Henry KL, Lawyer BL, Rizzo M, et al. Neurologists 2004: AAN member demographic and practice characteristics. St. Paul (MN): American Academy of Neurology; 2005, with permission.)

Regarding how many medical students are choosing neurology as a specialty, **Fig. 2**[19] shows a slight upward trend, albeit with a recent dip, in the number of neurologists in residency training programs between 1987 and 2008, along with a small increase in the proportion of international medical graduates. **Fig. 3** shows a positive trend in the number of ABPN certifications in adult neurology between 1985 and 2007, with the number of certifications in child neurology being almost flat (Dorthea Juul, ABPN, personal communication, 2008).

## FUTURE PREDICTIONS FOR THE NEUROLOGY WORKFORCE: INCREASED DEMAND

Although no precise or reliable figure exists for the number of clinical neurologists actively practicing in the United States, a reasonable and perhaps excessive estimate would be 14,000. Assuming an even distribution of neurologists over a typical 35-year practice career, 400 neurologists would be retiring each year, approximately equal to the number (see **Fig. 3**) of new neurology certifications per year. However, according to the AAN survey from 2004, 34% of all currently practicing neurologists at that time were between 50 and 60 years of age, compared with the expected 28.6% each decade, if evenly distributed. Therefore, the attrition rate in neurology (or lack of AAN member neurologists participating in the survey) over the next decade would significantly exceed the rate of neurologists entering into practice. These estimates, when combined with the aging patient population and the prevalence of neurologic disorders with increasing age, suggest that there will be higher demand for the estimated supply of adult neurologists, especially in already underserved areas.

Child neurologists will likely be in even greater demand. A 2005 workforce analysis by Polsky and colleagues[20] noted a decline in child neurology training program enrollment, predicting that "unless more child neurologists are trained in the near future, there will be no growth in the number of child neurologists relative to the projected number of children." The authors also noted an uneven distribution of child neurologists in the United States, with double the number per 100,000 population in the Northeast, compared with the West and South.

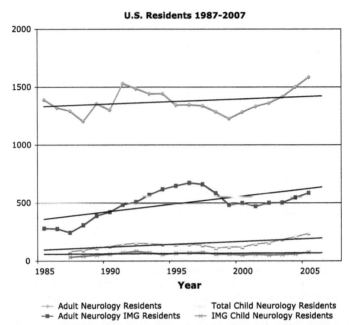

**Fig. 2.** Number of Residents in Neurology, 1987–2007. (*Data from* Annual Education Issues. JAMA 2008;300:1228–43; 2007;298:1081–96; 2006;296:1154–69; 2005;294:1129–43; 2004;292:1099–113; 2003;290:1234–48; 2002;288:1151–64; 2001;286:1095–107; 2000;284:1159–72; 1999;282: 893–906;1998; 280:836–45; 1997;278:775–84; 1996;276:739–48; 1995;274:755–62; 1994;272:725–32; 1993;270:1116–22; 1992;268:1170–76; 1991;266:933–43; 1990;264:822–32; 1989;262:1029–37; 1988;260:1093–101; 1987;258:1031–40.)

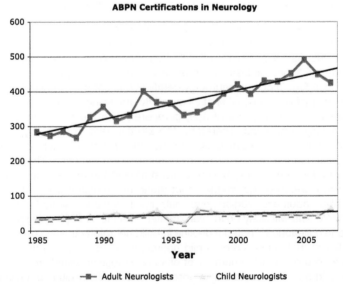

**Fig. 3.** ABPN Certifications in Neurology, 1985–2007. (*Courtesy of* Jennifer Vollmer, ABPN, personal communication, 2009.)

In the current outpatient practice of neurology in the United States, approximately 63% are group or solo practice (see **Table 1**), with the remainder split among multispecialty clinics, full-time university-based groups, government hospitals or clinics, staff-model HMOs, and other clinics or hospitals. Most neurologists see outpatients and inpatients with approximately equal frequency across multiple practice settings (**Table 2**),[18] with work hours varying depending on practice (**Table 3**).[18] In some groups, all the members rotate inpatient, outpatient, and procedure assignments, whereas other groups may have permanent assignments according to training, expertise, and interest.

## HISTORY PREDICTS MORE FUTURE SUBSPECIALISTS IN NEUROLOGY

In the past decade, seven new subspecialties of neurology have achieved certification status by the American Board of Psychiatry and Neurology (ABPN): Clinical Neurophysiology, Pain Medicine, Neurodevelopmental Disabilities, Vascular Neurology, Sleep Medicine, Neuromuscular Disease, and Hospice and Palliative Medicine. Additionally, the United Council of Neurologic Subspecialties (UCNS) offers subspecialty certification for autonomic neurology, behavioral neurology and neuropsychiatry (dementia), clinical neuromuscular pathology, geriatric neurology, headache, neurocritical care, neuroimaging, and neuro-oncology.

Furthermore, subspecialties exist within neurology self-defined, including epilepsy, movement disorders, multiple sclerosis and neuroimmunology, neuro-ophthalmology, neuro-otology, and neurorehabilitation. Recently, neurologic care has been dividing into inpatient and outpatient styles of practice, with "neurohospitalists" emerging similar to their medical hospitalist predecessors some 10 years earlier.[21–23] The "practice specialty or focus" reported by AAN member neurologists is shown in **Table 4** from the 2004 AAN survey.[18]

## FUTURE OF OUTPATIENT (AMBULATORY) NEUROLOGY: "MORE WORK, LESS TIME WITH PATIENTS"
### Outpatient Practice

In this country, multiple factors will shape and inform the future provision of outpatient neurologic care, including the demographics and uneven geographic distribution of neurologists already seen in 2004,[18] an essentially level or declining number of new neurologists, the increased subspecialization of those new neurologists, and the economic, regulatory, and legal pressures and constraints of the health care system itself, as they apply to a cognitive specialty with few procedures. The nature of outpatient, nonacute care neurologic practice will continue to evolve over the next 5 to 10 years, according to the expected changes in overall health care delivery and provider reimbursement systems.

Within the past decade, an aggregate shift of medical subspecialties has occurred away from solo and two-physician practices in favor of large single-specialty groups and nonowner, multispecialty clinics and institutions.[24] As shown in **Table 5**,[24] the shifts in neurologic practices showed a similar trend, although the number of neurologists surveyed was insufficient for statistical significance.

The Center for Studying Health System Change (CSHSC) survey[24] documented a trend toward larger and nonowner groups among older physicians, partly because so few physicians aged 40 years and younger were in solo or two-physician groups at the start of the period. The overall trend was stronger toward mid-sized single-specialty practices than multispecialty groups. CSHSC reasoned that it was easier for specialists to decrease practice expenses and enhance revenue from profitable services in

**Table 2**
**Patient events by practice setting**

| Practice Setting[a] | Mean Number of Patient Events Per Week | | | | | | |
| | Outpatient Evaluation | | Inpatient Evaluation: Attending | | Inpatient Evaluation: Consulting | | Total |
| | New | Follow-up | New | Follow-up | New | Follow-up | |
|---|---|---|---|---|---|---|---|
| Solo practice (n = 229) | 19.9 | 37.4 | 1.8 | 2.7 | 7.4 | 9.7 | 78.9 |
| Neurology group (n = 242) | 18.9 | 41.3 | 3.2 | 5.4 | 9.3 | 16.0 | 94.1 |
| Multispecialty group (n = 110) | 23.4 | 37.8 | 1.9 | 5.5 | 5.1 | 8.1 | 81.8 |
| University-based group (n = 176) | 9.4 | 15.9 | 4.1 | 7.2 | 4.0 | 5.0 | 45.6 |
| Government hospital or clinic (n = 44) | 14.4 | 19.1 | 2.6 | 4.7 | 4.9 | 3.2 | 48.9 |
| Staff-model HMO (n = 8) | 24.9 | 33.8 | 3.6 | 2.9 | 5.6 | 6.1 | 76.9 |
| Other public or private hospital or clinic (n = 45) | 14.9 | 16.2 | 4.0 | 7.4 | 5.0 | 4.8 | 52.4 |
| All practice settings (n = 854) | 17.4 | 32.0 | 2.9 | 5.1 | 6.7 | 9.7 | 73.8 |
| Results from 2000 (n = 759) | 16.5 | 31.7 | 2.7 | 5.2 | 6.0 | 9.4 | 71.5 |
| Results from 1998 (n = 1148) | 16.2 | 29.6 | 4.4 | 8.3 | 6.0 | 9.2 | 73.7 |
| Results from 1996–1997 (n = 1065) | 16.1 | 28.8 | 4.5 | 8.6 | 6.3 | 9.7 | 74.0 |

[a] Practice settings as determined from response to the 2003 Member Census.
Data from Henry KL, Lawyer BL, Rizzo M, et al. Neurologists 2004: AAN member demographic and practice characteristics. St. Paul (MN): American Academy of Neurology; 2005.

**Table 3**
Hours per week in practice

| Practice Setting[a] | Mean (Median)[b] Number of Hours Per Week | | | | | |
|---|---|---|---|---|---|---|
| | Patient Care | Administration | Teaching | Medical Research | Other | Total |
| Solo practice (n = 233) | 49.5 (50) | 4.1 (1) | 1.5 (0) | 1.5 (0) | 2.1 (0) | 58.7 (56) |
| Neurology group (n = 244) | 49.5 (50) | 4.2 (2) | 2.4 (5) | 2.5 (0) | 1.4 (0) | 59.9 (60) |
| Multispecialty group (n = 110) | 46.7 (50) | 3.4 (1) | 2.4 (0) | 2.4 (0) | 1.2 (0) | 56.1 (55) |
| University-based group (n = 181) | 26.6 (25) | 7.4 (5) | 7.7 (5) | 14.8 (10) | 2.4 (0) | 58.8 (55) |
| Government hospital or clinic (n = 45) | 24.8 (25) | 9.5 (5) | 6.1 (5) | 9.2 (5) | 1.4 (0) | 51.1 (50) |
| Staff-Model HMO (n = 8) | 43.1 (40) | 1.9 (1.5) | 2.4 (2) | 0.3 (0) | 1.3 (0) | 48.9 (45.5) |
| Other public or private hospital or clinic (n = 47) | 38.3 (40) | 4.7 (3) | 5.9 (5) | 6.3 (2) | 3.7 (0) | 59.0 (54) |
| All practice settings (n = 869) | 42.4 (40) | 5.0 (2) | 3.7 (1) | 5.3 (0) | 1.9 (0) | 58.3 (55) |
| Results from 2000 (n = 778) | 40.6 (40) | 5.7 (3) | 4.0 (2) | 6.2 (0) | 1.7 (0) | 58.2 (57) |
| Results from 1998 (n = 1193) | 44.7 (45) | 5.1 (3) | 3.6 (2) | 5.6 (0) | 2.1 (0) | 61.0 (50) |
| Results from 1996–1997 (n = 1032) | 42.1 (40) | 5.6 (4) | 4.0 (2) | 4.7 (0) | 2.2 (0) | 58.5 (58) |
| Results from 1993–1994 (n = 1203) | 43.3 (45) | 3.1 (0) | 4.4 (2) | 5.4 (0) | 2.3 (1) | 58.5 (50) |
| Results from 1991–1992 (n = 1367) | 42.3 (45) | 1.9 (0) | 4.6 (2) | 6.1 (0) | 2.6 (1) | 57.5 (50) |

[a] Practice settings as determined from response to the 2003 Member Census.
[b] The median may be a more accurate measure of responses due to skewed distributions.
Data from Henry KL, Lawyer BL, Rizzo M, et al. Neurologists 2004: AAN member demographic and practice characteristics. St. Paul (MN): American Academy of Neurology; 2005.

**Table 4**
**Practice specialty or focus reported by the American Academy of Neurology**

| Practice Focus | Count[a] | Percent of Respondents[a] |
|---|---|---|
| General neurology | 3561 | 56.5% |
| Headache | 2916 | 46.3% |
| Epilepsy | 2700 | 42.9% |
| Electromyography | 2570 | 40.8% |
| Cerebrovascular disease | 2519 | 40.0% |
| EEG | 2297 | 36.5% |
| Aging/dementia | 2281 | 36.2% |
| Movement disorders | 2094 | 33.2% |
| Multiple sclerosis/neuroimmunology | 2059 | 32.7% |
| Neuromuscular disorders | 1755 | 27.9% |
| Chronic pain | 1296 | 20.6% |
| Spine-related conditions | 1071 | 17.0% |
| Sleep disorders | 934 | 14.8% |
| Behavioral neurology | 877 | 13.9% |
| Critical care | 732 | 11.6% |
| Worker's compensation | 704 | 11.2% |
| Central nervous system infectious diseases | 649 | 10.3% |
| Neurohabilitation | 457 | 7.3% |
| Neuroimaging | 454 | 7.2% |
| Other | 392 | 6.2% |
| Neuro-ophthalmology | 322 | 5.1% |
| Neuro-oncology | 283 | 4.5% |
| Neuropharmacology | 223 | 3.5% |
| Interventional neurology | 114 | 1.8% |
| Neuroepidemiology | 87 | 1.4% |
| Total respondents | 6298 | |

[a] Because most respondents chose more than one response, the count adds up to more than 6804 and the percentages add up to more than 100%.
*Modified from* Henry KL, Lawyer BL, Rizzo M, et al. Neurologists 2004: AAN member demographic and practice characteristics. St. Paul (MN): American Academy of Neurology; 2005, with permission.

single-specialty practices, despite the greater opportunity to use information technology payment systems and better economies of scale in multispecialty settings.

Neurology and most of its subspecialties are primarily cognitive rather than procedural; therefore, they may have a greater degree of "fungibility" or replaceability than would be present in procedure-oriented medical subspecialties such as cardiology, gastroenterology, and pulmonary medicine. The unique historical role of the clinical neurologist, as the sole possessor of neurologic knowledge and clinical acumen, will be increasingly altered by information technology (including Internet medical resources and databases and open access to peer reviewed journals), broad availability of clinical guidelines, practice parameters, and treatment protocols.

These factors, including the reduced production of neurologists relative to the increasing need for neurologic services within the aging population, compounded

**Table 5**
**Neurologist practice size**

| | Solo to 2-Physician Practices | | 3- to 5-Physician | | >6 Physician Practices | | Other[c] | |
|---|---|---|---|---|---|---|---|---|
| | 1996–1997 | 2004–2005 | 1996–1997 | 2004–2005 | 1996–1997 | 2004–2005 | 1996–1997 | 2004–2005 |
| Medical specialists | 38.1 | 26.1[a] | 9.6 | 7.4[a] | 17.3 | 24.1[a] | 351 | 42.5[a] |
| Neurology (90) | 49.9 | 42.1 | 8.2 | 6.9[b] | 11.4 | 15.2[b] | 30.5 | 35.9 |

[a] Change from 1996–1997 is statistically significant (P<.05).
[b] Estimates are not reliable because they have a relative standard of error of greater than 30%.
[c] Includes physicians employed by medical schools, HMOs, hospitals (including those in office-based practices), community health centers, free-standing clinics, and other settings, and contractors.

*Adapted from* Liebhaber A, Grossman JM. Physicians moving to mid-sized, single-specialty practices. Supplementary Table 1, Center for Studying Health System Change. Available at: http://www.hschange.com/CONTENT/941/#ib8. Accessed November 23, 2009.

by trends toward subspecialization within neurology, will likely lead to consolidation of solo practices and smaller groups into larger group practices. Furthermore, larger group practices tend to hire physician extenders, helping fuel that trend. Over time, the use of standardized practices and protocols may lead to a more uniform type of neurologic practice than has been seen previously (eg, use of rtPA for eligible patients who have experienced ischemic stroke has grown substantially since its introduction in the 1990s).

What will occur with the geographic distribution of neurologists in the future? Historically, neurology practices are heavily concentrated in populous states and metropolitan areas.[18] Neurologists are specialists who need referrals and a sufficient population of patients to justify their income and overhead expenses. They have little incentive to practice in rural and underserved areas, despite some governmental fellowships and programs. Based on this information, little evidence suggests that neurology will change from an urban-predominant pattern of geographic distribution in the future. Unless some dramatic incentive comes from national health care reform, a shortage of neurologists similar to that of other specialists in underserved and rural areas is likely to continue.

Given the aging population and the likelihood for acute stroke care evaluation and management by neurologists, rural and underserved settings will be greatly challenged. One possibility to help meet this supply-and-demand mismatch for urgent neurologic opinion is telemedicine (ie, teleneurology). Neurology remains one of the most history and examination-intense specialties; one that may be especially well suited to a teleneurology approach. For example, teleneurology can help bring the neurologist to patients in rural and underserved areas who have experienced acute stroke.[25–27]

Teleneurology could address and improve several deficiencies, including those listed by Patterson[25]:

1. Patients admitted to hospital with acute neurologic symptoms rarely see a neurologist
2. Acute stroke treatment (eg, rtPA) is often delayed because of lack of neurology opinion
3. Suboptimal management of epilepsy
4. Unproductive travel time for neurologists
5. Poor access to a neurologist for doctors in the developing world
6. Long waiting times to see a neurologist.

In the future, because the demand for neurologists is expected to increase despite a fixed supply, teleneurology has the greatest potential to help underserved and rural areas.

### Physician Extenders (Nonphysician Providers) on the Rise

The use of physician extenders or nonphysician providers (NPPs) in neurology practice has become increasingly prevalent in recent years.[28,29] In 2004, almost 25% of all neurology practices reported using physician extenders or nonphysician providers (ie, physician assistants or nurse practitioners), more so in university settings (42%) than in private group (21%) or solo (9%) practice settings.[18] In the AAN survey of practices in 2004,[18] the percentage of respondents using physician assistants or nurse practitioners was 21.8% in 1998, 28.0% in 2000, and 23.6% in 2004. In the most recent survey, they were most commonly used in university-based or institutional settings (average of 37%), less so in neurology or multispecialty groups (22%), and least in solo practice (9%). The trend in NPPs seems to be increasing, albeit slowly, at university and private group settings, but this may be misleading and caused by sampling factors in the AAN surveys. If group practices increase and the number of solo practices decrease over the next 5 to 10 years, then the number of NPPs may grow accordingly.

What is fueling the growth of nonphysician providers? Part of the answer may just be supply and demand for neurologists (ie, more patients than neurologists or practices can see, especially in follow-up). A key driver, however, is reimbursement. With future private-sector and Medicare cuts, NPPs such as nurse practitioners may provide neurologists with more slots in which to see new and returning outpatients. Some practices have their NPP see only return-visit patients, with physicians focusing on new or complicated return patients. Other practices use NPPs at the hospital to help with consultations and call coverage.

As NPPs spend more time with patients, the neurologist spends even less time, which may signify a larger issue: an infringement on the hallowed one-on-one doctor–patient relationship, which was established and ingrained during the prior 2 centuries as the standard professional model. Is the "handwriting on the wall" for the American health care system because of declining reimbursements and the consequent economic pressures to see more patients in a reduced amount of time? Clearly, the patient–nonphysician provider relationship is emerging as an alternative model for health care in the United States, despite whether it is beneficial for care. This new paradigm may have other effects on the medical profession heritage, including changes in the way patients and the public perceive and respect physicians.

Part of the reason for the increase in NPPs is that they can do work similar to that of physicians, such as educating and counseling patients, writing or refilling prescriptions, and seeing follow-up patients independently. NPPs may also perform some billable procedures for which their time, assuming proper documentation, can be reimbursed. Although NPPs may generate more revenue through increasing clinic throughput, the costs of hiring physician extenders also have to be considered. Generally, however, the costs of hiring and length of training for nonphysician providers are less than hiring a neurologist, which may be another reason for their greater use, especially in group and university practice settings. Nonphysician providers may also be able to spend more time with patients, especially for counseling and education.

Neurology is rapidly evolving into a disease-oriented set of subspecialties, much like internal medicine, although many practicing neurologists still consider themselves competent to diagnose and treat a broad spectrum of neurologic diseases (see **Table 4**). More subspecialization is expected for the future, given the burgeoning of medical knowledge. According to one survey,[30] 60% of graduating neurology residents are now entering fellowships and further subspecialization. **Box 1** lists the fellowships available.

## FUTURE OF HOSPITAL NEUROLOGY: EMERGENCE OF NEUROHOSPITALISTS AND NEUROINTENSIVISTS

Hospitals and emergency departments (EDs) are stressed to the point of crisis[31] from increasing volumes of patients seeking urgent and primary care. Over the past decade, advances in medicine, such as tissue plasminogen activator (tPA) for acute ischemic stroke, require that hospitals and EDs provide rapid and high-quality care. However, hospital and physician reimbursements have steadily declined while litigation costs and malpractice premiums have continued on an upward trend. These

---

**Box 1**
**American Academy of Neurology list of fellowships**

Advanced clinical neurology

AIDS

Alzheimer's disease

Basic research

Behavioral neurology

Cerebrovascular disease/stroke

Clinical neurophysiology

Dementia

EEG

Electromyography

Epilepsy

Geriatric neurology

Headache

Interventional neurology

Movement disorders

Multiple sclerosis

Neuroepidemiology

Neurogenetics

Neuroimaging

Neuroimmunology

Neurologic critical care

Neuromuscular disorders

Neuro-oncology

Neuro-ophthalmology

Neuro-otology

Neuropathology

Neuropharmacology

Neurorehabilitation

Neurovirology

Pain

Sleep disorders

Spine

---

factors, coupled with the high potential legal risk inherent in tPA administration, have caused many neurologists to opt out of "stroke call."[32]

Because this reimbursement-versus-risk ratio continues to worsen, approximately 75% of EDs across the country lack specialist coverage in neurology.[31] Some neurologists have sought additional reimbursement from hospitals for stroke call, and the AAN has issued a position statement in its support.[33,34] Several hospitals without neurology consultation or a stroke specialty team start tPA after consulting with a referring stroke specialist, either by phone or telemedicine, and transfer the patient to the stroke center later. This policy, called *drip and ship*, remains controversial, particularly regarding reimbursement, because the shipping hospital may receive the full diagnosis related group (DRG) reimbursement from Medicare (from DRG 559 of $11,569) while assuming little of the risk associated with tPA or subsequent costs of managing these patients. Medicare is reportedly applying a V code to track this phenomenon to equalize reimbursements.

Outpatient neurologists lose revenue when they have to drop everything to evaluate an acute stroke patient for tPA in the ED. Additionally, costs are associated with time traveling to the ED from the outpatient neurologist's practice and lost revenue from procedures or outpatients who fail to return for appointments. Neurologists in solo practice face burnout in taking 24/7 ED coverage for stroke call, with little in the way of financial or other incentive.

Neurology group practices have tried various models to adapt to these pressures, including the rotation of ED call among practice members. Academic groups have often placed residents in-house to evaluate ED consults 24/7, but recent Accreditation Council for Graduate Medical Education (ACGME) duty-hour restrictions have cut resident manpower to the point where this option is less dependable.

### Neurohospitalists: Hospital-Based Neurologists

To combat these challenges, there has been a recent movement, similar to that of medicine hospitalists a decade ago, toward neurology hospitalists, or *neurohospitalists*,[21,22] who are site-specific neurology specialists. Neurohospitalists provide hospital and ED call coverage and handle ward floor consultations and hospital admissions similar to medicine hospitalists. Although not every practice or area can justify a neurohospitalist based on volume, a common observation is that once a neurohospitalist is in place, consultations from referring services may increase. Because neurohospitalists are situated at the hospital and do not see outpatients, they can provide more timely consultation to patients in the ED and hospital. Neurohospitalists add value to hospitals akin to that of medicine hospitalists through providing higher-intensity care (more tests or evaluation) during a shorter length of stay. **Box 2** lists the advantages and disadvantages of neurohospitalists.[21]

Neurohospitalists and hospitalists practice guideline-based care, leading to improved outcomes, improved patient safety, and improved quality care.[35–37] Neurohospitalists can also help bridge the work gap resulting from cuts in resident work hours, and some programs have proposed creation of a "neurohospitalist track" within residency to foster this career path.[38] The number of medicine hospitalists started out below 1000 in the mid-1990s, and is estimated to be approximately 30,000 by 2010.[39] The number of neurohospitalists is difficult to accurately quantify given the lack of uniform terminology (neurohospitalists often describe themselves as "stroke neurologists and neurointensivists") and the absence of a parent organization. However, in 2008, approximately 50 members rapidly identified themselves as neurohospitalists in one survey, and by May 2009 this group had grown to more than 250 members.[40] Additionally, the number of job positions has increased from 1 in 2005 to more than 20 in 2009 at the Dendrite AAN Web site.[41] The tremendous increase in medicine hospitalists within the past decade and the recent surge in neurohospitalists suggest significant growth in this subspecialty in the future.

### Neurointensivists: Intensive Care Unit Neurology Subspecialists

In a similar vein, and even more subspecialized within the hospital, are neurointensivists who are specific to the intensive care unit. Neurointensivists, also known as critical

---

**Box 2**
**Advantages and disadvantages of neurohospitalists**

*Advantages*

Improved emergency department (eg, stroke call) coverage and consultations

Shorter length of hospitalization compared with non-neurohospitalist model care

Improved neurology education of medical students and residents

Improved patient outcomes

Opportunity for inpatient neurologic research

Improved patient quality and safety

Outpatient neurology practice workflow unencumbered by emergency department consultation

*Disadvantages*

Discontinuity of care between outpatient neurologist and inpatient neurohospitalist

Costs of hiring neurohospitalist

*Modified from* Freeman WD, Gronseth G, Eidelman BH. Invited article: is it time for neurohospitalists? Neurology 2008;70(15):1282–8.

---

care neurologists, provide subspecialty care for patients who are critically ill with neurologic and neurosurgical disorders. The Neurocritical Care Society (NCS), for example, had 56 members in 2003 and has grown rapidly to 837 current members (Courtesy Tami Page, http://www.neurocriticalcare.org/). Starting in 2007, the NCS obtained subspecialty accreditation through the UCNS. Currently, more than 200 neurointensivists are UCNS-certified, and that number grows each year. Several NCS members argue that neurointensivists are not optional for stroke center designation, contrary to the original recommendation by the American Heart Association.[42]

Literature suggests that neurointensivists provide improved quality of care, reduced length of stay, improved documentation, reduced mortality, and better cost-of-care compared with the non-neurointensivist care model.[43–48] The practice of neurocritical care is conceived as a multidisciplinary subspecialty built among the specialties of neurology, neurosurgery, anesthesia, and critical care (**Fig. 4**). The UCNS board certification is based on core competencies in both general critical care and neurocritical care (www.neurocriticalcare.org). Based on the recent growth in this subspecialty and the increasing incidence of aging-related neurologic catastrophic disorders such as stroke, the demand for neurointensivists will likely increase in the next 5 to 10 years.

## TELEMEDICINE

Although telemedicine has not been proven to be equally efficacious as on-site treatment of stroke,[49] more hospitals, especially those that incur the associated liability of drip-and-ship acute stroke patients, are incorporating this technology. Based on similar arguments supporting the use of teleneurology in the outpatient sector,[25–27] an increase in the use of teleneurology is foreseeable at stroke centers that have little or no availability of specialty stroke neurologists, neurointensivists, or neurohospitalists. Because the United States has so many underserved and rural areas, the demand for teleneurology could be expanded significantly to help provide access to specialists until transfer to a specialized treating facility can be arranged. The authors predict increased use and further expansion of teleneurology in hospitals in the future.

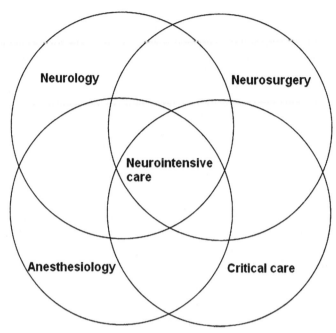

**Fig. 4.** Venn diagram of neurointensive care specialty (neurocritical care).

## FUTURE OF NEUROLOGY EDUCATION IN THE UNITED STATES: ASSAILED ON ALL SIDES

The number of future neurologists entering practice is dependent on the number of neurology residents in training, which in turn depends on the number of medical students entering neurology residency. Most medical students are exposed to neurology in medical school, but the amount of time spent in neurology education in medical school varies by location.[50] Regarding how many medical students enter neurology residency, **Fig. 2** shows a slight upward trend from 1985 to 2005, with minor fluctuations from approximately 1250 to 1500 residents per year. However, when these numbers are compared against the increase in United States population from 1995 to 2009 (from approximately 250 million in 1995 to more than 310 million in 2010),[51] this reflects a smaller fraction of the population going into neurology. In child neurology, the trend has essentially been flat (see **Fig. 2**) and no growth is projected over the next 20 years.[20]

Factors that could increase the number of neurologists (and trainees) would include (1) a marked increase in the number of neurology residencies, which is unlikely considering the complexity of starting a residency program and securing ACGME approval, and (2) an unexpected increase in current neurologists delaying retirement which, in any case, would be a short-lived effect.

The future of neurologic education, however, faces significant challenges, which could then negatively affect the pool of available neurologists. First, institutional support at academic centers with residencies faces harsh economic times. To compensate for this, and to improve the departmental bottom line, some academic institutions are asking teaching staff to see more clinic patients, taking time that was previously devoted to teaching. The ACGME and Neurology Residency Review Committee (RRC) reviews these issues at all sites designated for neurology residencies to maintain education quality.

Most of the RRC focus, however, is placed on extensive resident education documentation, rather than on the education delivered by staff. Second, the total time in which medical students are exposed to neurology is decreasing,[52] a factor that would tend to negatively affect the number of students choosing neurology as a specialty.

Arguably, the most significant factor altering the experience of resident education over the past decade has been the reduction in resident work hours by the ACGME, with further reduction being suggested by the Institute of Medicine (IOM).[53] The reduction in available resident work has translated to added costs[54] for institutions supporting residencies. These costs result from the hiring of additional staff (neurologists, neurohospitalists, hospitalists)[38] and physician extenders to do work previously performed by residents. This effect is compounded by the fact that reduction in resident hours has not translated into improved patient safety, as proposed by ACGME and IOM.[54] In an attempt to offset the manpower lost at the hospital from reduced duty hours, some neurology residencies have increased the number of inpatient months during residency.[55] However, this solution contradicts what 70% of residents and staff believe might improve education, which is more time on outpatient services.[55] Consequently, attending physician staff are doing more of the work that was previously performed by residents before their work hours were restricted, ironically putting patient safety at risk and increasing the likelihood of burnout.

Another unintended consequence of enforced reduction in duty hours is the dilution of the doctor–patient relationship caused by increased and earlier handoffs to other residents, and a lessening of perceived responsibility ("short-timers syndrome" not related to burnout).[56]

Despite the reduction in resident hours, the question of extending neurology residency[38] to ensure clinical competency similar to that of a prior "higher-intensity residency" (ie, pre-ACGME duty hours) has not been fully addressed.[57] Residents naturally oppose additional length of training (a fifth year).[55] Taxpayers doubtfully will be willing to shoulder the added costs of prolonged medical training or subsidize the rising indebtedness of medical students, which is concerning for future academic neurologists, who will earn less than their private practice counterparts.[58] Similar pressures also are affecting academic faculty development. [59]

Elkind[60] has written about the evolving demographics of younger generations of neurologists, and how these intergenerational differences result in new patterns of clinical training and acquisition of knowledge. The "democratization of knowledge," due in part to the ready availability of clinical data in real time (eg, using laptop computers and handheld devices) during physician-patient encounters in the clinic or at the bedside, has effectively broken down the traditional academic hierarchy in which information typically only flowed "downhill from attending to resident to medical student to patient."[60] Neurology residency and fellowship programs will have to develop models in which innovative and individualized methods of teaching take these paradigm shifts into account.

## FUTURE OF NEUROSCIENCE RESEARCH ON CLINICAL NEUROLOGY

The future landscape of neuroscience research remains bright well past the "Decade of the Brain" of the 1990s. The National Institute of Neurologic Diseases and Stroke (NINDS) held an expert panel brainstorming session in November 2007 to plan the next 15 years of neuroscience research.[61] The NINDS experts identified major trends in demographics, economics, and technologic innovations that will impact neuroscience research, and pivotal areas for neuroscience breakthroughs, termed *grand challenges*. They determined that the aging of the United States' population would lead to an increased burden of age-related conditions, such as stroke and neurodegenerative diseases, with its consequent increased economic costs to society. Areas of need this group identified included cost-effective strategies, given rising health care costs, and strategies to improve access to health care.

Telemedicine was also judged by this group to have an important role in the future of neuroscience research. It has the potential to replace or augment some face-to-face clinical encounters using Internet-based communication. The increasing use of electronic health records (EHRs) should create easier and more efficient data abstraction for clinical research. EHRs will facilitate data sharing, patient recruitment, and follow-up. Portable digital assistants (PDAs) or mobile phones with appropriate software could help interface the patient's record within the EHR, provide more continuous monitoring of disease signs and symptoms, and thus benefit research. Similar technology could improve patient education on personal health conditions and reduce economic long-term costs through disease prevention.

The NINDS group noted that worldwide increases in research and research funding are also occurring in other countries. This "globalization of science" affects scientific leadership within the United States by drawing the "best and brightest" minds away, especially when laws on the conduct of research continue to increase in complexity and pose difficulty for our researchers.

A major priority is to find new avenues to improve the United States' position in the global research market, and particularly to partner with other countries in research. The value of basic science research was reemphasized as being integral to fueling translational science. More physician–scientists in both basic and translational science will need to be recruited for clinical research. The future of recreational genomics and the ability of the public to purchase genomic testing both have widespread psychological, ethical, social, and economic implications. Approximately 2375 of human genes, of all the genes within the human genome, are expressed in brain.[62] This number of genes suggests considerable future work will be performed for discovery in neuroscience.

The planning group identified several grand challenges or aspirational goals to help guide future research efforts of the NINDS that they considered paramount for neuroscience over the next 15 years. These challenges included (1) mapping the connectivity of the nervous system; which would essentially be a wiring diagram of the brain, which to many is the "holy grail" of neuroscience research, and would require research into a large-scale *connectome* or map of interconnectivity of the brain; (2) development of a safe, effective treatment for one or more neurodegenerative diseases; (3) establishing biomarkers for monitoring and predicting disease progression and treatment outcomes; (4) healthy brain research into methods for sustaining healthy brain function throughout life, including research into the effects of diet, exercise, and lifestyle factors; (5) research into the biology of brain repair, including brain plasticity, or the brain's capability to change and adapt to injury, and the mechanisms the brain uses to repair itself; and (6) bridging the gap between the now separate disciplines of neurology and psychiatry.

Many disorders, such as stroke, epilepsy, and Parkinson's disease, present with depression, psychosis, or psychiatric overlap conditions. Understanding how these conditions interact will be fundamental to further breakthroughs and treatment and in understanding the unsolved mysteries of complex brain functions and even consciousness itself.

Basic science in neuroscience also gives way to translational research, especially within neurotherapeutics and pharmaceutical research. In the foreseeable future, major research will continue in areas such as brain injury, degenerative disorders (eg, Alzheimer's, Parkinson's disease, amyotrophic lateral sclerosis), and stroke. Since 1977, the NINDS has spent more than $200 million in clinical stroke trials, mostly within the past decade.[63]

## HYPOTHETICAL CONCERNS ABOUT THE FUTURE OF NEUROLOGY
### Is a Neurologist Really Needed?

In the classical neurology model, the one in which most currently practicing neurologists were trained and medical students were once taught, the history and detailed neurologic examination led to localization of the lesion at probable sites within the nervous system. From there, a short list of etiologic differential diagnoses could be narrowed down using a few ancillary tests, including lumbar puncture, radionuclide imaging, electrophysiological testing, and, less commonly, cerebral angiography and pneumoencephalography.

Before the advent of modern neuroimaging studies, the process of neurologic diagnosis almost always depended on this systematic, elegant process. However, advances in neuroimaging modalities, such as FLAIR MRI and functional MRI, along with advanced laboratory, electrophysiologic, and genetic studies, have fundamentally changed the traditional role of the neurologist, who is no longer the only one privy to the secrets of the nervous system. With the advent of online consultative resources (eg, www.WebMD.com, www.UpToDate.com, www.MDConsult.com), primary care (PCPs) and ED physicians can now make neuroradiographic diagnoses without much formal training in neurology. When combined with the advanced neurologic information that can be found in Internet resources readily available to PCPs and ED physicians, the degree to which neurologists will continue to add clinical value might become questionable.

Counterarguments abound against this hypothetical concern for neurology's future. First, insurance companies often deny outpatient MRIs of the nervous system to PCPs (except in emergent settings) as a cost-reduction effort (eg, a neurology Level 5 Medicare new patient office visit reimbursement is measured in a couple hundred dollars compared with an MRI reimbursed in the thousands of dollars).

Second, although a neuroradiologic diagnosis may seem to be evident from neuroimaging, the PCP or ED physician, having had minimal exposure to neurology in medical school and residency, and despite the online resources available to them, often will not be able to address all patient care concerns and questions efficiently because of their own time constraints.

Third, as long as subspecialists exist, the current medicolegal climate will continue to hold PCPs and ED physicians to a local standard of care that, in most areas, assumes a neurologist's level of care. Exceptions include underserved and rural areas in which no neurologists or neurology subspecialists practice. In areas with insufficient numbers of neurologists, teleneurology will presumably be used to an increasingly greater degree.

Recent trends toward a regulated medical environment could also be considered, in which treatment guidelines and standardized protocols based on evidence-based medicine are used, permitting practitioners to deviate from these standards only at professional and legal peril. The general neurologist will be increasingly required, when no neurologic subspecialist is readily available onsite, to use publicly available resources such as Internet databases, academic neurology Web sites, and teleneurology to meet subspecialty needs.

### Future of General Neurology: Vanishing Breed or Different Terminology?

Recently, concerns have been expressed about the future "extinction of the general neurologist" because of increasing subspecialization (see **Table 4**). General neurologists see patients who have varied neurologic problems, rather than a select subspecialty disease (eg, multiple sclerosis). The advent of outpatient subspecialists (eg, those who treat dementia or movement disorders, and inpatient subspecialists neurohospitalists and neurointensivists) is associated with a corresponding decrease in those who identify themselves as general neurologists (see **Table 5**). This perception may be somewhat artifactual, in the sense that neurologists have particular subspecialty interests but are still practicing in the generalist mode. However, the number of subspecialists continues to grow (see **Table 5**).

Furthermore, urban and highly populated areas with greater numbers of neurologists per patient population theoretically may have less demand for a general neurologist because of the presence of numerous subspecialists who see and follow up patients who have subspecialty neurologic problems. This model, however, may be too simplistic because of its dependence on the following assumptions: (1) that the patient is already diagnosed as having a subspecialty neurologic disease (eg, multiple sclerosis, Parkinson's disease), which is typically diagnosed by a neurologist; (2) that a general neurologist will refer the patient to a subspecialist; or that (3) that the PCP will refer the patient directly to a subspecialty neurologist. Each of these assumptions has flaws. In many cases, PCPs and ED physicians consult neurologists with a specific question (eg, whether a patient has myasthenia gravis), but other times the question is less focused or well defined (eg, why the patient is experiencing altered mental status or tremor), likely reflecting a lack of time or neurologic acumen necessary to formulate neurologic diagnosis the way it is taught in neurology residency or clerkships.

### Conclusions

Within the next 5 to 10 years, the demand for neurologists in clinical practice is expected to increase because of many factors, including a relatively static supply of neurology graduates, limitations on current immigration laws and international medical graduates, and an increased demand for neurologic services from an aging population, especially for common disorders such as stroke and neurodegenerative disease. Because of the estimated incidence of acute neurologic disorders, such as stroke, and rising American health care system pressures demanding timely neurologic care, increased demand for neurologic specialization is predicted at EDs and hospitals.

Hospitals in the United States face difficult times ahead because of urgent and primary care being sought within the ED, financial losses from care provided to uninsured/indigent patients, and increased expectations of similar or higher quality of care with shorter length-of-stay, despite heterogeneous patient populations and chaotic disease models. Hospitals will continue to be challenged financially by further Medicare reimbursement cuts and other insurance providers that base their reimbursements on the Medicare rates. The recent political appeals for a United States "health care overhaul" and "health care bill of rights" will substantially affect the future of neurology and health care in general. Because of the tumultuous and complex health care climate, a long-term vision for neurologic practice cannot be accurately forecasted.

Significant challenges confront neurologic education. Academic centers that face harsh financial pressures because of declining governmental and institutional support will increasingly require teaching staff to contribute more to the bottom line. Pressures from nongovernmental organizations, such as the IOM or ACGME, to increase time off for residents and reduce duty hours have a negative financial impact on academic institutions trying to fill the manpower in patient care previously provided by residents. Despite the reduction in resident hours, the question of extending residency to ensure clinical competency, similar to that which existed in the past with higher intensity residencies, has not yet been addressed. Whether the government and general public are willing to help finance the costs of medical education, thereby offsetting the rising average indebtedness of medical students and young physicians, is unclear. These issues have also served to diminish the recruitment of the best and brightest young minds into the medical profession, something that should be of great concern to society.

The future for neuroscience research remains a "blue sky" according to the NINDS. The NINDS leadership hopes to continue its emphasis on basic science neuroscience, translational neuroscience, increasing the number of physician-scientists, research into mapping the entire brain circuitry (*connectome*), discovering biomarkers of detecting disease and disease progression, brain repair/neuroplasticity, and bridging the gap of scientific research between neurology and psychiatry in areas of overlap.

## EPILOGUE

Notwithstanding the great uncertainties that face clinical neurology at the moment, neurologists possess unique training and expertise. They often stand between the real and the imaginary and must sort out incidental, false-positive, or misleading laboratory and imaging results. They are responsible for maintaining the diagnostic parsimony that is required in complex or difficult cases. It has been said that neurology is the one nonsurgical specialty that cannot be learned ad hoc for a particular clinical situation.

To survive in the coming years, neurology will have to present itself as the rightful owner of its specialty. It will need to fight for its territory, particularly the procedures that can be best performed and interpreted by neurologically trained physicians. Neurologists are considered the gatekeepers in many difficult cases but cannot be expected to continue to bear the major responsibility for the economic and legal burdens generated by these conditions. Especially in a field in which outcomes are frequently beyond the control of the practitioner, neurology should advocate strongly in the political arena for malpractice protection, and even immunity, when established clinical parameters and guidelines have been followed.

## SUMMARY

For the past 200 years, neurology has been deeply rooted in the history and neurologic examination, but 21st century advances in neurosurgery, endovascular techniques, and neuropathology, and an explosion in basic neuroscience research and neuroimaging have added exciting new dimensions to the field. Neurology residency training programs face intense governmental regulatory changes and economic pressures, making it difficult to predict the number of neurology residents being trained for the future. The future job outlook for neurologists in the United States, based on recent survey and trends, suggests an increased demand because of the prevalence of neurologic diseases within the aging population, particularly in underserved urban and rural areas. Telemedicine and "teleconsultation" offer a potential solution to bringing virtual subspecialists to underserved areas. The future for neurology and neuroscience research in the United States remains a high priority according to NIH-NINDS, but this may be affected in the long run by budgetary constraints and a growing deficit.

## ACKNOWLEDGMENTS

Rollin J. Hawley, MD (Christiansburg, VA), and David A Nye, MD (Eau Claire, WI), provided invaluable input and advice in the preparation of this article. The authors also want to thank Katherine A. Purcell, MA, (Mayo Clinic, Jacksonville, FL) for her meticulous academic support.

## REFERENCES

1. Martin JB. The integration of neurology, psychiatry, and neuroscience in the 21st century. Am J Psychiatry 2002;159(5):695–704.
2. Spillane JD. Hughlings Jackson lecture: Hughlings Jackson's American contemporaries: the birth of American neurology. Proc R Soc Med 1976;69(6):393–408.
3. Dandy W. Roentgenography of the brain after the injection of air into the spinal canal. Ann Surg 1919;70:397–403.
4. Doby T. Cerebral angiography and Egas Moniz. AJR Am J Roentgenol 1992; 159(2):364.
5. Sneader W. Drug discovery: a history. Hoboken (NJ): Wiley-Interscience; 2005.
6. Merritt H, Putnam TJ. Sodium diphenyl hydantoinate in the treatment of convulsive disorders. JAMA 1938;111:1068–75.
7. Glazko A. The discovery of phenytoin. Ther Drug Monit 1986;8(4):490–7.
8. Monheit DB. Use of prednisone in myasthenia gravis in a diabetic. N Y State J Med 1958;58(24):4033–4.
9. Goldstein M. The neurologist as a health resource. Facts, estimates, and aspirations for the supply of neurologists. Neurology 1977;27(10):901–4.
10. Menken M. The coming oversupply of neurologists in the 1980s. Implications for neurology and primary care. JAMA 1981;245(23):2401–3.
11. Kurtzke JF, Bennett DR, Berg BO, et al. On national needs for neurologists in the United States. Neurology 1986;36(3):383–8.
12. Kurtzke JF, Bennett DR, Berg BO, et al. Neurologists in the United States–past, present, and future. Neurology 1986;36(12):1576–82.
13. Engstrom JW, Hauser SL. Future role of neurologists. West J Med 1994;161(3): 331–4.
14. Menken M, Munsat TL, Toole JF. The global burden of disease study: implications for neurology. Arch Neurol 2000;57(3):418–20.
15. Murray CJ, Lopez AD. Mortality by cause for eight regions of the world: global burden of disease study. Lancet 1997;349(9061):1269–76.
16. Murray CJ, Lopez A. Harvard school of public health. ea: the global burden of disease: a comprehensive assessment of mortality and disability from diseases, injuries, and risk factors in 1990 and projected to 2020. Cambridge (MA): Harvard University Press; 1996.
17. Janca A, Prilipko L, Costa e Silva JA. The World Health Organization's global initiative on neurology and public health. J Neurol Sci 1997;145(1):1–2.
18. Henry K, Lawyer B, Rizzo M. Members of the AAN member demographics subcommittee (2005). Neurologists 2004: AAN member demographic and practice characteristics. St. Paul (MN): American Academy of Neurology; 2004.
19. Annual Education Issues. JAMA 2008;300:1228–43; 2007;298:1081–96; 2006;296:1154–69; 2005;294:1129–43; 2004;292:1099–113; 2003;290:1234–48; 2002;288:1151–64; 2001;286:1095–107; 2000;284:1159–72; 1999;282:893–906; 1998;280:836–45; 1997;278:775–84; 1996;276:739–48; 1995;274:755–62;

1994;272:725–32; 1993;270:1116–22; 1992;268:1170–6; 1991;266:933–43; 1990;264:822–32; 1989;262:1029–37; 1988;260:1093–101; 1987;258:1031–40.

20. Polsky D, Weiner J, Bale JF Jr, et al. Specialty care by child neurologists: a workforce analysis. Neurology 2005;64(6):942–8.

21. Freeman WD, Gronseth G, Eidelman BH. Invited article: is it time for neurohospitalists? Neurology 2008;70(15):1282–8.

22. Josephson SA, Engstrom JW, Wachter RM. Neurohospitalists: an emerging model for inpatient neurological care. Ann Neurol 2008;63(2):135–40.

23. Titomanlio L. Pediatric neurohospitalists. Ann Neurol 2008;64(3):353 [author reply 53].

24. Liebhaber A, Grossman J. Physicians moving to mid-sized, single-specialty practices. Results from the community tracking study. Washington, DC: Center for Studying Health System Change; 2007.

25. Patterson V. Teleneurology. J Telemed Telecare 2005;11(2):55–9.

26. Kane RL, Bever CT, Ehrmantraut M, et al. Teleneurology in patients with multiple sclerosis: EDSS ratings derived remotely and from hands-on examination. J Telemed Telecare 2008;14(4):190–4.

27. Patterson V, Wootton R. How can teleneurology improve patient care? Nat Clin Pract Neurol 2006;2(7):346–7.

28. Taft JM, Hooker RS. Physician assistants and the practice of neurology. JAAPA 2000;13(3):97–100, 103–4, 106.

29. Taft JM, Hooker RS. Physician assistants in neurology practice. Neurology 1999; 52(7):1513.

30. Residency training outcomes by specialty for New York: a summary of responses to the 2007 New York resident exit survey. Albany (NY): School of Public Health, University at Albany, SUNY; 2007.

31. Valeo T. IOM reports say ERs are in crisis—neurointensivists respond. Neurology Today 2006;6(15):10–1.

32. Avitzur O. As public expectation for tPA grows, so too do lawsuits; how neurologists can reduce malpractice risks. Neurology Today 2006;6(9):31–2.

33. Avitzur O. Stipends for stroke call create new pressures, demands on neurologists. Neurology Today 2006;6(7):6–7.

34. On-call reimbursement for neurologists (position paper). American Academy of Neurology. Available at: http://www.aan.com/globals/axon/assets/2502.pdf. Accessed March 7, 2007.

35. Glick TH. The neurologist and patient safety. Neurologist 2005;11(3):140–9.

36. Stradling D, Yu W, Langdorf ML, et al. Stroke care delivery before vs after JCAHO stroke center certification. Neurology 2007;68(6):469–70.

37. Avitzur O. Neurohospitalists: a new term for a new breed of neurologist. Neurology Today 2005;5(10):44–5.

38. Naley M, Elkind MS. Outpatient training in neurology: history and future challenges. Neurology 2006;66(1):E1–6.

39. Society of Hospital Medicine. Available at: http://www.hospitalmedicine.org/. Accessed March 7, 2007.

40. Likosky D, Kirkland W, Restrepo L, et al. Current State of Neurohospitalist Practice. 2009. Available at: http://www.aan.com/globals/axon/assets/6317.pdf. Accessed December 8, 2009.

41. American Academy of Neurology. Dendrite. search terms: hospitalist or neurohospitalist or neurology hospitalist. Available at: http://www.aan.com/marketplace/opportunities/index.cfm. Accessed March 7, 2009.

42. Hemphill JC III, Bleck T, Carhuapoma JR, et al. Is neurointensive care really optional for comprehensive stroke care? Stroke 2005;36(11):2344–5.

43. Suarez JI, Zaidat OO, Suri MF, et al. Length of stay and mortality in neurocritically ill patients: impact of a specialized neurocritical care team. Crit Care Med 2004; 32(11).2311–7.
44. Sung GY. Outcomes of neurocritical care. Curr Neurol Neurosci Rep 2001;1(6): 593–8.
45. Varelas PN, Spanaki MV, Hacein-Bey L. Documentation in medical records improves after a neurointensivist's appointment. Neurocrit Care 2005;3(3):234–6.
46. Varelas PN, Conti MM, Spanaki MV, et al. The impact of a neurointensivist-led team on a semiclosed neurosciences intensive care unit. Crit Care Med 2004; 32(11):2191–8.
47. Mirski MA, Chang CW, Cowan R. Impact of a neuroscience intensive care unit on neurosurgical patient outcomes and cost of care: evidence-based support for an intensivist-directed specialty ICU model of care. J Neurosurg Anesthesiol 2001; 13(2):83–92.
48. Diringer MN, Edwards DF. Admission to a neurologic/neurosurgical intensive care unit is associated with reduced mortality rate after intracerebral hemorrhage. Crit Care Med 2001;29(3):635–40.
49. Meyer BC, Raman R, Rao R, et al. The STRokE DOC trial technique: 'video clip, drip, and/or ship'. Int J Stroke 2007;2(4):281–7.
50. Charles PD, Scherokman B, Jozefowicz RF. How much neurology should a medical student learn? a position statement of the AAN Undergraduate Education Subcommittee. Acad Med 1999;74(1):23–6.
51. U.S. Population Projections. U.S. Census Bureau. Released 2008 (Based on Census 2000). Available at: http://www.census.gov/population/www/projections/ summarytables.html. Accessed August 13, 2009.
52. Aminoff MJ. Training in neurology. Neurology 2008;70(20):1912–5.
53. Ulmer C, Wolman DM, Johns MME, editors. Resident duty hours: enhancing sleep, supervision, and safety. Washington, DC: National Institutes of Medicine; 2008. p. 428.
54. Nuckols TK, Bhattacharya J, Wolman DM, et al. Cost implications of reduced work hours and workloads for resident physicians. N Engl J Med 2009;360(21): 2202–15.
55. Ringel SP, Vickrey BG, Keran CM, et al. Training the future neurology workforce. Neurology 2000;54(2):480–4.
56. Stawicki SP. Short timers syndrome among medical trainees: beyond burnout. OPUS 12 Scientist 2008;2(1):30–2.
57. Watson JC. Resident work hours: distinguishing resident service issues from education and safety. Neurology 2008;71(5):375–6 [discussion: 376–7].
58. Pedley TA. The changing face of academic neurology: implications for neurologic education at the millennium. Neurology 1999;53(5):906–14.
59. Rizzo M, Mobley WC. An AUPN/ANA survey of department leader opinions on the health of US academic neurology. Neurology 2004;63(8):1354–6.
60. Elkind MS. Teaching the next generation of neurologists. Neurology 2009;72(7): 657–63.
61. A blue sky vision for the future of neuroscience. 2009. Available at: http://www. ninds.nih.gov/about_ninds/plans/strategic_plan/blue_sky_vision.htm. Accessed December 8, 2009.
62. Adams MD, Dubnick M, Kerlavage AR, et al. Sequence identification of 2,375 human brain genes. Nature 1992;355(6361):632–4.
63. Marler JR. NINDS-sponsored clinical trials in stroke: past, present, and future. Stroke 2002;33(1):311–2.

# Index

*Note:* Page numbers of article titles are in **boldface** type.

## A

AAN. See *American Academy of Neurology (AAN)*.
ABPN. See *American Board of Psychiatry and Neurology (ABPN)*.
Absence of coercion, 463
Accelerometers, in improving neurologic practice, 397
ACGME neurology review committee, 478–480
ACMPE. See *American College of Medical Practice Executives (ACMPE)*.
Adult neurology residency training, 476
Advocacy, on Internet, 392
Alerting responses, on Internet, 385–388
AMA. See *American Medical Association (AMA)*.
American Academy of Neurology (AAN)
    defined, 350
    on benchmarking, 365
American Academy of Neuroscience, on Internet, 392
American Board of Psychiatry and Neurology (ABPN), 483–485
American College of Medical Practice Executives (ACMPE), 373
American Medical Association (AMA), 511
    in model managed care contract, 359
    on benchmarking, 366
American Productivity & Quality Center (APQC), 366
American Quality Alliance, 355, 511
Angioplasty, malpractice liability related to, 448–449
Anticoagulation, malpractice liability related to, 448
APQC. See *American Productivity & Quality Center (APQC)*.
Association of American Medical Colleges, ERAS of, 476
Attitude, as factor in negotiating with payers, 358
Audit rights, defined, 360

## B

Babinski, J., in neurology history, 537
Back pain, low, patient education in, 528
Benchmarking, **365–384**
    AAN on, 365
    AMA on, 366
    categories for medical practices, 367
    described, 366
    external, 367, 373
    financial measures related to, 373–375

Neurol Clin 28 (2010) 563–572
doi:10.1016/S0733-8619(10)00030-7
0733-8619/10/$ – see front matter © 2010 Elsevier Inc. All rights reserved.

neurologic.theclinics.com

# Moving?

## Make sure your subscription moves with you!

To notify us of your new address, find your **Clinics Account Number** (located on your mailing label above your name), and contact customer service at:

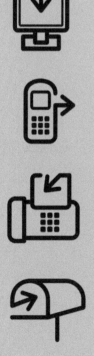

Email: **journalscustomerservice-usa@elsevier.com**

**800-654-2452** (subscribers in the U.S. & Canada)
**314-447-8871** (subscribers outside of the U.S. & Canada)

**Fax number: 314-447-8029**

**Elsevier Health Sciences Division**
**Subscription Customer Service**
**3251 Riverport Lane**
**Maryland Heights, MO 63043**

*To ensure uninterrupted delivery of your subscription, please notify us at least 4 weeks in advance of move.

ELSEVIER

Printed and bound by CPI Group (UK) Ltd, Croydon, CR0 4YY

03/10/2024

01040448-0005